Updates and Advances in Cardiovascular Nursing

Editor

LESLIE L. DAVIS

NURSING CLINICS
OF NORTH AMERICA

www.nursing.theclinics.com

Consulting Editor
BENJAMIN SMALLHEER

September 2023 • Volume 58 • Number 3

ELSEVIER

1600 John F. Kennedy Boulevard ● Suite 1800 ● Philadelphia, Pennsylvania, 19103-2899

http://www.theclinics.com

NURSING CLINICS OF NORTH AMERICA Volume 58, Number 3
September 2023 ISSN 0029-6465, ISBN-13: 978-0-443-18248-8

Editor: Kerry Holland
Developmental Editor: Isha Singh

Nursing Clinics of North America (ISSN 0029-6465) is published quarterly by Elsevier Inc., 360 Park Avenue South, New York, NY 10010-1710. Months of issue are March, June, September, and December. Periodicals postage paid at New York, NY and additional mailing offices. Subscription price per year is, $163.00 (US individuals), $557.00 (US institutions), $275.00 (international individuals), $680.00 (international institutions), $231.00 (Canadian individuals), $680.00 (Canadian institutions), $100.00 (US and Canadian students), and $135.00 (international students). To receive student/resident rate, orders must be accompanied by name of affiliated institution, date of term, and the signature of program/residency coordinator on institution letterhead. Orders will be billed at individual rate until proof of status is received. Foreign air speed delivery is included in all *Clinics* subscription prices. All prices are subject to change without notice. **POSTMASTER:** Send address changes to *Nursing Clinics*, Elsevier Health Sciences Division, Subscription Customer Service, 3251 Riverport Lane, Maryland Heights, MO 63043. **Customer Service: Telephone: 1-800-654-2452** (U.S. and Canada); **1-314-447-8871 (outside U.S. and Canada). Fax: 1-314-447-8029. E-mail: journalscustomerservice-usa@ elsevier.com** (for print support) and **journalsonlinesupport-usa@elsevier.com** (for online support).

Nursing Clinics of North America is covered in *EMBASE/Excerpta Medica, MEDLINE/PubMed (Index Medicus), Social Sciences Citation Index, Current Contents, ASCA, Cumulative Index to Nursing, RNdex Top 100,* and Allied Health Literature and International Nursing Index (INI).

Contributors

CONSULTING EDITOR

BENJAMIN SMALLHEER, PhD, RN, ACNP-BC, FNP-BC, CCRN, CNE, FAANP
Assistant Dean, Master of Science in Nursing Program, Associate Professor, School of Nursing, Duke University, Durham, North Carolina

EDITOR

LESLIE L. DAVIS, PhD, RN, ANP-BC, FAAN, FAANP, FACC, FPCNA, FAHA
Associate Professor, PhD Division, School of Nursing, The University of North Carolina at Chapel Hill, Chapel Hill, North Carolina

AUTHORS

ANTHONY M. ANGELOW, PhD, ACNPC, ACNP-BC, AGACNP-BC, CEN, FAEN, FAANP, CRNP
Associate Clinical Professor and Chair, Advanced Practice Nursing, Division of Graduate Nursing, Drexel University, College of Nursing and Health Professions, Philadelphia, Pennsylvania

SUSAN ASHCRAFT, DNP, APRN, ACNS-BC, CCRN-K, SCRN, FAHA
Neurocritical Care Clinical Nurse Specialist, Novant Health, Inc, Charlotte, North Carolina

JENNIFER BALLARD-HERNANDEZ, DNP, FNP-BC, AG ACNP-BC, FAHA, FACC, FAANP
Cardiology Division, Department of Medicine, Department of Veterans Affairs, VA Long Beach Healthcare System, Long Beach, California

JOHN R. BLAKEMAN, PhD, RN, PCCN-K
Assistant Professor, Mennonite College of Nursing, Illinois State University, Normal, Illinois

CIANTEL A. BLYLER, PharmD
Smidt Heart Institute, Cedars-Sinai Medical Center, Los Angeles, California

MARGARET T. BOWERS, DNP, FNP-BC, AACC, FAANP, FAAN
Clinical Professor, Duke University School of Nursing, Duke Health Division of Cardiology, Durham, North Carolina

ANDERSON BRADBURY, MSN, RN, AGNP-C
Nurse Practitioner, Department of Cardiac Electrophysiology, The University of North Carolina at Chapel Hill, Chapel Hill, North Carolina

BILLY A. CACERES, PhD, RN, FAHA, FAAN
Assistant Professor of Nursing, Center for Sexual and Gender Minority Health Research, Columbia University School of Nursing, New York, New York

TONYA CARTER, DNP, MSN, FNP-BC
University of North Carolina Health, Chapel Hill, North Carolina

JENNIFER COATES, DNP, MBA, ACNPC, ACNP-BC
Associate Clinical Professor and Track Director, Adult-Gerontology Acute Care Nurse Practitioner Program, Drexel University, College of Nursing and Health Professions, Philadelphia, Pennsylvania

CRYSTAL CUSIN, DNP, AG-ACNP-BC
Acute Care Nurse Practitioners, Henry Ford Hospital, Structural Heart Disease, Henry Ford Health, Heart and Vascular Service Line, Detroit, Michigan

LESLIE L. DAVIS, PhD, ANP-BC, FAAN, FAANP, FACC, FAHA, FPCNA
Associate Professor, PhD Division, School of Nursing, The University of North Carolina at Chapel Hill, Chapel Hill, North Carolina

DANNY DOAN, MPH
Research Coordinator, Center for Sexual and Gender Minority Health Research, Columbia University School of Nursing, New York, New York

ANN L. ECKHARDT, PhD, RN
Associate Chair of Clinical Education, Department of Graduate Nursing, College of Nursing and Health Innovation, The University of Texas at Arlington, Arlington, Texas

DAYNA GJUROVSKI, DNP, AG-ACNP-BC
Acute Care Nurse Practitioners, Henry Ford Hospital, Structural Heart Disease, Henry Ford Health, Heart and Vascular Service Line, Detroit, Michigan

RÉMI M. HUECKEL, DNP, CPNP-AC, FAANP
Associate Professor, Duke University School of Nursing, Pediatric Acute Care NP, Duke Children's Hospitals and Clinics, Durham, North Carolina

DEBRA KOHLMAN-TRIGOBOFF, RN, MS, ACNP-BC, CVN
Nurse Practitioner for Duke Heart and Vascular, Department of Cardiology, Duke University Medical Center, Fayetteville, North Carolina

CHRISTY LEYLAND, MSN, PED-BC, CNL, CPNP-AC
Part Time Faculty, Northeastern University Bouvé School of Nursing Charlotte Campus, Pediatric Acute Care NP, Atrium Health Levine Children's, Midland, North Carolina

CARRIE PALMER, DNP, RN, ANCC. ANP-BC
Associate Professor, The University of North Carolina at Chapel Hill School of Nursing, Chapel Hill, North Carolina

ELIZABETH RADCHIK, PharmD
Smidt Heart Institute, Cedars-Sinai Medical Center, Los Angeles, California

JAMES SALL, PhD, FNP-BC
Evidence-Based Practice Program, Veterans Health Administration, Washington, DC

SARAH E. SCHROEDER, PhD, ACNP-BC, MSN RN, AACC
Mechanical Circulatory Support Nurse Practitioner and Program Manager, Bryan Heart, Lincoln, Nebraska

YASHIKA SHARMA, MSN, RN
PhD Candidate, Center for Sexual and Gender Minority Health Research, Columbia University School of Nursing, New York, New York

DAVID LÓPEZ VENEROS, MA, RN
PhD Student, Center for Sexual and Gender Minority Health Research, Columbia University School of Nursing, New York, New York

T. JENNIFER WALKER, MSN, RN, ANP-BC
Nurse Practitioner, Department of Cardiac Electrophysiology, The University of North Carolina at Chapel Hill, Chapel Hill, North Carolina

SUSAN E. WILSON, DNP, ANP-BC, FAHA
Professor, Department of Neurology, Director, Neurosciences Clinical Trials Unit, The University of North Carolina at Chapel Hill, Chapel Hill, North Carolina

JANET F. WYMAN, DNP, ACNS-BC
Director of Structural Heart Clinical Services, Henry Ford Hospital, Structural Heart Disease, Henry Ford Health, Heart and Vascular Service Line, Detroit, Michigan

Contents

Focus on Cardiovascular and Stroke Conditions

> An acute elevation of blood pressure (BP) greater than 180/120 mm Hg associated with target organ damage is considered a hypertensive emergency. Patients with a hypertensive emergency need intravenous medications and close monitoring in the intensive care unit. Whereas an acute elevation of BP greater than 180/120 mm Hg without evidence of target organ damage is a hypertensive urgency. Patients with a hypertensive urgency are treated with oral medications and generally discharged home with outpatient follow-up. Patients with either condition need a thorough evaluation to determine cause of the acute increase in BP and education to optimize the treatment regimen long-term.

> Nurses play a key role in promoting successful transitions of patients with heart failure (HF) from the hospital to the ambulatory setting. Engaging patients and caregivers in discharge teaching early in the hospitalization can enhance their understanding of HF as a clinical syndrome and identify precipitants of decompensation. Effective transitional care interventions for patient with HF include a phone call within 48 to 72 hours and a follow-up appointment within 7 days. Early symptom identification and treatment are key aspects of HF care to improve quality of life and minimize risk of hospitalization.

> Cardiovascular disease (CVD) is the leading cause of morbidity and mortality in the United States. The development and progression of atherosclerotic CVD are largely dependent on a multitude of modifiable and nonmodifiable risk factors. Current therapeutic strategies involve risk factor modification, especially dyslipidemia. The treatment of dyslipidemia continues to be dynamic, and in this paper, we review the current strategies for risk assessment, diagnosis, and treatment. As treatments for the management of dyslipidemia continue to evolve with ever-increasing options for therapeutic targets, an understanding of lipid-lowering therapies remains an essential topic of understanding for all health care providers.

> Within the United States, someone will have a stroke approximately every 40 seconds. Eighty-five percent of strokes are ischemic, with 15% classified as either intracranial or subarachnoid hemorrhage. Stroke care is complex, and nurses play a critical role in identification, assessment, management, and coordination throughout the stroke continuum of care. This article will explore the nursing care of the patient with ischemic and hemorrhagic stroke during the first 24 hours.

> When a patient develops wide complex tachycardia, it is important to determine the cause quickly and accurately. This article will help the bedside nurse understand different causes, determine the most probable cause, and provide appropriate first-line treatment.

> This article focuses on peripheral arterial disease (PAD) of the lower extremities. There is a higher incidence of myocardial infarction, stroke, and cardiovascular death, resulting in higher rates of all-cause mortality compared with patients without PAD. Thus, the presence of PAD is a marker for systemic atherosclerotic disease and can lead to the early detection and treatment of coronary artery disease or cerebrovascular disease. This article reviews the latest information about the prevalence, symptoms, classification, diagnosis, and treatment of PAD. Monitoring and detection of PAD are also discussed, including implications for nursing care.

> Over the last few decades, there have been dramatic advances in the understanding of the mechanisms of valvular heart disease and development of percutaneous treatment options. These innovations have resulted in the need for a multidisciplinary heart team approach for quality patient outcomes, a team in which nursing is an integral member. This update provides an overview of the major valve diseases, current guideline recommendations, catheter-based treatment options and key elements of nursing care: physical examination, diagnostic testing, pre- and post-procedure care protocols, and patient education elements.

Focus on Treatment (Drug and Device Updates)

> Cardioembolic stroke from atrial fibrillation causes substantial death and disability in the United States. Treatment with oral anticoagulants provides safe and effective stroke prevention for high-risk patients. This article

reviews strategies for the use of anticoagulation and highlights the nurse's role in patient education.

Pharmacologic agents are a key part of the medical armamentarium aimed at reducing the significant morbidity and mortality caused by cardiovascular disease (CVD). In recent years, the landscape of CVD treatment has evolved with the development of new medication classes and the repurposing of existing medications for new indications. This article provides nurses with a pharmacologic update on new and emerging therapies for the treatment of hypertrophic cardiomyopathy, familial hypercholesterolemia, and heart failure. The authors review clinical indications, pharmacology, practical considerations for the safe and appropriate use of these medications, and implications for nurses.

Although the concepts of pacing have been around for more than half a century, technological advances in cardiac implantable electronic devices (CIEDs) have changed the landscape for patients in need of pacing support or sudden death prevention. Nurses encounter patients with CIEDs in all aspects of the health care setting. Because exciting CIED therapies are on the horizon, nurses must stay up-to-date to promote optimal outcomes for CIED patients. This essential guide provides nurses with a comprehensive overview of the principles of pacing and implantable cardioverter defibrillators (ICDs), as well as innovative technologies such as leadless cardiac pacemakers and subcutaneous ICDs.

Mechanical circulatory support (MCS) includes temporary and durable mechanical devices used for two sets of indications: 1. acute heart failure (HF) secondary sepsis, a myocardial infarction, or pulmonary emboli, and 2. for chronic end-stage HF secondary to worsening cardiomyopathy despite guideline driven medical treatment. This article is to aide cardiac intensive care unit (ICU) nurses in understanding the history of MCS therapy, the care of the MCS patient in the cardiac ICU, the critical and collaborative role of transplant teams with MCS therapy, educational needs for a successful discharge, and implications for education and shared decision-making when placing these devices.

Special Populations

Cardiovascular disease (CVD) is the leading cause of death in women but is often underrecognized and undertreated. Women are more likely to experience delay in treatment and worse outcomes, even though they experience similar symptoms as men. Women are more likely to experience ischemia related to microvascular dysfunction, which is not readily diagnosed by commonly used diagnostic tests. Nurses are ideally positioned to be patient advocates and use evidence-based guidelines to encourage primary prevention and ensure prompt treatment. This paper provides an update on CVD in women for clinical nurses based on the latest research evidence.

This article summarizes existing evidence on cardiovascular disease (CVD) risk and CVD diagnoses among sexual and gender minority adults and provides recommendations for providing nursing care to sexual and gender minority adults with CVD. More research is needed to develop evidence-based strategies to care for sexual and gender minority adults with CVD.

Many healthy children may be found to have a murmur on physical exam. Whether this murmur is discovered at a routine health maintenance visit or as a result of a focused exam on a child with illness, it is just one finding and must be considered in the context of the child's history and other physical exam findings. Murmurs associated with heart defect or dysfunction occur most often in infancy. Most murmurs discovered in children, especially after infancy, between ages 3 to 6 and in young-adulthood, are innocent or benign murmurs and less likely a symptom of cardiac dysfunction or defect.

NURSING CLINICS

SERIES OF RELATED INTEREST

Advances in Family Practice Nursing
www.advancesinfamilypracticenursing.com

THE CLINICS ARE AVAILABLE ONLINE!
Access your subscription at:
www.theclinics.com

Foreword

The New Edge of Cardiovascular Care

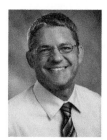

Benjamin Smallheer, PhD, RN, ACNP-BC, FNP-BC, CCRN, CNE, FAANP
Consulting Editor

Progression in health care has consistently required roles and responsibilities of nurses to advance year after year. These can be seen across all care settings and patient populations. Care of the cardiovascular patient is no exception to this occurrence. Within the progression of health care, these phenomena have been witnessed through the following:

- Changes in the understanding of pharmacogenomic research, fueling revolutionary approaches to both short- and long-term anticoagulation management.
- Advances in anticoagulation reversal agents and updated coagulation monitoring technology.
- Surgical procedures, previously viewed as the gold standard and often a patient's only option to maintain a meaningful quality of life, are now being replaced by minimally invasive procedures.
- Patients who just years ago may have been faced with conversations surrounding end-of-life care now have additional options to extend quality and quantity of life.
- Mechanical support, which often accompanies surgical interventions, has crossed over from the inpatient and critical care environments to the outpatient and long-term care arena.
- Devices are smaller, more durable, less dangerous, and more consistent with a patient's expectations.
- Disease management previously requiring inpatient interventions now has more options available, including outpatient therapy and monitoring.

The delivery of care across the spectrum of the patient's is receiving increased attention for deficiencies of social justice and equitable care. Social injustice, social determinates of health, and health inequity have contributed to increasing cardiovascular

Nurs Clin N Am 58 (2023) xiii–xiv
https://doi.org/10.1016/j.cnur.2023.06.008
0029-6465/23/© 2023 Published by Elsevier Inc.

nursing.theclinics.com

disease mortality.[1] The need and responsibility to advance care for sexual- and gender-minority populations, such as cisgender women, the transgender (eg, transwomen and transmen) community, communities of color, pediatric patients, and other at-risk populations, are on the forefront to decrease social injustice and health care inequities.[2] By directing attention outward toward communities of need, the discipline of nursing is well poised to move toward training an advancing workforce of health care providers and positively impacting cardiovascular-related mortality.

Numerous experts have come together in this issue of *Nursing Clinics of North America*, to disseminate updated guidelines for care and advances in cardiovascular nursing. This issue serves as a resource for the care of specific acute and chronic conditions, updated pharmacologic therapy, advances in device therapy and management, and key information addressing care for special populations in 2023 and beyond.

Benjamin Smallheer, PhD, RN, ACNP-BC, FNP-BC, CCRN, CNE, FAANP
Assistant Dean- Master of Science in Nursing Program
Associate Professor, School of Nursing, Duke University
307 Trent Drive, Box 3322, Office 3117
Durham, NC 27710, USA

E-mail address:
benjamin.smallheer@duke.edu

REFERENCES

1. Powell-Wiley TM, Baumer Y, Baah FO, et al. Social determinants of cardiovascular disease. Circ Res 2022;130(5):782–99.
2. Bureau of Population, Refugees, and Migration. (ND). US Department of State: at-risk populations. Available at: https://www.state.gov/other-policy-issues/at-risk-populations/. Accessed June 13, 2023.

Preface

Tackling Cardiovascular and Stroke Disease in 2023 and Beyond

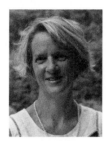

Leslie L. Davis, PhD, RN, ANP-BC, FAAN, FAANP, FACC, FPCNA, FAHA
Editor

Cardiovascular diseases remain the leading cause of death globally, with ischemic heart disease and ischemic stroke ranking as the top two causes of cardiovascular disease deaths, respectively.[1] Despite improved evidence-based treatment options being available to reduce mortality and morbidity associated with cardiovascular diseases, patients continue to experience recurrent events. Thus, an essential component of disease prevention and health promotion is to address common cardiovascular risk factors. Worldwide, common cardiovascular risk factors include elevated systolic blood pressure, dietary risks, smoking, high body mass index, low physical activity, elevated low-density lipoprotein cholesterol, and high fasting plasma glucose.[1] As nursing is the largest professional discipline worldwide, nurses are in an ideal position to lead efforts to prevent and manage cardiovascular risk factors.[2] Many health care systems have adopted a team-based approach, including nurses and other professionals from various disciplines to optimize patient outcomes.[3] As part of a team, nurses can be instrumental in empowering patients to modify health-related lifestyle behaviors to serve as the cornerstone of primary and secondary prevention efforts.[3] Nurses have an obligation and an opportunity to lead efforts to improve patient outcomes, especially when educating patients and caregivers about self-care activities.

Many updates have occurred in the past decade in the field of cardiovascular and stroke care, such as advancements in prevention, disease and symptom management, and treatment options. These advancements have implications for nursing practice in hospital and community settings. In this issue of *Nursing Clinics of North America*, a breadth of topics related to various conditions (eg, hypertensive emergencies, chronic heart failure, dyslipidemia, stroke, wide complex tachycardias, peripheral arterial disease, and valvular heart disease), new drug and device therapies (eg, chronic oral anticoagulation, newly approved novel drug therapies, pacemakers,

Nurs Clin N Am 58 (2023) xv–xvi
https://doi.org/10.1016/j.cnur.2023.06.007
0029-6465/23/© 2023 Published by Elsevier Inc.

defibrillators, and mechanical assist devices), and special populations (women, sexual and gender minorities, and pediatric patients) are covered. Authors discuss the latest evidence and clinical practice guidelines and share pearls to help guide nurses as they care for patients living with or at risk for cardiovascular diseases. This issue will equip practicing nurses and other clinicians with the knowledge and skills to ultimately improve care delivery for this vulnerable patient population for 2023 and beyond.

Leslie L. Davis, PhD, RN, ANP-BC, FAAN, FAANP, FACC, FPCNA, FAHA
School of Nursing
University of North Carolina at Chapel Hill
4007 Carrington Hall
Campus Box # 7460
Chapel Hill, NC 27599-7460, USA

E-mail address:
LLDavis@email.unc.edu

REFERENCES

1. Vaduganathan M, Mensah GA, Turco JV, et al. The global burden of cardiovascular diseases and risk: a compass for future health. J Am Coll Cardiol 2022;80(25): 2361–71. https://doi.org/10.1016/j.jacc.2022.11.005.
2. Hayman LL, Fletcher B, Miller NH, et al. The global cardiovascular nursing leadership forum: promoting optimal cardiovascular health worldwide. J Cardiovasc Nurs 2023;38(2):111–3. https://doi.org/10.1097/JCN.0000000000000971.
3. Commodore-Mensah Y, Turkson-Ocran RA, Dennison Himmelfarb CR. Empowering nurses to lead efforts to reduce cardiovascular disease and stroke risk: tools for global impact. J Cardiovasc Nurs 2019;34(5):357–60. https://doi.org/10.1097/JCN.0000000000000606.

Focus on Cardiovascular and Stroke Conditions

Hypertensive Emergencies: Implications for Nurses

Leslie L. Davis, PhD, NP-BC, FAAN, FAANP, FACC, FAHA, FPCNA

KEYWORDS

- Hypertension • Hypertensive emergencies • Hypertensive urgency
- Hypertensive crisis • Nursing

KEY POINTS

- Blood pressure (BP) treatment goals vary depending on the target-organ damage and treatment ordered by the medical team.
- The BP treatment goal in the first hour is typically different than the more gradual reduction of BP in the hours and days following the first hour of treatment.
- Intraarterial BP monitoring is the most accurate way to measure BP in patients with a hypertensive emergency.
- Placement of an intraarterial line for BP monitoring should not delay starting the medication ordered to reduce BP in patients with a hypertensive emergency.

INTRODUCTION

Approximately one-half of all adults in America with hypertension (HTN) do not meet their blood pressure (BP) treatment goal.[1] One complication of uncontrolled HTN is an acute, marked increase in BP, a relatively common condition in adults evaluated in the emergency department or admitted to the hospital. A *hypertensive crisis* describes the spectrum of acute, severe uncontrolled HTN conditions and is defined as a systolic BP of greater than 180 mm Hg or a diastolic BP of greater than 120 mm Hg.[2] A hypertensive crisis can be categorized as either a *hypertensive emergency* or a *hypertensive urgency*. A hypertensive emergency is defined as an acute increase of BP greater than 180/120 mm Hg that is associated with new or worsening target organ damage (eg, neurologic, cardiovascular, or renal manifestations).[3] Whereas a hypertensive urgency is defined as the same BP parameters, yet no evidence of acute target organ damage. The overall prevalence for patients presenting to the emergency department for a suspected hypertensive emergency is approximately 1 in 200 persons (0.5%), which generally does not vary globally.[4] When examining prevalence of each type of a hypertensive crisis, hypertensive urgencies are

University of North Carolina at Chapel Hill, School of Nursing, 4007 Carrington Hall, CB # 7460, Chapel Hill, NC, USA
E-mail address: LLDavis@email.unc.edu

Nurs Clin N Am 58 (2023) 271–281
https://doi.org/10.1016/j.cnur.2023.05.011
0029-6465/23/© 2023 Elsevier Inc. All rights reserved.

nursing.theclinics.com

more common than hypertensive emergencies (approximately 1 in 100 adults vs 1 in 300 adults, respectively).[5]

Hypertensive emergencies, as the name implies, are associated with a high death rate especially if not treated. For example, the median survival for a patient experiencing a hypertensive emergency if untreated is 10.4 months.[3] It is not the actual (high) BP value that requires emergent treatment to immediately reduce the BP as much as it is the rapidity in which the marked BP increase occurs that places patients in acute danger[3]; this is because many patients with uncontrolled HTN tolerate much higher levels of BP on a daily basis as compared with those who are normotensive.[3] In fact patients with a hypertensive urgency do not require immediate reduction of the BP, referral to the emergency department, and/or hospitalization.[3] These patients often have their BP medication restarted (if it had been discontinued by the patient or provider) or intensified (if they require additional medication for better BP control) as an outpatient with regular follow-up care scheduled.[3]

The purpose of this paper is to discuss the workup for a patient with suspected hypertensive emergency including the initial evaluation (history, physical examination, and diagnostic testing) to determine the likely cause of the acute increase in BP, first-line treatment based on suspected cause, priorities for nursing care in the acute care setting, and implications for patient and family education.

PATHOPHYSIOLOGY

Hypertensive crises, whether they are a hypertensive urgency or an emergency, are a heterogeneous group of conditions, with variation in cause and clinical manifestations. Most of the patients with a hypertensive crisis have underlying uncontrolled essential (primary) HTN.[4] In fact, the prevalence of underlying HTN in patients with hypertensive emergencies and hypertensive urgencies are 82.5% and 78%, respectively.[5] For these patients, the most common reason for a hypertensive crisis is nonadherence to the treatment regimen and/or the use of sympathomimetics. Notably, some patients with preexisting HTN are unaware of their condition, largely due to the asymptomatic nature of elevated BP. A smaller percentage of patients with a hypertensive crisis (about 20%–40%) have a secondary cause for their underlying HTN (most commonly

Table 1	
Potential causes of a hypertensive crisis	
Possible Causes of Acute Increase in BP	**Secondary Causes of Uncontrolled BP**
• Nonadherence, especially if abrupt withdrawal of antihypertensive agents (eg, clonidine or β-blockers) • Dietary indiscretion • Medications (eg, steroids, NSAIDs, cyclosporin, sympathomimetics, antiangiogenic therapy) • Drug-drug interactions (eg, monoamine oxidase inhibitors and tricyclic antidepressants, antihistamines, or tyramine) • Interfering substances (eg, cocaine, amphetamines, phencyclidine [PCP], stimulant diet supplements)	• Cardiovascular (coarctation of the aorta) • Renal (kidney disease, renal artery stenosis) • Endocrine (pheochromocytoma, Cushing syndrome, hyperthyroidism, primary hyperaldosteronism) • Pregnancy-related (preeclampsia or eclampsia) • Neurologic (eg, head or spinal cord injuries, ischemic stroke, hemorrhagic stroke, brain tumor) • Collagen vascular disorders (eg, systemic lupus erythematosus)

Abbreviations: BP, blood pressure; NSAIDs, nonsteroidal antiinflammatory agents.

glomerulonephritis or renal artery stenosis).[4] **Table 1** displays potential causes of a hypertensive crisis.

Regardless of the cause, the exact pathophysiological mechanism underlying a hypertensive crisis in patients with or without preexisting HTN is not fully understood. However, interrelated mechanisms thought to contribute to the development of a hypertensive crisis include overactivation of the renin-angiotensin-aldosterone system, pressure-induced natriuresis (a maladaptive diuretic response resulting in increased sodium excretion by the kidneys), and an abrupt increase in systemic vascular resistance.[4] Microvascular damage associated with these mechanisms creates a viscous cycle interfering with normal autoregulatory function, resulting in target organ damage from the sudden abrupt increase in BP. As discussed, presence of target organ damage is what differentiates a hypertensive emergency from a hypertensive urgency (no target organ damage).

ASSESSMENT
History Taking

History taking for patients presenting with a hypertensive crisis should focus on assessment of symptoms and potential causes associated with the acute increase in BP. Symptoms vary greatly among patients, with some being asymptomatic to others experiencing life-threatening symptoms associated with target organ damage. Based on a 2020 meta-analysis of 8 studies with a combined sample of 1970 hypertensive emergencies and 4983 urgencies the most common symptoms for patients presenting with a hypertensive emergency were neurological symptoms (35%) and dyspnea (31%) followed by nonspecific symptoms (24%),[5] whereas the most common symptoms for patients presenting with a hypertensive urgency were nonspecific symptoms (48%) followed by headache (22%).[5] Other symptoms associated with a hypertensive crisis may include chest pain or palpitations, visual disturbances, dizziness, gastrointestinal symptoms (abdominal pain, nausea, vomiting, anorexia), and epistaxis, among others.[6]

Beyond symptoms, assessment of patients with a hypertensive emergency should include whether the patient has a history of HTN, and if so, what their treatment regimen is and how adherent they are to their regimen. History should also include questions related to possible causes of the acute increase of BP, especially for patients with preexisting uncontrolled HTN.

Physical Examination

The physical examination for a patient with a hypertensive crisis begins with a baseline assessment of vital signs including temperature, respiratory rate, heart rate, and BP. The BP should be taken with an automated BP cuff with an appropriately sized BP cuff. Use of a BP cuff that is too small may result in a falsely elevated reading. Likewise, a BP cuff that is too large may result in a falsely lower BP reading. Initially BP measurements should be taken in both arms. Most patients have BP readings that differ between their arms, usually less than 10%. Otherwise, a more marked difference between the arms could suggest aortic dissection, which could be associated with a hypertensive emergency. In addition, as tolerated by the patient, the nurse should obtain BPs in different positions: supine (lying), sitting, and standing to evaluate the patient for volume depletion. After these initial vital signs are obtained, repeated BP and heart rate measurements are needed to monitor for changes over time.

After obtaining vital signs, a focused physical examination should include assessment of cardiovascular, pulmonary, and neurological function. Starting with the head and neck, the nurse should inspect the neck for jugular vein distention, which, if present, may represent acute heart failure associated with a hypertensive emergency. The nurse should then auscultate heart and lung sounds. The optimal positioning for assessment of heart sounds includes auscultating at the aortic (second intercostal space to the right of the sternum), pulmonic (second intercostal space to the left of the sternum), tricuspid (fourth intercostal space to the left of the sternum), and mitral (fifth intercostal space, midclavicular line) valve areas, in addition to Erb point (third intercostal space to the left of the sternum). When auscultating heart sounds the nurse should identify S1 (the first heart sound) that is synchronous with the carotid pulse and S2 (the second heart sound) to determine the heart rate, rhythm, and presence (or absence) of extra heart sounds (gallops), murmurs, or rubs. An extra heart sound after S2 (an S3) best heard in the mitral area could represent pulmonary edema, whereas a new diastolic murmur heard best at Erb point at the end of expiration while the patient is sitting up and leaning forward may represent aortic regurgitation that could be associated with acute aortic dissection.

Lung sounds should be auscultated in all lung fields with a full cycle (inspiration and expiration) in each area, primarily assessing for bibasilar crackles (rales) that may represent acute pulmonary edema. Moving to the extremities, the nurse should assess for absent or delayed peripheral pulses (potentially indicative of aortic dissection), for the presence of peripheral edema (often associated with heart failure), and for bilateral movement, sensation, and muscle strength in the arms and legs. A more thorough neurological examination (eg, cranial nerve examination, cerebellar and gait testing), abdominal examination (to assess for masses and bruits), and a fundoscopic (dilated) eye examination (to assess for soft exudates, hemorrhages, papilledema) are completed by the provider (physician, nurse practitioner, or physician assistant). Refer to **Table 2** for the possible target organ dysfunction, associated clinical findings, and corresponding diagnostic testing that may be ordered by the medical team.

TREATMENT
Goals of Care

After determining that the patient is experiencing a hypertensive emergency (vs urgency), treatment goals include (1) identifying the likely cause of the acute increase in BP, (2) controlling the extent of the target organ damage through reduction of BP, and (3) monitoring the patient for adverse effects of medications in addition to worsening signs of vital organ perfusion. Patients experiencing a hypertensive emergency should be admitted to the intensive care unit for prompt initiation of intravenous medications to induce rapid BP reduction and to allow for close hemodynamic monitoring.[3]

BP treatment goals vary depending on the type of target organ damage the patient is experiencing and how quickly the target BP should be reached. Unfortunately, there are no data from randomized controlled trials to provide evidence for how rapidly or how much to lower the BP in patients with a hypertensive emergency.[3] However, 3 compelling conditions require *very rapid* lowering of systolic BP within the first hour of presentation, namely aortic dissection, severe preeclampsia or eclampsia, and pheochromocytoma with hypertensive crisis.[3] Specifically, during the first hour of treatment, patients with severe preeclampsia or eclampsia and pheochromocytoma with hypertensive crisis should have their systolic BP reduced to less than 140 mm Hg, whereas patients with aortic dissection to less than 120 mm Hg.[3]

Otherwise, the primary treatment goal is to decrease systolic BP *no more than 25%* in the first hour.[3] Reducing BP too rapidly can result in ischemia to the brain, coronary

Table 2
Target-organ dysfunction, associated clinical findings, diagnostic tests

Target Organ Damage	Possible Clinical Findings	Possible Diagnostic Testing
Neurologic (~45% prevalence) • Cerebral infarction • Hemorrhagic stroke • Hypertensive encephalopathy	*Symptoms:* headache, visual disturbances, nausea *Signs:* altered mental status, focal neurologic deficits, unsteady gait, seizures, cortical blindness, visual field deficits	CT or MRI of the brain
Cardiovascular (~49% prevalence) • Acute coronary syndrome • Acute heart failure/pulmonary edema	*Symptoms:* chest pain or pressure radiating to jaw, epigastrium, shoulders, arms; dyspnea, orthopnea, paroxysmal nocturnal dyspnea; cough; fatigue; palpitations. *Signs:* jugular vein distension; edema; basilar lung crackles; third heart sound; new-onset murmur.	12-lead ECG, chest radiograph; cardiac troponin if ACS suspected, BNP if acute heart failure suspected; echocardiogram
Renal (~10% prevalence) • Acute kidney injury/failure	*Symptoms:* hematuria or oliguria	*Laboratory tests:* urinalysis; serum creatinine, sodium, potassium, BUN *Imaging:* renal ultrasound
Vascular (~6.5% prevalence) • Eclampsia • Acute aortic dissection (type A or B)	*Symptoms of eclampsia:* dyspnea; visual disturbances; headache. *Signs of eclampsia:* pregnant > 20 wk; seizures *Symptoms of aortic dissection:* syncope; chest pain with or without radiation to the back *Signs of aortic dissection:* neurologic deficits; limb ischemia; new-onset murmur; asymmetry of pulse and blood pressure between arms.	*Eclampsia:* electrolytes, serum creatinine, urinalysis, liver function tests *Aortic dissection:* chest radiograph; CT angiography of chest and abdomen; transesophageal echocardiography

Abbreviations: ACS, acute coronary syndrome; BNP, brain natriuretic peptide; BUN, blood urea nitrogen; CT, computed tomography; ECG, electrocardiogram; MRI, magnetic resonance imaging.

arteries, or the kidneys. Further reduction of BP to a systolic BP of 160 mm Hg and/or diastolic BP of 100 mm Hg within the next 2 to 6 hours is recommended with outpatient goals to be reached within 24 to 48 hours.[3] An exception to these rules is with patients who are having an ischemic or hemorrhagic stroke (which require BP to be lowered more slowly). Notably, specific timelines and treatment goals vary among countries. Thus, these values serve as a general guide. The medical team will provide orders for the patient's specific BP goal during these time intervals. **Table 3** displays the target BP based on timeline and commonly used medications for each clinical presentation based on target organ damage.

First-Line Pharmacologic Therapy

First-line therapy given to lower BP depends on the specific target organ dysfunction associated with the hypertensive emergency and the patient's comorbidities that may be potential contraindications for the medication. The intravenous administration route is most commonly used due to rapid onset of action, relatively short half-life, ease of titration, and shorter duration if the patient experiences an adverse event from the medication.

Table 4 displays intravenous medications commonly used for treating patients with hypertensive emergencies.

IMPLICATIONS FOR NURSING CARE

All patients with a hypertensive emergency should be admitted to the intensive care unit and have an intraarterial intravenous line (to monitor BP) and continuous cardiac monitoring (to assess for dysrhythmias). Noninvasive BP readings (obtained by a BP cuff and an automated BP machine) tend to run lower than more invasive intraarterial BP readings in patients who are hypertensive. Beyond better accuracy, intraarterial BP monitoring offers the advantage of assessing BP in real time for patients who are being treated with intravenous anti-HTN medications. However, treatment of these patients should not be delayed while waiting on placement of an intraarterial line.

Nurses should anticipate BP changes in response to treatment so should monitor the BP, heart rate, and rhythm closely, watching for sudden changes that may induce cerebral, cardiac, or renal ischemia. If the patient is pregnant, then fetal monitoring will also likely be ordered by the medical team. In addition, the patient should be monitored for a change in orientation status, mood, level of consciousness, vision changes, nausea, vomiting, and a change in intake and output, which could signal a change in perfusion to vital organs. The patient should be kept as comfortable as possible. Pain and increased anxiety can increase BP, thus should be addressed as quickly as possible.

Discharge planning should begin before the date/time of the actual discharge. Nurses should assess social factors that can impede the patient's ability to follow the treatment regimen posthospitalization. For example, the nurse should assess whether the patient has access to stable housing, heart-healthy food and clean drinking water, physical and mental health care, social support, and affordable, reliable transportation.[7] Nurses can advocate for a simplified medication regimen (once daily, generic medications) as appropriate to improve adherence. Discharge teaching should include when the first follow-up appointment is and with whom. In addition, patients should be instructed who to call if they experience side effects related to their medications after leaving the hospital. Patients who have experienced extensive target organ damage (eg, stroke, myocardial infarction, heart failure) should have a referral to cardiac rehabilitation. **Box 1** displays priorities for patient and family education.

Table 3
Blood pressure treatment goals for patients with a hypertensive emergency

Target Organ Damage	Timeline for Reaching Goal	Acute BP Goal	Common Treatment (Not in Order of Priority)
Encephalopathy	Immediate	↓ MAP by 20%–25%[3,4]	Labetalol, nicardipine, nitroprusside[4]
Acute aortic dissection	Immediate	SBP < 120 mm Hg[3,4] and heart rate < 60 beats per minute[4]	Esmolol, labetalol,[3] or nitroglycerin, nicardipine, or metoprolol[4]
Acute coronary syndrome	Immediate	SBP < 140 mm Hg[3,4]	Esmolol, labetalol, nicardipine, nitroglycerin[3,4]
Acute pulmonary edema	Immediate	SBP < 140 mm Hg[3,4]	Clevidipine, nitroglycerin, nitroprusside[3,4] in addition to loop diuretic[4]
Eclampsia/severe preeclampsia	Immediate	SBP < 140 mm Hg[3] and DBP < 105 mm Hg[4]	Hydralazine, labetalol, nicardipine[3]
Acute hemorrhagic stroke	Immediate	SBP < 180 mm Hg[4] (while avoiding sudden BP drops)	Labetalol, nicardipine, urapidil[4]
Acute ischemic stroke	Within 1 h	<185/110 mm Hg before giving thrombolysis or thrombectomy[4]; after receiving thrombolysis BP goal < 180/105 mm Hg for next 24 h Otherwise, initial BP < 220/120 mm Hg can be considered with a gradual ↓ of MAP by15% over 24–48 h (unless other comorbidities require lower BP goals)[2]	In addition to thrombolytic therapy (if appropriate), labetalol, nicardipine, nitroprusside[4]

Abbreviations: BP, blood pressure; DBP, diastolic BP; MAP, mean arterial pressure; SBP, systolic BP.

Table 4
Medications used to treat hypertensive emergencies

Drug Class	Example	Onset and Duration of Action[4]	Usual Dose Range[3,4]	Comments
Adrenergic blockers	Esmolol (beta$_1$ blocker)	1–2 min; 10–30 min	0.5–1 mg/kg/min IV bolus over 1 min; 5–200 μg/kg/min infusion. Bolus may be repeated.[3]	• Contraindicated in severe bradycardia, second or third degree heart block, decompensated HF, or cocaine toxicity. Labetalol contraindicated in reactive airway disease or COPD. • Monitor for bradycardia and worsening HF (all listed); bronchospasm (labetalol); and flushing, tachyarrhythmias, and chest pain (phentolamine).[4]
	Labetalol (alpha$_1$, beta$_1$, beta$_2$ blocker)	5–10 min; 3–6 h	0.3–1.0 mg/kg dose (maximum 20 mg) slow IV injection every 10 min or 0.4–1.0 mg/kg IV infusion up to 3 mg/kg/h. Adjust to cumulative dose of 300 mg. May repeat every 4–6 h[3]	
	Metoprolol (beta$_1$ blocker)	1–2 min; 5–8 h	2.5–5 mg IV bolus over 2 min; may repeat every 5 min to max dose of 15 mg[4]	
	Phentolamine (nonselective alpha blocker)	1–2 min; 10–30 min	0.5–1 mg/kg IV bolus or 50–300 μg/kg/min IV infusion[4]	
	Urapidil (alpha$_1$ blocker, serotonin agonist)	3–5 min; 4–6 h	12.5–25 mg IV bolus, 5–40 mg/h infusion[4]	
Angiotensin converting enzyme inhibitor	Enalaprilat	5–15 min; 4–6 h	0.625–1.25 mg IV over 5 min. May increase up to 5 mg every 6 h as needed to reach BP goal[3,4]	• Contraindicated if history of angioedema, pregnancy, bilateral renal artery stenosis, acute myocardial infarction.[3] • Relatively slow onset of action compared with other options.[3] • Monitor for headache, nausea, vomiting, hyperkalemia, or worsened kidney function.
Calcium channel blockers-dihydropyridines	Clevidipine	2–3 min; 5–15 min	2 mg/h IV infusion, increase 2 mg/h every 2 min until at BP goal.[3,4] Max dose 32 mg/h; max duration 72 h[3]	• Nicardipine contraindicated in liver failure. • Monitor for headache, reflex tachycardia including atrial fibrillation.
	Nicardipine	5–15 min; 30–40 min	5 mg/h IV infusion, increasing every 5 mg by 2.5 mg/h to max 15 mg/h[3]	

Class	Drug	Onset; duration	Dosing	Notes
Dopamine₁ receptor agonist	Fenoldopam	5–15 min; 30–60 min	0.1–0.3 μg/kg/min IV, increase 0.05–0.1 μg/kg/min every 15 min until at goal BP.[3,4] Max infusion rate 1.6 μg/kg/min[3]	• Contraindicated if increased intraocular pressure (glaucoma), intracranial pressure, or sulfite allergy. • Monitor for headache, reflex tachycardia or bradycardia, dizziness, hypokalemia, increased intraocular pressure.
Vasodilators	Hydralazine (direct vasodilator)	10–30 min; 2–4 h	10–20 mg slow IV infusion to start; repeat every 4–6 h as needed.[3]	• For hydralazine, BP starts to drop within 10–30 min and continues for 2–4 h. Less predictable BP response and prolonged duration.[3]
	Nitroglycerin (nitric oxide–dependent vasodilator)	1–5 min; 3–5 min	5 μg/min; increase by 5 μg/min every 3–5 min to max of 20 μg/min[3]	• For nitroglycerin only use if acute coronary syndrome or acute pulmonary edema. Do not use in patients with volume depletion, cerebral hemorrhage, or closed-angle glaucoma.[3]
	Sodium nitroprusside (nitric-oxide dependent vasodilator)	Immediate; 1–2 min	0.3–0.5 μg/kg/min to start; increase by 0.5 μg/kg/min to reach BP goal; max 10 μg/kg/min[3]	• For nitroprusside, duration of treatment should be as short as possible. If infusion rates ≥ 4–10 μg/kg/min may administer thiosulfate to avoid cyanide toxicity.[3] • Monitor for headache, reflex tachycardia, flushing.

Abbreviations: BP, blood pressure; COPD, chronic obstructive pulmonary disease; HF, heart failure; hr, hours; IV, intravenous; max, maximum; mg, milligrams; min, minutes; μg, micrograms

---

Box 1
Priorities for patient and family education

- Treatment of HTN is lifelong.
- Elevated BP is not typically associated with symptoms, thus ongoing monitoring of BP is essential.
- Importance of adherence to nonpharmacologic and pharmacologic therapy to control BP.
- Lifestyle modifications to obtain/maintain BP control (including DASH eating plan, reduction in dietary sodium, daily physical activity, moderation of alcohol, weight reduction in those with overweight or obese, adequate sleep, and tobacco cessation).
- Benefits of home BP monitoring and how to implement home BP monitoring once discharged from the hospital.
- Importance of follow-up care with primary care provider and specialty provider.
- How to access a pharmacy assistance program or social worker if financial challenges or other social determinants of health are present, which influences the patient's ability to follow the treatment regimen.

Abbreviations: BP, blood pressure; DASH, dietary approaches to stop hypertension; HTN, hypertension.

SUMMARY

An acute increase in BP that is greater than 180/120 mm Hg associated with new or worsening target organ damage is indicative of a hypertensive emergency. These patients require admission to the intensive care unit for invasive monitoring of BP (intra-arterial BP monitoring) and intravenous medication to lower BP. Reducing BP too quickly (or too slowly) is associated with increased risk. Thus, the presenting signs and symptoms, extent of target organ damage, and the patient's comorbidities are taken into consideration to determine how quickly to lower the BP and specific medication to be administered. Nurses need to be knowledgeable about how to start and titrate intravenous medications. In addition, nurses can be instrumental in detecting symptom changes and possible side effects that require prompt communication with the medical team to optimize patient outcomes.

CLINICS CARE POINTS

- Patients experiencing an acute increase in BP of greater than 180/120 mm Hg should be worked up for a suspected hypertensive emergency.
- A complete history and physical examination, including diagnostic testing, should be done to determine possible causes of the acute BP increase and whether there are associated signs of target organ damage.
- Patients with signs of target organ damage need ongoing BP monitoring through an arterial line in the intensive care unit in addition to intravenous medication to get the BP to the goal based on the cause of the hypertensive emergency.
- Nurses need to be knowledgeable of titrating intravenous BP medications to monitor the patient for adequacy of response and potential side effects.
- Nurses are in an ideal position to educate patients and their family members about the treatment being provided and implications for care after hospital discharge.

DISCLOSURE

The author has no commercial or financial conflicts of interest or any funding sources to disclose.

REFERENCES

1. Tsao CW, Aday AW, Almarzooq ZI, et al. Heart Disease and Stroke Statistics-2023 Update: A Report From the American Heart Association. Circulation 2023; 147(8):e93–621.
2. Sharma K, Mathews EP, Newton FCE. Hypertensive Emergencies: A Review. Am J Nurs 2021;121(10):24–35.
3. Whelton PK, Carey RM, Aronow WS, et al. 2017 ACC/AHA/AAPA/ABC/ACPM/AGS/APhA/ASH/ASPC/NMA/PCNA Guideline for the Prevention, Detection, Evaluation, and Management of High Blood Pressure in Adults: A Report of the American College of Cardiology/American Heart Association Task Force on Clinical Practice Guidelines. Hypertension 2018;71(6):e13–115.
4. van den Born BH, Lip GYH, Brguljan-Hitij J, et al. ESC Council on hypertension position document on the management of hypertensive emergencies. Eur Heart J Cardiovasc Pharmacother 2019;5(1):37–46.
5. Astarita A, Covella M, Vallelonga F, et al. Hypertensive emergencies and urgencies in emergency departments: a systematic review and meta-analysis. J Hypertens 2020;38(7):1203–10.
6. Saladini F, Mancusi C, Bertacchini F, et al. Diagnosis and treatment of hypertensive emergencies and urgencies among Italian emergency and intensive care departments. Results from an Italian survey: Progetto GEAR (Gestione dell'Emergenza e urgenza in ARea critica). Eur J Intern Med 2020;71:50–6.
7. The vital role of nurses in supporting social determinants of health. https://www.healthify.us/healthify-insights/the-vital-role-of-nurses-in-supporting-social-determinants-of-health. Accessed May 11, 2023.

Heart Failure
Priorities for Transition to Home

Margaret T. Bowers, DNP, FNP-BC, AACC[a],*,
Tonya Carter, DNP, MSN, FNP-BC[b]

KEYWORDS

- Heart failure • Transitions • Discharge teaching • Patient education

KEY POINTS

- In patients with heart failure (HF), health literacy must be addressed before engaging patient and family/caregiver in discharge education.
- Discharge teaching should be focused on self-management and early recognition of HF symptoms.
- Hospital follow-up telephone calls by nurses identify gaps in care including medication issues, changes in weight and HF symptoms.

INTRODUCTION

As the prevalence of heart failure (HF) increases, nurses should be aware of how best to support patients who are hospitalized because they transition to the ambulatory setting. This starts on the day of admission with identification of precipitants of HF, educating the patient and family or caregiver(s) about HF and preparing for the transition to home. During the hospital stay, nurses have the opportunity to engage the patient and their family/caregiver(s) in education to enhance their understanding of this clinical syndrome of HF and learn how to manage their care postdischarge. Early symptom identification and treatment are key aspects of HF care to improve quality of life and minimize risk of hospitalization.

HEART FAILURE HOSPITALIZATION

Annually a diagnosis of HF is one of the most common reasons for hospitalization and with more than 1 million new cases identified each year and an aging population, hospitalization rates may be increasing.[1] These hospitalizations are associated with increased cost, and it is anticipated that by 2030 costs will exceed US$70 billion

[a] Department of Medicine, Duke University School of Nursing, 307 Trent Drive, Durham, NC 27710, USA; [b] University of North Carolina Health, 160 Dental Circle Drive, CB# 7075, Chapel Hill, NC 27599, USA
* Corresponding author.
E-mail address: Margaret.bowers@duke.edu

Nurs Clin N Am 58 (2023) 283–294
https://doi.org/10.1016/j.cnur.2023.05.001
0029-6465/23/© 2023 Elsevier Inc. All rights reserved.

per year with HF readmissions accounting for a significant portion of this cost.[2] Annually in the United States (US), HF readmission rates are estimated to be 25% and up to 40% of these readmissions may be avoidable.[3] Nurse-led transitional care interventions have been implemented to address this elevated utilization of health-care resources. In a meta-analysis conducted by Li and colleagues after screening more than 3000 articles, 25 articles including 22 randomized controlled clinical trials (RCTs) and 3 cluster RCTs were reviewed to determine the effects of nurse-led transitional care interventions in patients with HF.[3] Overall results described varying degrees of reduced readmissions were associated with nurse-led transition care interventions in patients with HF compared with usual care.[3] This highlights the key role that nurses play in facilitating successful care transitions.

Nurses are knowledgeable in disease management and provide patients with the skills for self-management. When caring for patients admitted with HF, nurses are in an ideal position to explore factors that may have contributed to the HF decompensation and make an impact on the trajectory of illness. Early recognition of the reason for an HF hospitalization must be addressed to mitigate future preventable readmissions. Potential precipitating events are listed in **Table 1**.

RISK FOR READMISSION

A diagnosis of HF is associated with a poor prognosis and the chronicity of the illness is associated with symptom exacerbations that affect quality of life and loss of productivity.[4,5] For patients with HF, readmission risk is tracked at 30 days and risk can remain high for up to 90 days postdischarge.[6] Many of the precipitants listed in **Table 1** are also risks for HF readmission. Identifying factors that are associated with an increased risk of HF readmission before discharge from the hospital affords an opportunity to mitigate this risk. Nurses play a key role in addressing patient issues that may contribute to the risk for readmission. Once the patient-specific risks are identified, the nurse can discuss strategies to reduce them. For example, to address nonadherence to medications using a daily pillbox may be a simple approach to lessen the number of days medications are missed.

Patient and family/caregiver education are key in preventing readmission, and it is important to consider health literacy and reading level when providing this education. Health literacy is a key component to assess before delivering patient education. In

Table 1 Reasons for readmission	
Precipitant for Readmission	**Diagnosis and Findings**
Ischemia	Acute coronary syndrome—chest discomfort
Dysrhythmias	Atrial fibrillation, atrial flutter, ventricular tachycardia, frequent premature ventricular contractions
Uncontrolled hypertension	Elevated systolic and/or diastolic blood pressure
Acute infection	Pneumonia, sepsis, myocarditis, elevated white blood count
Thyroid disorders	Hypothyroidism or hyperthyroidism
Anemia	Reduced hemoglobin and hematocrit
Nonadherence	Medication reconciliation is inaccurate Dietary recall indicates high-sodium foods
Medications that contribute to decompensation	Nonsteroidal anti-inflammatory drugs, verapamil, and other negative inotropes

2018, the American Heart Association published a scientific statement focused on health literacy and the relationship to both primary and secondary prevention of cardiovascular disease.[7] Health literacy refers to an individual's ability to access, assimilate, and evaluate health information to make educated decisions.[8] There are a variety of tools available to measure health literacy. To evaluate an individual's health literacy, the nurse must first be able to communicate clearly and in plain language with the patient/caregiver(s). The nurse should verify understanding when providing the patient and family/caregiver(s) with health-care information, not just once but at multiple time points. Because reading text may not always be easy for the patient or family/caregiver(s), consider alternative forms of delivering health-care information including videos, images, or podcasts.

Patient and family/caregiver education are key in preventing readmission, and it is important to consider the format in which this education is delivered. The American Medical Association recommends that written documents should be at a sixth grade reading level and should be available in multiple languages based on the patient population seen in your region.[9] In routine practice printed educational materials and videos and or links focused on HF education are shared with the patient and family/caregiver(s).[10] Research has shown that although more than 50% of patients interviewed in one qualitative study preferred printed materials, they did not want "large volumes" and preferred a single page with discharge instructions.[10]

Patient and family/caregiver education, effective discharge planning, follow-up within 7 days of discharge, medication monitoring, and outpatient titration of medications are all common transitional themes and modifiable factors that can reduce 30-day readmissions.[11,12]

PREPARING FOR DISCHARGE

Goals of a hospitalization for HF include symptomatic improvement including decongestion, titration of guideline-directed medical therapy, and performing diagnostic studies to guide the course of treatment. Preparation for discharge should start at the day of admission as the nurse works with the patient and their family/caregiver(s) to identify goals of care and collaborates with the health-care team to facilitate achievement of these goals. A variety of personnel may need to be included as part of the transition team including case management, physical therapy, and occupational therapy to ensure that the patient has the resources to successfully rehabilitate at home.

There are system-level transitional care interventions that need to be in place to meet regulations from the Joint Commission. These include a postdischarge telephone call and a follow-up clinic appointment within 7 days scheduled before leaving the hospital.[13] This telephone call should take place between 24 and 48 hours after discharge and address key aspects of the discharge plan. The focus of all nursing interventions should be empowering patients to engage in self-care.

PATIENT/FAMILY EDUCATION

When preparing a patient for discharge, education should focus on assessment of health literacy, symptom management, adherence to medication regimen, weight monitoring, limiting dietary sodium, and scheduling a follow-up appointment. **Table 2** describes the specific patient and family/caregiver education topic areas that should be included in discharge teaching.

This educational content can be overwhelming and needs to be broken up into smaller pieces of information as to not overwhelm the patient or their family/

Table 2
Patient and family/caregiver education topics

Issue to be Addressed	Nursing Intervention
Health literacy	Assess patient literacy by asking the patient to repeat back to you the information you have shared
Symptom monitoring	Describe signs and symptoms of HF decompensation including worsening dyspnea, orthopnea, or paroxysmal nocturnal dyspnea (PND), increase in lower extremity or abdominal edema, development of chest pain or palpitations
Emergency contact information	Provide information about when and who to contact if they develop worsening HF symptoms
Weight monitoring	Instruct patient to weigh at the same time each day after emptying bladder and wearing the same type of clothing. Report an increase in weight of 0.9- 1.3 kg overnight or 2.2 kg in 1 wk
Medication management	Review medication list and verify medications that were started, stopped, or changed
Limited sodium diet	Discuss limiting dietary sodium to <2000 mg/d. Focus on eating fresh or frozen vegetables to limit sodium intake
Follow-up appointment	Assist in obtaining a postdischarge follow-up appointment within 7 d

caregiver(s). Once the nurse assesses health literacy, they can prioritize areas that align with the patient's goals of care then discuss the remaining topics. As part of inter-professional practice, the nurse can consult other disciplines such as nutrition/dietary services or pharmacy to provide patient and family/caregiver education in their specialties.

SYMPTOM MONITORING

Patients with HF may present with a variety of symptoms. During discharge teaching, the nurse should inform the patient and caregivers of these potential symptoms (**Table 3**).

EMERGENCY CONTACT INFORMATION

The nurse should provide the patient with information on who to contact after discharge if they develop HF symptoms during a time when their primary care or cardiology office is closed. This is another effective strategy to empower the patient and their family/caregiver(s) in managing their symptoms and avoid an unnecessary hospitalization or emergency department visit.

WEIGHT MONITORING

There are key aspects of daily weight monitoring that the nurse should describe when providing patient education. The first instruction is to weigh at the same time each day, in the same type of clothing. The scale should be on a flat surface, not on carpet. If using a digital scale, make sure it is zeroed before standing on the scale to weigh. Patients should report a weight gain of 2 to 3 lbs overnight or 5 lbs in 1 week.

Table 3
Symptoms associated with heart failure

Symptoms	Description/Pathophysiology	Associated Signs on Examination
Chest pressure	Discomfort described as pressure, tearing, burning, or aching Imbalance between myocardial oxygen supply and myocardial oxygen demand	Dyspnea
Dyspnea	Sensation of running out of air Elevated pressures in the blood vessels around the lung due to the hearts decreased ability of the heart to fill and empty	Breathlessness Exertional With position changes
Early satiety	Accumulation of fluid around the liver and digestive system	Anorexia
Exercise intolerance	Due to multiple factors such as reduced perfusion of skeletal muscles and peripheral vasculature	Reduced activity level
Fatigue	Due to the decreased pumping ability of the heart, less blood reaches the muscles and tissues Blood is diverted away from less vital organs	Daytime sleepiness
Nocturnal cough	Back flow of fluid into the lungs Fluid triggers a cough as the body tries to get rid of it	Orthopnea
Edema	Disruption in pressure forces between extravascular and intravascular fluid spaces Loss of pumping power of the right side of the heart allowing for congestion (fluid buildup)	Abdominal swelling (ascites) Third heart sound (S3 Gallop) Jugular vein distension (with patient laying at 45°) Scrotal edema Subconjunctival edema Peripheral edema Weight gain
Pain	Discomfort of congestion and fluid retention in the liver and gut	Abdominal Deep visceral
Rapid or irregular heart rate	Abnormal impulse formation, impulse conduction or both	Arrhythmias such as atrial fibrillation Tachycardia

MEDICATION RECONCILIATION

The transition period from hospital to outpatient setting is a critical time for medication reconciliation. During this vulnerable phase, drug omission as well as deviations in dosage, frequency, and strength are various types of medication discrepancies that can cause potential harm to patients.[5,14] The purpose of completing a comprehensive medication reconciliation is to verify current medications and resolve any inconsistencies.[5] This allows for the creation of the most accurate list of medications that the patient is taking and can reveal challenges in getting prescriptions filled. Patients with limited finances may not be able to afford new prescriptions, and there may be an alternative or less-expensive option available. Before discharge, nurses can collaborate with the pharmacist to explore discounted options for obtaining medications. The patient and family/caregiver can meet with the social worker to discuss pharmacy assistance programs and/or help with getting medication vouchers. In addition to possible financial barriers, nurses should ask about the patient's ability to access the pharmacy and if this is an obstacle for obtaining medications. If getting to the pharmacy to pick up medications is an impediment, then the nurse can explore options for pharmacies that provide delivery services. Completion of a comprehensive medication reconciliation provides an opportunity to ensure medications that were discontinued are no longer in the pillbox and identify and prevent potential adverse drug events.[15]

DIETARY SODIUM RESTRICTION

One of the main reasons to reduce sodium intake is to reduce the development of hypertension, stroke, kidney disease, or additional cardiovascular diseases.[16] In addition to providing written materials, nurses may consult with a dietician to provide detailed information on how to limit dietary sodium. On average, Americans consume greater than 3 g of sodium per day.[16]

Therefore, it is recommended that patients with HF reduce their dietary sodium intake to between 2 and 3 g/d. The first step is removing the saltshaker from the table. Reading labels to look for sodium content that is less than 300 mg/serving and adhering to serving size. Fresh vegetables are recommended when in season and frozen vegetables are preferred over canned foods. If a salt substitute is used, the label should be checked to ensure no sodium present, and the amount of potassium is noted. Patients with elevated serum potassium should avoid salt substitutes with potassium. In patients on potassium sparing diuretics such as spironolactone or eplerenone, using a salt substitute may increase the serum potassium level and serum potassium should be monitored.

FOLLOW-UP

The nurse should prepare the patient for the type of follow-up that occurs after discharge including a telephone call as well as a scheduled appointment. Early communication is helpful in assessing the patient's belief in the treatment plan. Patients who think their treatment was ineffective are less likely to maintain medication adherence and are at increased risk for readmission.[17] Transitional care follow-up calls are an affordable way to provide patient-centered support. Nurse-driven callback programs within 48 to 72 hours of discharge allows for early assessment of the patient, their understanding of after-care instructions and an opportunity to address patient concerns. It also allows for triage of symptoms, vital signs, and improves subjective quality of care transition. Applying strong assessment, communication, and clinical judgment allows the nurse to identify early signs of HF exacerbation allowing for opportunity to intervene before symptoms become severe enough to require admission to hospital. It also increases the rate of successful early follow-up visits.[18] A structured telephone questionnaire template should be utilized (**Table 4**).

Early in-person clinic follow-up, within 7 days after discharge, is associated with lower 30-day readmission rates and provides an opportunity to evaluate how the patient is doing in their home environment.[19] These early follow-up visits allow for recognition of gaps in medication reconciliation, symptom monitoring, and clarification of discharge instructions and is a meaningful strategy, which can improve the disease trajectory. Another important component of early clinic follow is the introduction of nursing in supporting patients in the mastery of self-monitoring. A nurses' patient-centered perspective encourages patients to engage in reflection on their own and developing body awareness. Building this outpatient support system helps patients with HF cope with feelings of powerlessness and constraints.[20] During the transition period, patients often struggle with negative emotions, self-care regime, and the ability to adapt.[21] The nurse–patient relationship, established thorough telephone calls and in-clinic visits, provide checkpoints that ensures patient safety.[22] It promotes more effective health-care consumptions and builds capacity for treatment and self-care.

CARDIAC REHABILITATION

As part of the discharge plan, cardiac rehabilitation may be ordered. The nurse must understand the benefits of cardiac rehabilitation and describe these benefits to the patient and their family in a meaningful way. (**Table 5**) Currently, cardiac rehabilitation is approved for those with an ejection fraction of 35% or less and future options may expand to include patients with other ejection fractions.

Cardiac rehabilitation is a physician-supervised program consisting of prescribed exercise, psychosocial assessment, cardiac risk reduction modification, and outcome assessment.[23] Cardiac rehabilitation remains underused in patients with HF despite confirmation of efficacy, safety, improvements in quality of life, and reductions in hospitalizations. Key factors contributing to underuse include lack of referral, patient adherence, payer coverage, and overall awareness. Implementing cardiac rehabilitation in patients with HF has been associated with reversal of ventricular remodeling, improvement in ventricular filling pressures, vasomotor and skeletal muscle function.[23] There are ongoing efforts to increase the cutoff for heart failure with reduced ejection fraction (HFrEF) to 40% or less and include patients with heart failure with preserved ejection fraction (HFpEF) (ejection fraction greater than or equal to 50%).

TRAJECTORY

All stages of symptomatic chronic HF carry high morbidity and mortality rates. Nurses need to be aware of this chronic illness, which has both acute and chronic episodes so that they can prepare patients and families for these exacerbations. Despite regularly updated European and American position articles, advanced HF is still underestimated. The categorical HF classification that is based solely on left ventricular ejection fraction presents a limited, often unrealistic view of how a patient is actively engaged in their day-to-day activities. When patients are first diagnosed with HF, the New York Heart Association Class (NYHA) functional status is used to describe symptom severity. Nurses have an opportunity to discuss this functional class, which is a fluid classification system so that patients can understand when symptoms are worsening.

Table 4
Sample of a structured telephone questionnaire

Sample Questionnaire	
Patient identifiers	• Name • Date of birth • Medical record number
General information	• Discharge date • Discharging facility • Cardiologist name • Primary care provider name
Diagnostic data	• Ejection fraction • Laboratories (last date of completion)
Fluid restrictions	• What is your instructed fluid limit? • How many liters per day can you consume? • How do you plan to track your fluid restriction? • Assess understanding of examples of fluid *Ex: 8 ounces = 1 cup = 240 mL*
Dietary restrictions	• What does the phrase "low-sodium diet" mean to you? • What is your sodium limit per day? • How do you plan to take your sodium intake per day? • What are alternative flavorful salt alternatives? • Do you need assistance from a nutritionist?
Weight	• What was your discharge weight? • What is your goal dry weight? • Do you have a scale at home that you can weigh daily? • Have you been weighing yourself daily? • What time during the day do you weigh yourself? • Do you have a weight diary that you can use to record your weight? • What is your plan of action if you gain 2–3 lbs within 48 h?
Review of HF medications	Write down name and dosage of the following: • ARNI or ACEI/ARB • Beta blocker • Aldosterone antagonist • SGLT-2 inhibitor • Diuretic • Anticoagulation (for patients with arrhythmia or mechanical valve) • Potassium supplementation • Magnesium supplementation
	Do you have prescription medications? • Day's supply and refills? What pharmacy do you plan to use for refills? • Name of pharmacy_____ Can you afford to buy your medications? • Do you need help filling out application for patient support programs?
Review of social habits	Do you smoke? • If you smoke, were you offered smoking-cessation counseling? Do you consume any alcohol? • If consumes, should be advised to stop. Do you use any illicit drugs? • If uses illicit drugs, were you offered counseling?

(continued on next page)

Table 4 (*continued*)	
Sample Questionnaire	
Exercise	• Where you offered information about cardiac rehabilitation services?
Review of coming up appointments	• Review upcoming appointment dates and time • Review transportation for these appointments
Questions	
	Further actions or interventions to be completed
Closing out telephone call	Give contact information: • Name • Telephone number • Instructions for telemedicine communication
Date/time completed	
Name of interviewer	

Abbreviations: ACEI, angiotensin converting enzyme inhibitors; ARB, angiotensin receptor blockers; ARNI, Angiotensin-receptor-neprilysin inhibitors.
Adapted from Hollenberg et al.[19]

Guideline-directed medical therapy is often underutilized.[24] Most eligible patients do not receive targeted doses and few patients have medications increased over time.[25] Angiotensin-receptor-neprilysin inhibitors (or angiotensin converting enzyme inhibitors or angiotensin receptor blockers), mineralocorticoid antagonist receptors, beta blockers (BBs), and sodium-glucose cotransporter-2 inhibitors are the cornerstones of HF management, reducing all-cause morbidity and mortality in patients with HFrEF.[24] Notably, with the exception of BBs, all of these medication classes are now also approved for patients with HFpEF. Medications are uptitrated slowly to reach patient-specific maximally tolerated dosing. One or more medication from each drug class may be initiated during a hospitalization and the nurse provides instructions about which home medications should be stopped and those that may be continued at a new dose. When completing a medication reconciliation before

Table 5	
Effects of cardiac rehabilitation and exercise raining in patients with heart failure	
Body System	**Effect**
Cardiac	Increased cardiac output Decreased filling pressures and resting heart rate
Respiratory	Increased respiratory muscle strength and minute ventilation Decreased dyspnea
Autonomic	Increased vagal tone Decreased sympathetic tone
Endothelial function	Decreased left ventricular (LV) afterload, vasoconstriction, and hypertension
Musculoskeletal	Increased muscle strength, mass, and function Increased oxygen extraction
Kidney function	Decrease renin, angiotensin, and aldosterone
Endocrine	Decreased hyperlipidemia and insulin resistance

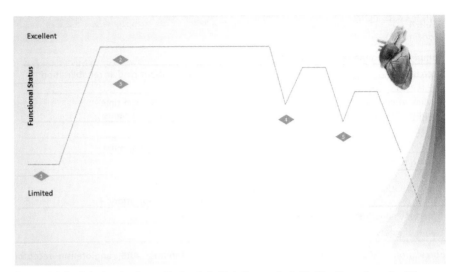

Fig. 1. Original design by AgapeTechs. 1. Initial diagnosis. 2. Uptitration of medical therapy. 3. Possible placement of ICD or cardiac resynchronization therapy device (CRT-D) 4. Intropic support. 5. Mechanical Support—LVAD or Heart transplantation.

discharge, the nurse has the opportunity to ensure that the patient is aware of the significance of these medications and how they improve symptoms and mortality. If specific guideline-directed medical therapy medications are not on the medication list and there is no documented reason for holding or stopping the medication, the nurse should discuss this with the provider. Ensuring that the patient is receiving evidence-based medical treatment is another strategy for the nurse to use to ensure a smooth discharge transition.

During the hospitalization, patients may have discussed additional therapeutic interventions with the health-care team. These interventions include both implantable cardioverter defibrillator (ICD) and/or cardiac resynchronization therapy (CRT). If the ejection fraction remains 35% or less despite guideline-directed medical therapy, consideration is given to the placement of ICD or CRT. ICD therapy is recommended for primary prevention of sudden cardiac death.[26] CRT is indicated for patients with left bundle-branch block with a QRS duration of 150 ms or greater.[26] As the nurse providing discharge teaching, being familiar with the indications for these devices is important, so that you are able to provide clarification for questions that are asked.

Over time as patients progress along the expected HF spectrum, ambulatory use of inotropes may be used to improve NYHA functional class through symptom management and reduction in hospitalizations.[27] It is important to understand that inotropes are used for palliative care and are not curative.[28] They may be used while awaiting mechanical circulatory support or to provide symptomatic relief as the patient reaches end of life.

An established treatment option for end-stage HF is left ventricular assist devices (LVAD) or heart transplantation. Nurses need to be aware of these interventions and be able to clarify patient questions regarding what their life would be like after receiving once of these treatment options. **Fig. 1** describes the trajectory of HF and provides a visual representation for the clinical course. Interventions along this timeline can reduce the disease progression and improve quality of life.

CLINICS CARE POINTS

- Identify potential precipitants of an HF hospitalization to assist the patient in mitigating these factors.
  - Provide resources to assist with medication adherence.
  - Collaborate with a dietician to identify lower sodium food choices.

- Nurses play a pivotal role in preventing readmission through effective discharge teaching.
  - Discharge education should include daily weight monitoring, medication adherence, dietary sodium limits, and identification of HF symptoms.
  - When possible, caregivers and family members should be included in discharge teaching.

- Inform patients, families, and caregivers that HF is a "forever" illness with acute exacerbations and chronic stages and a variety of treatments available in each phase.

DISCLOSURE

The authors have nothing to disclose.

REFERENCES

1. Benjamin E, Muntner P, Alonso A, et al. Virani, S. and on behalf of the American Heart Association Council on Epidemiology and Prevention Statistics Committee and Stroke Statistics Subcommittee. Circulation 2019;139(10):e56–528.
2. Urbich M, Globe G, Pantiri K, et al. A systematic review of medical costs associated with heart failure in the USA (2014–2020). Pharmacoeconomics 2020; 38(11):1219–36.
3. Li M, Li Y, Meng Q, et al. Effects of nurse-led transitional care interventions for patients with heart failure on healthcare utilization: A meta-analysis of randomized controlled trials. PLoS One 2021;16(12):e0261300.
4. Charais C, Bowers M, Do OO, et al. Implementation of a Disease Management Program in Adult Patients With Heart Failure. Prof Case Manag 2020;25(6): 312–23.
5. Waters S, Giblin E. Acute Heart Failure: Pearls for the First Posthospitalization Visit. J Nurse Pract 2019;15(1):80–6.
6. Khan M, Sreenivasan J, Lateef N, et al. Trends in 30- and 90-day readmission rates for heart failure. Circulation: Heart Fail 2021;14:e008335.
7. Magnani JW, Mujahid MS, Aronow HD, et al. Health Literacy and Cardiovascular Disease: Fundamental Relevance to Primary and Secondary Prevention: A Scientific Statement From the American Heart Association. Circulation 2018;138(2): e48–74.
8. Van der Heide I, Poureslami I, Mitic W, et al. Health literacy in chronic disease management: a matter of interaction. J Clin Epidemiol 2018;102:134–8.
9. Athilingam P, Jenkins B, Redding BA. Reading Level and Suitability of Congestive Heart Failure (CHF) Education in a Mobile App (CHF Info App): Descriptive Design Study. JMIR Aging 2019;2(1):e12134.
10. Gatto D, Newcomb P. Impressions of Conventional Bedside Discharge Teaching Among Readmitted Heart Failure Patients. J Nurs Adm: 2022;52(9):479–85.
11. Heidenreich PA, Bozkurt B, Aguilar D, et al. AHA/ACC/HFSA Guideline for the Management of Heart Failure: A Report of the American College of Cardiology/ American Heart Association Joint Committee on Clinical Practice Guidelines. Circulation 2022;145(18):e895–1032 [published correction appears in Circulation.

2022 May 3;145(18):e1033] [published correction appears in Circulation. 2022 Sep 27;146(13):e185].

12. Palazzuoli A, Evangelista I, Ruocco G, et al. Early readmission for heart failure: An avoidable or ineluctable debacle? Int J Cardiol 2019;277:186–95.

13. Mai Ba H, Son YJ, Lee K, et al. Transitional Care Interventions for Patients with Heart Failure: An Integrative Review. Int J Environ Res Public Health 2020;17(8):2925.

14. Almanasreh E, Moles R, Chen T. The medication discrepancy taxonomy (Med-Tax): The development and validation of a classification system for medication discrepancies identified through medication reconciliation. Res Soc Adm Pharm 2020;16(2):142–8.

15. Anderson Sarah L, C Marrs Joel. A Review of the Role of the Pharmacist in Heart Failure Transition of Care. Adv Ther 2018;35(3):311–23.

16. Patel Y, Joseph J. Sodium Intake and Heart Failure. Int J Mol Sci 2020;21(24): 9474.

17. Turrise S. Illness Representations, Treatment Beliefs, Medication Adherence, and 30-Day Hospital Readmission in Adults With Chronic Heart Failure: A Prospective Correlational Study. J Cardiovasc Nurs 2016;31(3):245–54.

18. Lee KK, Thomas RC, Tan TC, et al. The Heart Failure Readmission Intervention by Variable Early Follow-up (THRIVE) Study: A Pragmatic Randomized Trial. Circ Cardiovasc Qual Outcomes 2020;13(10):e006553.

19. Hollenberg S, Warner Stevenson L, Ahmad T, et al. ACC Expert Consensus Decision Pathway on Risk Assessment, Management, and Clinical Trajectory of Patients Hospitalized With Heart Failure. J Am Coll Cardiol 2019;74(15):1966–2011.

20. Matsukawa R, Masuda S, Matsuura H, et al. Early follow-up at outpatient care after discharge improves long-term heart failure readmission rate and prognosis. ESC Heart Fail 2021;8(4):3002–13.

21. Taniguchi C, Seto N, Shimizu Y. Outpatient nursing support for self-monitoring in patients with chronic heart failure. PLoS One 2021;16(7):e0254019.

22. Li CC, Chang SR, Shun SC. The self-care coping process in patients with chronic heart failure: A qualitative study. J Clin Nurs 2019;28(3–4):509–19.

23. Nordfonn OK, Morken IM, Lunde Husebø AM. A qualitative study of living with the burden from heart failure treatment: Exploring the patient capacity for self-care. Nurs Open 2020;7(3):804–13.

24. Long L, Mordi IR, Bridges C, et al. Exercise-based cardiac rehabilitation for adults with heart failure. Cochrane Database Syst Rev 2019;1(1):CD003331.

25. Burnett H, Earley A, Voors AA, et al. Thirty Years of Evidence on the Efficacy of Drug Treatments for Chronic Heart Failure With Reduced Ejection Fraction: A Network Meta-Analysis. Circ Heart Fail 2017;10(1):e003529.

26. Greene SJ, Fonarow GC, DeVore AD, et al. Titration of Medical Therapy for Heart Failure With Reduced Ejection Fraction. J Am Coll Cardiol 2019;73(19):2365–83.

27. Yancy CW, Jessup M, Bozkurt B, et al. ACC/AHA/HFSA Focused Update of the 2013 ACCF/AHA Guideline for the Management of Heart Failure: A Report of the American College of Cardiology/American Heart Association Task Force on Clinical Practice Guidelines and the Heart Failure Society of America. Circulation 2017;136(6):e137–61.

28. Graffagnino JP, Avant LC, Calkins BC, et al. Home Therapies in Advanced Heart Failure: Inotropes and Diuretics. Curr Heart Fail Rep 2020;17(5):314–23.

Dyslipidemia Update

Jennifer Ballard-Hernandez, DNP, FNP-BC, AG ACNP-BC[a,b,*],
James Sall, PhD, FNP-BC[c]

KEYWORDS

- Dyslipidemia • Hyperlipidemia • Cardiovascular risk reduction

KEY POINTS

- The foundation of cardiovascular risk reduction for primary and secondary prevention is lifestyle management.
- Statins remain the cornerstone of pharmacologic therapy in the management of dyslipidemia.
- Traditional and novel nonstatin pharmacologic therapies may be considered for specific patient populations to reduce cardiovascular risk further.

INTRODUCTION

Cardiovascular disease (CVD) is the leading cause of morbidity and mortality in the United States.[1,2] The development of atherosclerotic cardiovascular disease (ASCVD) is largely dependent on a multitude of modifiable and nonmodifiable risk factors. Control and reduction of CVD risk factors, including elevated blood pressure, elevated blood glucose levels, tobacco use, poor dietary habits, a sedentary lifestyle, and high cholesterol levels, can contribute to a reduction in CVD morbidity and mortality. Elevated serum cholesterol is a well-established independent risk factor in the development of ASCVD and remains a major target for cardiovascular risk reduction. Importantly, the isolated management of dyslipidemia has shifted to managing dyslipidemia in the context of overall risk for CVD in the latest professional guidelines for the management of cholesterol. Cholesterol guidelines are published by a multitude of professional societies, including the American College of Cardiology (ACC)/American Heart Association (AHA),[3] the US Preventive Services Task Force (USPSTF),[4] the Department of Veterans Affairs (VA)/Department of Defense (DoD),[5] the Canadian Cardiovascular Society (CCS),[6] and the European Society of Cardiology (ESC).[7]

[a] Cardiology Division, Department of Medicine; [b] Department of Veterans Affairs, VA Long Beach Healthcare System, 5901 East 7th Street, Long Beach, CA 90822, USA; [c] Evidence-Based Practice Program, Veterans Health Administration, 811 Vermont Avenue, Northwest, Washington, DC 20420, USA
* Corresponding author.
E-mail address: JHernandezNP@yahoo.com

Nurs Clin N Am 58 (2023) 295–308
https://doi.org/10.1016/j.cnur.2023.05.002
0029-6465/23/Published by Elsevier Inc.

The current treatment milieu for dyslipidemia focuses on lifestyle changes and lipid-lowering drugs. The management of dyslipidemia continues to be dynamic and, at times, controversial. Although some clinical practice guidelines from various professional societies are often aligned in their recommendations, others are often nuanced, with subtle differences and sometimes conflicting guidance. The purpose of this article is to display the similarities and highlight areas of discordance and the need for future research.

MEASUREMENT OF LIPOPROTEINS

The biochemistry of lipids and lipoproteins is multifaceted and complex. Lipoproteins vary in size and density and are classified by their density in plasma, gauged by floatation in an ultracentrifuge.[8] Serum cholesterol and its lipoprotein carriers are implicated in the progression of ASCVD.[7] The primary serum lipoproteins include chylomicrons, very low-density lipoprotein, intermediate-density lipoprotein, low-density lipoprotein cholesterol (LDL-C), and high-density lipoprotein (HDL-C). Advanced lipid testing, including LDL particle size and composition, may be evaluated in special populations to evaluate additional cardiovascular risk. Emerging evidence associates lipoprotein a [Lp(a)] and apolipoprotein B (apoB) levels with additional cardiovascular risk for ASCVD and may be measured in specific high-risk populations.[3]

The serum lipid panel, measured via a peripheral blood draw, is an easily accessible set of clinical data that nurses and other clinicians can utilize in cardiovascular risk assessment. In general, dyslipidemia has traditionally been defined as any abnormal level of lipoproteins and is frequently evidenced in one or more of the following: LDL-C $\geq$130 mg per deciliter (mg/dL), HDL-C <40 mg/dL, or triglycerides (TGs) $\geq$200 mg/dL.[5] The most commonly measured indices in the standard lipid panel include total cholesterol, TGs, LDL-C, and HDL-C. Although LDL-C is a focal point in professional society guidelines, it is rarely measured directly and typically is measured using the Friedewald equation LDL-C = (TC)-(TG/5)-(HDL-C). The Friedewald equation can be inaccurate if the TGs are elevated.[9]

Traditionally, serum sampling for lipid analysis has recommended a fasting state. Recent evidence has shifted the paradigm and it is generally agreed upon by the contemporary clinical practice guidelines that a nonfasting panel is appropriate for screening in the general population.[3–6] There are 2 notable exceptions where a fasting lipid panel is recommended including those being evaluated for a family history of premature ASCVD or genetic hyperlipidemia and individuals who have consumed a high-fat meal in the previous 8 hours.[3,5] The initial age for screening for lipid disorders and the longitudinal monitoring frequency recommendations differ slightly by each respective professional society guidelines; however, the ACC/AHA cholesterol guideline recommends that either a fasting or a nonfasting plasma lipid profile is effective in estimating ASCVD risk and documenting baseline LDL-C for adults aged 20 years or more who are not on lipid-lowering therapy.[3]

PATIENT MANAGEMENT GROUPS
Primary and Secondary Prevention

Identification of appropriate patient populations for risk stratification is imperative to provide accurate risk assessment and appropriate therapeutic treatment. Primary prevention of ASCVD refers to efforts to prevent disease before it occurs.[10] Several professional societies endorse that the most important way to prevent ASCVD development is to promote a healthy lifestyle throughout life.[3,7,9] Secondary prevention refers to efforts that treat known ASCVD and focus on preventing the progression of ASCVD or ASCVD events. Those with known ASCVD are at the highest risk of recurrent events.[3,7,9]

Familial Hypercholesterolemia

Familial hypercholesterolemia (FH) is a genetic disorder resulting from a genetic mutation of one or more genes for LDL-C catabolism. This results in elevated LDL-C levels and a predisposition to premature ASCVD. A variety of diagnostic criteria schemas can be used diagnose FH, but a commonly used definition is that the AHA's criteria for clinical diagnosis are an LDL-C of > 190 mg/dl and a first-degree relative with an LDL-C of > 190 mg/dl or known premature ASCVD.[11] Heterozygous FH (HeFH) is one of the most common genetic disorders and affects approximately 1 in 311 individuals.[12] Patients typically present with premature ASCVD from long-term exposure to elevated LDL-C levels. Homozygous FH (HoFH), however, is a rare genetic condition causing severe, premature ASCVD with associated high mortality before age 20.[13]

CARDIOVASCULAR RISK ASSESSMENT

Assessment of ASCVD risk is the foundation of primary prevention.[9] Cardiovascular risk in the primary prevention population can be calculated using a variety of validated risk calculators. There is significant variation in the recommended use of different risk estimators in professional society guidelines.[3–6] Endorsed by the 2018 AHA/ACC Cholesterol Guidelines and the USPSTF Statin Use for the Primary Prevention of Cardiovascular Disease in Adults statement, the Pooled Cohort Equation (PCE) has become the most commonly utilized risk calculator in the United States.[3,4] The PCE estimates the 10 year and lifetime risk of subsequent ASCVD events using a variety of factors, including the nonmodifiable risk factors of age, sex, and race, and the modifiable risk factors of total cholesterol, HDL cholesterol, LDL cholesterol, blood pressure, diabetes status, smoking status, and statin, aspirin, and blood pressure lowering medication use.

The 10 year ASCVD risk can serve as a framework and allow for a shared decision-making conversation and recommended interventions, including lipid management. Although developed and validated to predict population risk, the PCE can over or underestimate risk in certain patient subgroups, such as race.[3] PCE risk estimates must be used in context of the patient's specific circumstances when deciding to implement statin therapy. The PCE should only be used to estimate risk in primary prevention efforts and should not be used to estimate risk in patients for the secondary prevention of ASCVD. For primary prevention, in patients where statin treatment decisions are uncertain, nurses and other clinicians can consider obtaining a coronary artery calcium score to help stratify ASCVD risk and facilitate decision-making.[3]

RISK ENHANCING FACTORS

In addition to LDL-C, several other factors are associated with higher ASCVD risk and are known as risk-enhancing factors. The 2018 ACC/AHA Cholesterol Guidelines recommend the evaluation of major risk factors and risk-enhancing factors to serve as the framework in the decision to initiate and adjust the intensity of LDL-lowering therapy.[3] These risk-enhancing factors include family history of premature ASCVD (men <55 years old; women < 65 years old), primary hypercholesterolemia (LDL-C 160–189 mg/dL, non-HDL-C 190–219 mg/dL), metabolic syndrome, chronic kidney disease, chronic inflammatory conditions, history of premature menopause, high-risk races/ethnicities, and lipids/biomarkers associated with ASCVD, including elevated high-sensitivity C-reactive protein ($\geq$2.0 mg/L), elevated Lp(a) ($\geq$50 mg/dL), elevated apoB ($\geq$130 mg/dL), or Ankle-Brachial Index < 0.9.[3]

LIFESTYLE THERAPIES

Healthy lifestyle habits have been the cornerstone of cardiovascular risk reduction for primary and secondary prevention. All professional society guideline recommendations highlight the critical role that a healthy lifestyle plays in ASCVD risk reduction and prevention of recurrent events.[3–6] Healthy lifestyle habits include diet, physical activity, maintaining a healthy weight, maintaining normal blood pressure, and avoiding tobacco use and secondhand smoke.[3–6] Key lifestyle habits are outlined in **Fig. 1**. Intensive lifestyle change has the potential to lower lipids and the associated ASCVD risk factor burden.[3]

Diet

Nutrition plays a pivotal role in the prevention of ASCVD. Both through reducing circulating blood lipid levels and direct action on cardiovascular risk factors, dietary factors influence the development of ASCVD. To decrease ASCVD risk, the ACC/AHA Primary Prevention of Cardiovascular Disease Guideline recommends a diet rich in fruits, vegetables, nuts, legumes, whole grains, and fish.[9] Given the association of increased CV mortality in observational studies, sugar, low-calorie sweeteners, high and low carbohydrate diets, *trans* fats, saturated fat, sodium, and red and processed meats should be avoided or minimized.[9] The Mediterranean diet has proven, through randomized control trials, to be effective in reducing CV events in primary and secondary prevention.[14–16] The Mediterranean dietary pattern includes a high unsaturated fat/saturated fat ratio, a substantial increase in fiber from plant-based foods, an increased intake of fish, a moderate intake of low-fat dairy products, and low-to-moderate red wine intake for those who drink alcohol.[5] The VA/DoD guideline authors also recommend registered dietitian-led medical nutrition therapy for the management of dyslipidemia because lipid outcomes have shown improvement with this intervention.[5]

Bodily Weight

Maintaining a healthy body weight is a necessary healthy lifestyle behavior for the primary prevention of ASCVD. Weight target goals for CVD prevention include a body

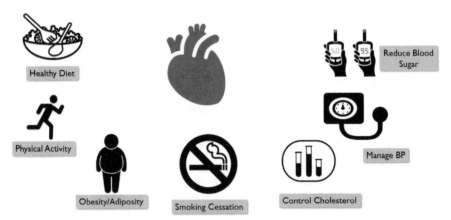

Fig. 1. Key concepts for CV prevention.

mass index of 20 to 25 kg/m^2 and a waist circumference < 94 cm in men and <80 cm in women.[7] Being overweight, obesity, and abdominal obesity are often important risk factors for the development of dyslipidemia and cardiovascular risk.[7] Body weight reduction for those who are overweight or have obesity, even in modest amounts, has been shown to improve lipid abnormalities as well as positively impact other CV-related risk factors.[17]

Physical Activity

The benefits of physical activity in primary and secondary prevention of CVD are abundant. Physical activity can improve CV outcomes by positively altering lipid profiles, in addition to improving other risk factors that can contribute to cardiovascular risk. Multiple professional societies recommend at least 150 minutes per week of moderate-intensity or 75 minutes per week of vigorous-intensity aerobic physical activity to reduce ASCVD risk.[3,5,7,9] Although data are lacking from randomized control studies, there is an expansive body of observational data to demonstrate associations between recommended physical activity levels and a reduction in CV mortality in the primary and secondary prevention populations.[18,19]

PHARMACOLOGIC THERAPIES

Pharmacologic treatment is one of the key foundations in the management of dyslipidemia to reduce ASCVD events in primary and secondary prevention.[3,5,7,9] The primary emphasis of lipid-lowering therapy is to achieve LDL-C reduction with subsequent reductions in ASCVD-related events and mortality.[9] In recent years, specific LDL-C goals and targets have been a matter of intense debate in professional society guidelines; however, the overarching theme and consensus across all guideline recommendations is that elevated LDL-C is associated with cardiovascular risk, and lowering the LDL-C reduces ASCVD events and mortality.[3,5,7,9]

Statin Therapy

Statins, inhibitors of 3-hydroxy-3-methylglutaryl-coenzyme A (HMG-CoA) reductase, are the primary pharmacologic therapy used in the management of hypercholesterolemia. Statins reduce cholesterol synthesis in the liver by competitively inhibiting HMG-CoA reductase. This results in a reduction of intracellular cholesterol, promoting LDL receptor expression in the hepatocytes, increasing uptake of LDL, and augmenting LDL clearing capacity. Statins efficiently reduce plasma cholesterol. Beyond LDL lowering, statins possess anti-inflammatory effects, especially at the site of endothelial dysfunction and atheroma, resulting in the stabilization of plaque.[20,21] Statins lower LDL-C in a dose-response manner, although variation in response may occur because of various factors including genetics, biologic availability, baseline LDL-C levels, and medication adherence.[8]

Statins are the cornerstone of pharmacotherapy treatment of dyslipidemia in the management of cardiovascular risk reduction. Evidence shows that statins lower ASCVD events, CV mortality, and all-cause mortality in secondary prevention and select primary prevention populations.[3,5,7,9] An area of discordance among contemporary professional society guidelines is variation in statin treatment group approaches and dosing recommendations for moderate to high-risk patient groups. These differences are outlined in **Table 1**. Statin intensity and dosing recommendations are outlined in **Table 2**.

Statins are generally well tolerated, and although there are known risks associated with statin use, the benefits outweigh the potential risks in targeted guideline-

Table 1
Recommendations for statin treatment for primary and secondary prevention based on professional guidelines

	ACC/AHA 2018[3]	CCS 2021[6]	ESC/EAS 2019[7]	USPSTF 2022[4]	VA/DoD 2020[5]
For Primary Prevention	a. *Borderline Risk* > 5% to < 7.5% with risk enhancers: moderate intensity statin b. *Intermediate Risk* ≥ 7.5% to < 20%: moderate intensity to reduce LDL-C 30%–49% c. *High Risk* ≥ 20%: initiate statins to reduce LDL-C ≥ 50%	a. Intermediate Risk 10%–19.9%: Initiate statin with additional risk factors present b. *High Risk* ≥ 20%: initiate statin c. Statin indicated conditions: Most patients with diabetes, chronic kidney disease	d. *Moderate Risk* ≥ 1% to <5% e. *High Risk* ≥ 5%- <10% f. *Very High Risk* ≥ 10% ᵃTreatment groups and statin doses depend on untreated LDL-C levels	a. Age 40–75: 7.5% to < 10% and 1 or more CVD risk factor; moderate dose statin in select patients after risk discussion b. Age 40–75: risk ≥ 10% and 1 or more CVD risk factor moderate dose statin c. Age > 75: Insufficient evidence for recommendation	a. Risk 6%–12%: Risk discussion, then moderate for select patients b. Risk > 12%: moderate intensity statin
For Secondary Prevention	Clinical ASCVD *not at very high risk:* a. Age ≤ 75: High intensity statin b. Age > 75: Moderate or high intensity statin is reasonable ASCVD high risk: a. High intensity or maximally tolerated statin	Maximally tolerated statin dose	Maximally tolerated statin dose to achieve target treatment goal	Not addressed	Moderate intensity statin, but high intensity for higher risk ASCVD patients

ᵃ All risks calculated using a 10 y ASCVD risk calculator.

Table 2
Statin intensity and dosing

Level of Intensity	High Intensity	Moderate Intensity	Low Intensity
Estimated LDL-C lowering	≥50%	30%–49%	<30%
Agent and dosing[a]	Atorvastatin 40–80 mg Rosuvastatin 20–40 mg	Atorvastatin 10–20 mg Rosuvastatin 5–10 mg Simvastatin 20–40 mg Pravastatin 40–80 mg Lovastatin 40–80 mg Fluvastatin XL 80 mg (or Fluvastatin 40 mg BID) Pitavastatin 1–4 mg	Simvastatin 10 mg

[a] All are daily doses unless indicated.
Adapted from Grundy SM, Stone NJ, Bailey AL, et al. 2018 AHA/ACC/AACVPR/AAPA/ABC/ACPM/ADA/AGS/APhA/ASPC/NLA/PCNA Guideline on the Management of Blood Cholesterol: A Report of the American College of Cardiology/American Heart Association Task Force on Clinical Practice Guidelines. Circulation. 2019;139(25):e1082-e1143.

recommended populations.[3,5,7,9] However, studies of primary and secondary prevention suggest that higher dose statin use increases the potential adverse event risk.[5] Risks involved with statin therapy include myalgia (infrequent), myositis/myopathy (rare), statin-associated autoimmune antibodies (rare), rhabdomyolysis (rare), new onset diabetes mellitus (rare), transaminase elevation (infrequent), and liver failure (rare).[5] Reassuringly, the SAMSON randomized clinical trial evaluating side effects of statins showed patient-reported symptom scores were no different between months on statins versus placebo.[22] Thus, when a patient reports statin-associated side effects, it is imperative for the nurse and provider to perform a thorough assessment of symptoms to identify perceived side effects versus side effects that require immediate follow-up and intervention.

Ezetimibe

Ezetimibe is an LDL-C-lowering agent primarily utilized to lower LDL-C as an add-on therapy in patients who are not achieving target LDL-C despite maximally tolerated statin therapy. This medication can be used as a statin add-on therapy or as a monotherapy in patients with partial or complete intolerance to statins. Ezetimibe targets intestinal absorption by inhibiting Niemann-Pick C1-like 1 receptors, a protein in the gastrointestinal tract that is critical for cholesterol absorption.[7] As a result, biliary cholesterol absorption is inhibited at the level of the brush border of the intestine.[7] Ezetimibe reduces the amount of cholesterol delivered to the liver, and in response, the liver upregulates LDLR expression, increasing LDL clearance from the blood.[7] Ezetimibe is well tolerated with few adverse effects as monotherapy.[7] The most common complaints are fatigue and gastrointestinal side effects, including abdominal pain and diarrhea.

Ezetimibe, when added to ongoing statin therapy, has been shown to lower LDL-C and reduce cardiovascular events for secondary prevention of ASCVD. The clinical efficacy of ezetimibe has been demonstrated in multiple trials. In the IMProved Reduction of Outcomes: Vytorin Efficacy International Trial (IMPROVE-IT), ezetimibe was added to simvastatin in patients with acute coronary syndrome.[23] The IMPROVE-IT trial showed that ezetimibe, in combination with simvastatin, decreased LDL-C and improved cardiovascular outcomes. The 2018 ACC/AHA Cholesterol Guidelines recommend the addition of ezetimibe for high risk ASCVD patients with an LDL-C ≥70 mg/dL despite maximally tolerated statins (Class IIa indication).[3] Similarly, the 2020 VA/DoD dyslipidemia guideline also recommends the addition of ezetimibe to moderate-intensity statin to high-intensity statin in higher risk patients.[5] At this time, there is a paucity of evidence to support the use of ezetimibe in the primary prevention of ASCVD. Dosing recommendations are outlined in **Table 3**.

Proprotein Convertase Subtilisin/Kexin Type 9 Inhibitors

The proprotein convertase subtilisin/kexin type 9 inhibitors (PCSK9 inhibitors) monoclonal antibody drug class has demonstrated potent LDL-C lowering capability, regardless of background therapy, in a wide variety of patients. PCSK9 is a protein that regulates the expression of low-density lipoprotein receptors (LDLR) on the hepatocyte, thus reducing deregulation of the LDLR.[7] This deregulation allows LDLRs to clear LDL-C from the circulation, resulting in lower LDL-C levels.[7]

Randomized clinical trials have demonstrated the ability of PCSK9 inhibitors to reduce LDL-C and ASCVD events in the FOURIER and ODYSSEY OUTCOMES trials.[24–26] The 2018 ACC/AHA cholesterol guideline indicates that it is reasonable to add a PCSK9 inhibitor for patients at high risk for ASCVD and an LDL-C ≥70 mg/dL despite maximally tolerated statins and ezetimibe (Class IIa indication).[3] Similarly, the 2020 VA/DoD Dyslipidemia Guideline also suggests the addition of a PCSK9 inhibitor to a maximally tolerated statin dose with ezetimibe in patients at higher risk for ASCVD.[5] Given the uncertain long-term safety data with PCSK9 inhibitors and cost, ACC/AHA and VA/DoD professional guidelines recommend shared decision-making discussions with patients about the net benefit, safety, and cost.[3,5] Dosing recommendations are outlined in **Table 3**.

Inclisiran

Inclisiran is a novel, first in-class of small interfering RNA (siRNA)-based therapeutic to receive FDA approval in December 2021 for the treatment of HeFH or hyperlipidemia in patients with ASCVD who have not reached optimal LDL levels despite treatment with statins.[7] Inclisiran inhibits the synthesis of PCSK9 by targeting its mRNA.[7] Inclisiran binds to specific receptors that are highly expressed on the hepatocyte surface and within the intracellular milieu and binds to the RNA-induced silencing complex, thus inhibiting its expression and lowering circulating LDL-C in the bloodstream.[7]

Although PCSK9 inhibitors have been an important addition to a variety of approaches to lowering LDL-C and ASCVD risk, their cost and frequency of administration (every 2–4 weeks) pose challenges for implementation in the real world. One of the potential benefits of inclisiran is that it requires less frequent dosing (initial dose, quarterly, then semiannually). The ORION-9, ORION-10, and ORION-11 studies evaluated inclisiran administration in patients with HeFH and ASCVD on maximally tolerated statins with or without ezetimibe. Inclisiran led to a near 50% reduction in LDL-C.[26,27] Studies from the patient-level pooled analysis of ORION-9, ORION-10, and ORION-11 suggest potential CV benefits of lowering LDL-C with inclisiran, with potential benefits for MACE reduction.[27] Dosing recommendations are outlined in **Table 3**.

Bempedoic Acid

Bempedoic acid is a novel, first-in-class LDL-C-lowering oral agent that gained FDA approval in February 2020 for the treatment of adults with HeFH or established ASCVD who require additional lowering of LDL-C. Bempedoic acid is an adenosine triphosphate-citrate lyase (ACL) inhibitor that lowers LDL-C by inhibiting cholesterol

Table 3
Non-statin pharmacologic agents

Drug Category	Drug	Dose and Route	Potential Adverse Drug Reactions	Outcomes
Cholesterol absorption inhibitors	Ezetimibe	10 mg daily orally	• Diarrhea • Arthralgia • Myalgia • Hepatitis (rare)	Reduces nonfatal CV events in secondary prevention in addition to statin
PCSK9 inhibitors	Alirocumab	75 mg once every 2 wk OR 300 mg once every 4 wk Max: 150 mg every 2 wk subcutaneous	• Injection site reactions • Nasopharyngitis • Influenza • Angioedema • Myalgia • Musculoskeletal pain	Reduces nonfatal CV events in secondary prevention in addition to maximally tolerated statin ± ezetimibe
	Evolocumab	140 mg once every 2 wk OR 420 mg once monthly subcutaneous	• Injection site reactions • Nasopharyngitis • Influenza • Cough • Rash • Arthralgia • Fatigue	Reduces nonfatal CV events in secondary prevention in addition to maximally tolerated statin ± ezetimibe
PCSK9 siRNA	Inclisiran	284 mg at initiation, 3 mo after initiation, then every 6 mo subcutaneous	• Injection site reactions • Arthralgia • Diarrhea • Urinary tract infectious disease • Bronchitis	• Near 50% reduction in LDL-C • Effect on cardiovascular morbidity and mortality not yet established
ACL inhibitors	Bempedoic acid	180 mg daily orally	• Hyperuricemia • Gout • Abdominal pain • Increased liver enzymes • Bronchitis • Rupture of tendon	• Used in combination with maximally tolerated statin • Can be used in statin intolerant patients • Reduces risk of MACE

(continued on next page)

Table 3
(continued)

Drug Category	Drug	Dose and Route	Potential Adverse Drug Reactions	Outcomes
Omega-3 fatty acids	Icosapent ethyl	2 gm twice daily with meals orally	• Arthralgia • Peripheral edema • constipation • Gout • Hemorrhage • Atrial fibrillation • Musculoskeletal pain • Potential for allergic reactions in patients with fish allergy	CV mortality and morbidity in patients treated for secondary prevention on statins with persistently elevated TG (>150 mg/dL)

synthesis in the liver.[7] Bempedoic acid is a prodrug activated in the liver, potentially mitigating statin-associated muscle complaints.[28]

Bempedoic acid has demonstrated robust LDL-C-lowering capabilities. The CLEAR Outcomes trial evaluated patients who have statin intolerance and compared bempedoic acid to placebo against a no-statin background.[29] In this randomized trial, bempedoic acid was associated with a lower risk of MACE, including death from CV causes, nonfatal myocardial infarction, and nonfatal stroke.[29] Additionally, small clinical trials evaluating bempedoic acid have signaled that its use slightly increases in gout, tendon rupture, atrial fibrillation, and benign prostatic hypertrophy.[28] Several factors may contribute to implementation challenges with bempedoic acid, including cost and a lack of long-term studies identifying the appropriate patient populations and safety data. Dosing recommendations are outlined in **Table 3**.

Icosapent Ethyl

Icosapent ethyl is a purified ethyl ester of the omega-3 fatty acid eicosapentaenoic acid. It is generally thought that the primary mechanism of benefit from omega-3 fatty acid therapy is because of the reduction of TGs, although anti-inflammatory properties may play a role.[30] In the Reduction of Cardiovascular Events With Icosapent Ethyl-Intervention Trial (REDUCE-IT) trial, treatment with icosapent ethyl, when compared to placebo, reduced fatal and nonfatal MI, fatal and nonfatal stroke, and cardiovascular death.[31] The 2019 EAS/ESC dyslipidemia guidelines recommend the addition of icosapent ethyl 2 g twice daily in high-risk patients with elevated TG levels (135–499 mg/dL) in addition to statin therapy.[7] Dosing recommendations are outlined in **Table 3**.

Low-Density Lipoprotein Apheresis

Apheresis is a treatment option where Apo B-containing lipoproteins are directly removed from the bloodstream using weekly extracorporeal filtration to directly lower LDL-C.[28] This therapy is generally reserved for individuals with HoFH and HeFH who have failed traditional medical therapy. Because apheresis is a specialized procedure, it is often performed in a lipid center of expertise, and treatment accessibility may be limited. Additional limitations to the use of apheresis include time, cost, and patient preference.

ADHERENCE

Patient adherence to lifestyle measures and pharmacologic therapy are imperative factors in the successful management of dyslipidemia. It is well established that suboptimal adherence limits the projected benefits of dyslipidemia treatment.[7] The 2018 ACC/AHA Cholesterol Guideline stresses the importance of ASCVD risk discussions, including adherence to a healthy lifestyle.[3] Additionally, follow-up LDL-C monitoring should be assessed by a fasting lipid test 4 to 12 weeks after statin initiation or dose adjustment to assess adherence and the adequacy of statin therapy.[3] Nurses and other clinicians should use a multifaceted approach to promote adherence, including verbal dialogue, advocating for once daily dosing of medications, the use of automated reminders, and pharmacist and nursing-led interventions.[3,7]

NURSE'S ROLE IN STRATEGIES FOR PRESCRIBING

Nurses play a key role in the pharmacologic and nonpharmacologic management of dyslipidemia to prevent CVD. Nurse-led interventions may encompass a wide variety of treatment approaches, including cardiovascular risk assessment, lifestyle counseling, and education about medications and potential side effects. When compared to usual care, nurse-led interventions have been found to improve the application of guideline-directed medical therapy and adherence to medication.[32–36] With clearly defined training and medication management protocols, nurses can play a pivotal role in the primary and secondary prevention of CVD.

SUMMARY

Dyslipidemia is a significant risk factor in the development and progression of ASCVD, ultimately contributing to adverse cardiovascular outcomes. In recent years, the paradigm has shifted from treating LDL-C targets to a focus on overall ASCVD risk factor reduction. Despite a well-rounded arsenal of pharmacologic and nonpharmacologic therapies to reduce LDL-C and ASCVD, treatment application challenges still exist. The management of dyslipidemia is best approached through a multidisciplinary team-based model of care, including registered nurses. Because research continues to rapidly progress and novel therapeutics become readily available for the management of dyslipidemia, nurses need to stay abreast of the rapidly changing treatment landscape. Nurses and other clinicians can significantly impact cardiovascular risk by practicing in a systematic, guideline-directed manner.

CLINICS CARE POINTS

- The management of dyslipidemia is best approached through a multidisciplinary team-based model.
- A nonfasting serum lipid panel is appropriate for dyslipidemia screening in the general population.
- Cardiovascular risk assessment should be estimated using a validated risk calculator.

DISCLOSURE

The authors have nothing to disclose.

REFERENCES

1. Heron M. Deaths: Leading causes for 2017. Natl Vital Stat Rep 2019;68(6):1–77.
2. Tsao CW, Aday AW, Almarzooq ZI, et al. Heart Disease and Stroke Statistics-2023 Update: A Report From the American Heart Association. Circulation 2023; 147(8):e93–621.
3. Grundy SM, Stone NJ, Bailey AL, et al. 2018 AHA/ACC/AACVPR/AAPA/ABC/ACPM/ADA/AGS/APhA/ASPC/NLA/PCNA Guideline on the Management of Blood Cholesterol: A Report of the American College of Cardiology/American Heart Association Task Force on Clinical Practice Guidelines. Circulation 2019;139(25):e1082–143.
4. Mangione CM, Barry MJ, Nicholson WK, et al. Statin Use for the Primary Prevention of Cardiovascular Disease in Adults: US Preventive Services Task Force Recommendation Statement. JAMA 2022;328(8):746–53.
5. VA/DoD clinical practice guideline for the management of dyslipidemia for cardiovascular risk reduction. Washington, DC: U.S. Government Printing Office; 2020.
6. Pearson GJ, Thanassoulis G, Anderson TJ, et al. 2021 Canadian Cardiovascular Society Guidelines for the Management of Dyslipidemia for the Prevention of Cardiovascular Disease in Adults. Can J Cardiol 2021;37(8):1129–50.

7. Mach F, Baigent C, Catapano AL, et al. 2019 ESC/EAS Guidelines for the management of dyslipidaemias: lipid modification to reduce cardiovascular risk. Eur Heart J 2020;41(1):111–88.
8. Libby P, Bonow R, Mann DL, et al. Braunwald's heart disease : a textbook of cardiovascular medicine. 12th edition. Philadelphia, PA: Elsevier-Saunders; 2022.
9. Arnett DK, Blumenthal RS, Albert MA, et al. 2019 ACC/AHA Guideline on the Primary Prevention of Cardiovascular Disease: A Report of the American College of Cardiology/American Heart Association Task Force on Clinical Practice Guidelines. Circulation 2019;140(11):e596–646.
10. Short L, La VT, Patel M, et al. Primary and Secondary Prevention of CAD: A Review. Int J Angiol 2022;31(1):16–26.
11. Stone NJ, Robinson JG, Lichtenstein AH, et al. 2013 ACC/AHA guideline on the treatment of blood cholesterol to reduce atherosclerotic cardiovascular risk in adults: a report of the American College of Cardiology/American Heart Association Task Force on Practice Guidelines. J Am Coll Cardiol 2014;63(25 Pt B): 2889–934.
12. Hu P, Dharmayat KI, Stevens CAT, et al. Prevalence of Familial Hypercholesterolemia Among the General Population and Patients With Atherosclerotic Cardiovascular Disease: A Systematic Review and Meta-Analysis. Circulation 2020; 141(22):1742–59.
13. Nohara A, Tada H, Ogura M, et al. Homozygous Familial Hypercholesterolemia. J Atheroscler Thromb 2021;28(7):665–78.
14. Estruch R, Ros E, Salas-Salvadó J, et al. Retraction and Republication: Primary Prevention of Cardiovascular Disease with a Mediterranean Diet. N Engl J Med 2013;368:1279–90. N Engl J Med. 2018;378(25):2441-42.
15. Sofi F, Macchi C, Abbate R, et al. Mediterranean diet and health status: an updated meta-analysis and a proposal for a literature-based adherence score. Public Health Nutr 2014;17(12):2769–82.
16. Grosso G, Marventano S, Yang J, et al. A comprehensive meta-analysis on evidence of Mediterranean diet and cardiovascular disease: Are individual components equal? Crit Rev Food Sci Nutr 2017;57(15):3218–32.
17. Zomer E, Gurusamy K, Leach R, et al. Interventions that cause weight loss and the impact on cardiovascular risk factors: a systematic review and meta-analysis. Obes Rev 2016;17(10):1001–11.
18. Hupin D, Roche F, Gremeaux V, et al. Even a low-dose of moderate-to-vigorous physical activity reduces mortality by 22% in adults aged ≥60 years: a systematic review and meta-analysis. Br J Sports Med 2015;49(19):1262–7.
19. Stamatakis E, Lee IM, Bennie J, et al. Does Strength-Promoting Exercise Confer Unique Health Benefits? A Pooled Analysis of Data on 11 Population Cohorts With All-Cause, Cancer, and Cardiovascular Mortality Endpoints. Am J Epidemiol 2018;187(5):1102–12.
20. Sukhova GK, Williams JK, Libby P. Statins reduce inflammation in atheroma of nonhuman primates independent of effects on serum cholesterol. Arterioscler Thromb Vasc Biol 2002;22(9):1452–8.
21. Tahara N, Kai H, Ishibashi M, et al. Simvastatin attenuates plaque inflammation: evaluation by fluorodeoxyglucose positron emission tomography. J Am Coll Cardiol 2006;48(9):1825–31.
22. Howard JP, Wood FA, Finegold JA, et al. Side Effect Patterns in a Crossover Trial of Statin, Placebo, and No Treatment. J Am Coll Cardiol 2021;78(12):1210–22.
23. Cannon CP, Blazing MA, Giugliano RP, et al. Ezetimibe Added to Statin Therapy after Acute Coronary Syndromes. N Engl J Med 2015;372(25):2387–97.

24. Sabatine MS, Giugliano RP, Keech AC, et al. Evolocumab and Clinical Outcomes in Patients with Cardiovascular Disease. N Engl J Med 2017;376(18):1713–22.
25. Schwartz GG, Steg PG, Szarek M, et al. Alirocumab and Cardiovascular Outcomes after Acute Coronary Syndrome. N Engl J Med 2018;379(22):2097–107.
26. Raal FJ, Kallend D, Ray KK, et al. Inclisiran for the Treatment of Heterozygous Familial Hypercholesterolemia. N Engl J Med 2020;382(16):1520–30.
27. Ray KK, Raal FJ, Kallend DG, et al. Inclisiran and cardiovascular events: a patient-level analysis of phase III trials. Eur Heart J 2022;44(2):129–38.
28. Lloyd-Jones DM, Morris PB, Ballantyne CM, et al. 2022 ACC Expert Consensus Decision Pathway on the Role of Nonstatin Therapies for LDL-Cholesterol Lowering in the Management of Atherosclerotic Cardiovascular Disease Risk: A Report of the American College of Cardiology Solution Set Oversight Committee. J Am Coll Cardiol 2022;80(14):1366–418.
29. Nissen SE, Lincoff AM, Brennan D, et al. Bempedoic Acid and Cardiovascular Outcomes in Statin-Intolerant Patients. N Engl J Med 2023;388(15):1353–64.
30. Mason RP, Libby P, Bhatt DL. Emerging Mechanisms of Cardiovascular Protection for the Omega-3 Fatty Acid Eicosapentaenoic Acid. Arterioscler Thromb Vasc Biol 2020;40(5):1135–47.
31. Bhatt DL, Steg PG, Miller M, et al. Cardiovascular Risk Reduction with Icosapent Ethyl for Hypertriglyceridemia. N Engl J Med 2019;380(1):11–22.
32. Zhu X, Wong FKY, Wu CLH. Development and evaluation of a nurse-led hypertension management model: A randomized controlled trial. Int J Nurs Stud 2018;77: 171–8.
33. Shaw R.J., McDuffie J.R., Hendrix C.C., et al., Effects of Nurse-Managed Protocols in the Outpatient Management of Adults with Chronic Conditions [Internet]. Washington (DC): Department of Veterans Affairs (US); 2013. Available at: https://www.ncbi.nlm.nih.gov/books/NBK241377/.
34. Persell SD, Karmali KN, Lazar D, et al. Effect of Electronic Health Record-Based Medication Support and Nurse-Led Medication Therapy Management on Hypertension and Medication Self-management: A Randomized Clinical Trial. JAMA Intern Med 2018;178(8):1069–77.
35. Parappilly BP, Field TS, Mortenson WB, et al. Effectiveness of interventions involving nurses in secondary stroke prevention: A systematic review and meta-analysis. Eur J Cardiovasc Nurs 2018;17(8):728–36.
36. Ogedegbe G, Plange-Rhule J, Gyamfi J, et al. Health insurance coverage with or without a nurse-led task shifting strategy for hypertension control: A pragmatic cluster randomized trial in Ghana. PLoS Med 2018;15(5):e1002561.

Stroke
Hospital Nursing Management Within the First 24 Hours

Susan E. Wilson, DNP, ANP-BC[a],*,
Susan Ashcraft, DNP, APRN, ACNS-BC, CCRN-K, SCRN[b]

KEYWORDS

- Acute hospital nursing care • Ischemic • Subarachnoid • Hemorrhage • Stroke

KEY POINTS

- Review nursing assessment and triage criteria.
- Identify emergent management of stroke and the nurse's role.
- Distinguish nursing interventions to reduce complications within the first 24 hours.
- Encourage nursing palliative care processes for all patients diagnosed with a stroke, regardless of prognosis.

A stroke is simply classified as either ischemic, when a clot forms in a vessel, or hemorrhagic, when there is rupture of a blood vessel. Approximately, 85% of strokes are ischemic, with 15% classified as either intracranial (bleeding within the brain) or subarachnoid hemorrhage (SAH) (bleeding within the subarachnoid space).[1] Both types of strokes are medical emergencies that interrupt blood flow to the brain, resulting in neural tissue death and neurological deficits. Within the United States, someone will have a stroke approximately every 40 seconds.[2] Stroke care is complex, and nurses play a critical role in identification, assessment, management, and coordination throughout the stroke continuum of care.[3,4] This article will explore the nursing care of the patient with ischemic and hemorrhagic stroke during the first 24 hours.

CASE STUDIES
Acute Ischemic Stroke

A 59 year old woman with a history of hypertension (HTN) and diabetes presents with sudden onset slurred speech, right-sided weakness, and numbness. Symptom onset

[a] Department of Neurology, University of North Carolina at Chapel Hill, CB# 7025, 170 Manning Drive, Chapel Hill, NC 27599-7025, USA; [b] Neurocritical Care Clinical Nurse Specialist, Novant Health, Inc., 1918 Randolph Road Suite LL175A, Charlotte, NC 28207, USA
* Corresponding author.
E-mail address: wilsons@neurology.unc.edu

Nurs Clin N Am 58 (2023) 309–324
https://doi.org/10.1016/j.cnur.2023.05.003
0029-6465/23/© 2023 Elsevier Inc. All rights reserved.

occurred 1 hour prior to presentation to the emergency department (ED). Blood pressure (BP) was 192/99 and blood glucose was 187 milligrams per deciliter (mg/dL).

Intracerebral Hemorrhage

A 71 year old man with a history of HTN and atrial fibrillation on a direct-acting oral anticoagulant (DOAC) presents with a sudden onset of nausea and headache followed by right-sided weakness.

Subarachnoid Hemorrhage

A 44 year old woman with complaints of the worst headache of her life, followed by a seizure and loss of consciousness.

Assessment and triage: nurse role

The diagnosis and treatment of stroke rely strongly on the presentation and time of the last known normal (LKN). Emergency nursing triage hastens identification and activates stroke treatment pathways.

HISTORY

During triage, the stroke type is unknown, and all aspects of care are time-sensitive. The nurse will perform an emergent assessment of the airway, breathing, and circulation. If stable, the nurse will obtain a brief focused history that identifies symptoms (**Table 1**), time of stroke symptom onset or LKN (obtained from the patient, family, and/or emergency medical services [EMS]), key medical history, and anticoagulant use. The use of standardized emergent stroke screening tools, such as the Recognition of Stroke in the Emergency Room (ROSIER) Scale (**Table 2**), aids in rapid identification and teasing out stroke mimics.[5] Activation of stroke code alerts/protocols engages providers in the ED (eg, physicians, nurse practitioners, and physician assistants), additional nurses, laboratory personnel, and radiology personnel, facilitating rapid diagnostic studies and neuro-imaging with the goal of minimizing time to treatment.

STAT LABORATORIES

A glucose level must be obtained to exclude hypoglycemia. During the placement of intravenous (IV) access, the nurse will draw stat laboratory tests or utilize point of care testing. In addition, for patients taking anticoagulants, a stat prothrombin time is necessary to determine thrombolysis eligibility or the need for reversal.

NEURO-IMAGING

Acute stroke protocols prioritize imaging, with many hospitals implementing direct transfer to computerized tomography (CT) from EMS if the patient is stable. The nurse is key in determining the safety of following such protocols and coordinating the workflow of the interdisciplinary team during the diagnostic work-up. An initial noncontrast CT is critical for excluding intracerebral or SAH.[3]

Advanced imaging is useful for accurate diagnosis, treatment, and prognosis. In acute ischemic stroke (AIS), perfusion imaging can assist in identifying patients that may benefit beyond the standard treatment window. CT perfusion (CTP) provides information on infarct core volume (irreversible), ischemic penumbra (salvageable tissue), and mismatch, indicating prompt intervention may provide reperfusion and improve outcomes[6] (**Fig. 1**).

Table 1
Recognition of stroke symptoms

Signs and Symptoms of Stroke	Ischemic Stroke	Intracerebral Hemorrhage Stroke	Subarachnoid Stroke
Sudden confusion	X	X	X
Sudden unilateral weakness or numbness	X	X	X
Sudden visual deficit	X	X	X
Sudden dizziness, gait disturbance, balance difficulty, or ataxia	X	X	X
Sudden language difficulties; aphasia, dysarthria	X	X	X
Sudden nausea and/or vomiting		X	X
Sudden severe headache with no known cause	X	X	X
Sudden severe "thunderclap" headache			X
Sudden loss of consciousness		X	X
Photophobia and/or nuchal rigidity			X
Seizure		X	X

Noncontrast CT is the imaging of choice to detect intracerebral or SAH because of the availability and speed for which it can be completed. Acute hemorrhage is seen as an area of high density (shades of white) and can detect blood as small as 2 mm in size. Brain matter is low density and appears in shades of gray. The location of high-density areas of blood on CT further describes the type of hemorrhage and location of the stroke. Intracerebral hemorrhage (ICH) may extend from the brain parenchyma into the ventricular system (**Fig. 2**). Subarachnoid hemorrhage is defined as blood within the subarachnoid space and may appear diffuse, involving the ventricular system (**Fig. 3**).

For patients with a diagnosis of hemorrhagic stroke, nurses should anticipate a follow-up CT scan 6 hours and 24 hours after presentation to monitor for hematoma expansion or the development of cerebral edema. In addition, CT angiography (CTA) within the first few hours may assist with determining patients at high risk for hematoma expansion or extension into the ventricular system.[7]

Digital subtraction angiography (DSA) is the gold standard for the diagnosis of aneurysmal SAH and should be completed early to determine size, location, and aneurysmal characteristics. Data obtained from DSA will assist in the decision of securement approaches.

Table 2
ROSIER: score > 0 indicates possible stroke[5]

Symptoms	Score
Loss of consciousness or syncope	Yes: −1, No: 0
Seizure activity	Yes: −1, No: 0
Asymmetric facial weakness	Yes: +1, No: 0
Asymmetric arm weakness	Yes: +1, No: 0
Asymmetric leg weakness	Yes: +1, No: 0
Speech disturbance	Yes: +1, No: 0
Visual field deficit	Yes: +1, No: 0

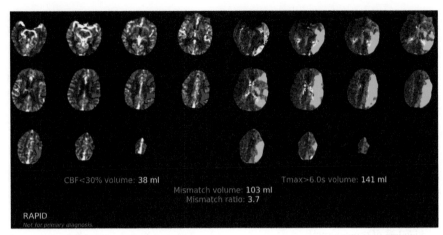

CBF<30% volume: **38 ml**   Tmax>6.0s volume: **141 ml**

Mismatch volume: **103 ml**
Mismatch ratio: **3.7**

RAPID
Not for primary diagnosis

Fig. 1. CTP of left MCA ischemic stroke.

NEUROLOGICAL EXAMINATION

The nurse should complete a brief but thorough neurological exam. The National Institutes of Health Stroke Scale (NIHSS) identifies stroke severity, predicts prognosis, may identify stroke location, determines treatment eligibility, assists with monitoring for improvement or deterioration, and promotes communication between the health care team.[8] The NIHSS ranges from 0 to 42, with higher scores associated with larger strokes and requiring training to ensure exam reliability.[9] The nursing guidelines provide a thorough NIHSS table of pearls assessing the aphasic, comatose, and intubated patient.[3]

The Glasgow Coma Scale (GCS) can be a useful assessment for patients with limited neurological exams and decreased level of consciousness (LOC) (**Table 3**).

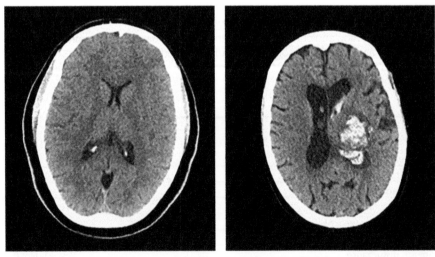

Fig. 2. Normal brain CT (image on the left) compared to CT of left basal ganglia and intraventricular hemorrhage (image on the right).

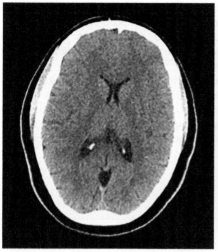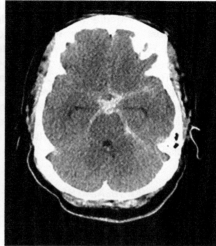

Fig. 3. Normal brain CT (image on the left) compared to CT of an aneurysmal subarachnoid hemorrhage (image on the right).

The nurse should use the GCS to trend improvements or declines in LOC and add components of the neurological assessment as the patient is able to participate.[7]

EMERGENT MANAGEMENT OF STROKE: NURSE ROLE
Initial blood pressure management

Blood pressure management depends on stroke type and treatment candidacy. In ischemic stroke, BP is often elevated to maximize perfusion and will spontaneously decline within the first 24 hours, returning to baseline over the next 4 to 7 days.[10] Because many patients have comorbid conditions, the guidelines recommend that for patients with severe elevations in their BP (≥220/120 mmHg) and not treated with thrombolysis, it is reasonable to decrease the BP by 15% during the first 24 hours.[11]

Table 3 Glasgow Coma Scale[7]	
Eye Opening	4 = spontaneous
	3 = to sound
	2 = to pressure
	1 = none
Verbal Response	5 = oriented
	4 = confused
	3 = words, but not coherent
	2 = sounds, but no words
	1 = none
Best Motor Response	6 = obeys commands
	5 = localizing
	4 = normal flexion
	3 = abnormal flexion
	2 = extension
	1 = none
Total	3–15

The optimal BP for thrombolysis eligibility is < 185/110, with the goal dropping to < 180/105 mmHg after treatment initiation.[11] Systolic blood pressure (SBP) management post endovascular recanalization (TICI 2b or 3) ranges from 120 to 160 mmHg. For nontreatment eligible patients or those that are not recanalized, a higher BP is allowed to support cerebral perfusion.[12]

Acute HTN is also common in ICH, and variability in control may contribute to hematoma expansion and poor outcomes. The target SBP goal for ICH is between 130 and 150 mmHg[7] and for SAH, guidelines recommend maintaining the SBP < 160 mmHg and avoiding aggressive lowering until the aneurysm is secured.[13] The use of fast acting and easily titratable medications is commonly used to provide rapid lowering and precise BP control.

ISCHEMIC STROKE TREATMENT
Thrombolysis

Treatment should be administered within 4.5 hours from symptom onset, and the sooner the better because every minute counts in preventing further brain tissue damage. For patients treated with thrombolysis, the nurse is a critical member of the treatment team, ensuring each step in the thrombolysis pathway is followed and a rapid treatment time is achieved. Once the decision is made to treat, nursing actions include:

- Ensure 2 large-bore IV lines are placed and patent
- Ensure the SBP is < 185 millimeters of mercury (mmHg)
- Calculate the dose based on the patient's actual body weight at 0.9 mg/kg (milligrams per kilogram) with a maximum dose of 90 mg
- Perform a 2 person sign-off to verify the correct dose
- Administer 10% of the dose as a bolus over 2 minutes and the remaining 90% via IV infusion over 1 hour
- After drug infusion, hang normal saline and flush at the same rate as the drug to ensure the dose is received

MONITORING DURING AND POST-THROMBOLYSIS

- Vital signs and neurological assessments are performed frequently, with standard protocols recommending every 15 minutes during and after drug infusion for 2 hours, every 30 minutes for 6 hours, and hourly until 24 hours after treatment.
- Maintain BP < 180/105.
- Assess for signs of systemic bleeding, which may present as blood leakage at catheter sites, gum bleeding, or bruising under BP cuffs. Symptomatic intracranial bleeding may present as a change in LOC, nausea and vomiting, headache, worsening of neurological symptoms, and increased BP.
- If symptoms of symptomatic intracranial bleeding occur, immediately stop the thrombolysis drug and notify the treating provider.
- Assess for signs of angioedema. Orolingual angioedema (OA) is uncommon, occurring in 0.9 to 5%, but can be life-threatening. OA risk is increased in patients taking ACE inhibitors. The nurse should assess for swelling of the tongue, lips, and tissue of the oropharynx. Because swelling may rapidly progress to upper airway obstruction, immediately stop the thrombolysis drug and notify the treating provider.[14]

ENDOVASCULAR

For patients eligible for endovascular intervention, the nurse will facilitate the timely transfer of the patient to the interventional radiology (IR) team. During transport, BP and oxygen level monitoring continue, ensuring a safe hand-off to the IR nurse.

Like thrombolysis, endovascular intervention is time sensitive, with goals for arterial puncture and first pass of the device at 60 minutes for direct transfers from outside hospitals and 90 minutes for ED to IR transfers. The ED or critical care nurse to IR nurse hand-off should include: (1) medical history and allergies, (2) treatment provided in the ED (thrombolysis, BP IV medications), and (3) current vital signs and neurological assessment.[3]

A neurological exam is performed by the IR nurse prior to the procedure because neurological changes may indicate further deterioration associated with the stroke or a procedural complication. During the procedure, the nurse monitors vital signs every 5 minutes, notifying the interventional team if the BP rises above 180/105 mmHg if treated with thrombolysis, or greater than 185/110 mmHg if no thrombolysis is received. In addition, potential allergic reactions to contrast, such as pruritus, rash, angioedema, shortness of breath, hypotension, and tachycardia, must be assessed.[5]

DIGITAL SUBTRACTION ANGIOGRAPHY AND ENDOVASCULAR TREATMENT FOR THROMBECTOMY, COILING, OR FLOW DIVERSION

Post-procedure requires close BP monitoring, a neurological exam, and arterial puncture site monitoring. Nursing interventions include:[15]

- Vital signs and neurological assessments every 15 minutes for 2 hours, every 30 minutes for 6 hours, every 1 hour for 16 hours
- Arterial puncture site assessment every 15 minutes for 1 hour, every 30 minutes for 1 hour, every 1 hour for 4 hours
  - Apply compression per institutional policy post sheath removal, ensuring the vessel is not occluded
  - Femoral arterial puncture requires leg immobilization
  - Assess for bleeding, hematoma, and bruising
  - Assess for poor perfusion: pain, change in skin color, decreased temperature, poor capillary refill, and decreased distal pulses

HEMORRHAGIC STROKE MANAGEMENT
Intracerebral Hemorrhage: Anticoagulation Reversal

Use of anticoagulant or antiplatelet agents increases the patient's risk of developing an ICH. Hematoma expansion and growth occur more often in patients anticoagulated with vitamin K antagonists (eg, warfarin). Communication between the care team is essential to ensuring timely ordering, preparation, and administration of anticoagulation reversal agents. Gathering the patient's present medication history in addition to the current lab values will assist in the selection of an anticoagulation reversal agent (refer to the reversal algorithm, page 301).[7] For patients with ICH, the use of platelet transfusions should be limited to those requiring emergency surgery or having severe thrombocytopenia.[7] Nurses should be prepared to immediately stop any anticoagulant medication and rapidly administer reversal therapy once available to minimize the patient's risk for further complications.

MANAGING INCREASED INTRACRANIAL PRESSURE
General Nursing Care

Noninvasive nursing measures should immediately be put into practice to manage the potential for or actual increases in intracranial pressure (ICP). These include patient positioning with elevation of the head of bed (HOB) to at least 30 degrees and the neck at midline. Additional nursing measures should target minimizing noxious stimuli, providing analgesia or sedation for pain or anxiety, and targeting normothermia and hemodynamic stability. Close monitoring and management of serum sodium and blood glucose levels to maintain normal serum osmolality and prevent hypoglycemia and hyperglycemia should be implemented.[16]

External Ventricular Device

Intraventricular hemorrhage (IVH) is common, with up to 50% of ICH patients developing hydrocephalus and increased ICP. Insertion of an external ventricular device (EVD) may be necessary to divert cerebral spinal fluid from the ventricles to manage ICP. Nursing care of patients with EVDs includes meticulous attention to infection prevention practices to prevent ventriculitis, in addition to proper leveling and safety practices to prevent misplacement or over drainage.[7]

Hyperosmolar Therapy

Hyperosmolar agents such as mannitol or hypertonic saline may be used to reduce cerebral edema in the surrounding hematoma area by creating an osmolar gradient and pulling water from the brain tissue into the vasculature, thus decreasing ICP. The choice of therapy depends on the speed of required action on the ICP in addition to other factors such as central line access (**Table 4**). Nursing responsibilities include close monitoring of the patient's neurological status, intake and output, and laboratory values to assess the effects of hyperosmolar therapy and prevent complications.[17]

Surgical Evacuation and Decompression

The decision for open surgical evacuation or use of a less invasive surgical approach to the space-occupying blood clot is made by the medical team, taking into consideration the size and location of the hematoma, the need for anticoagulation reversal, and the potential to rebleed. Providers must also consider the potential risk–benefit ratio of the procedure when discussing surgical options with the patient's family.[7]

Aneurysm Securement: Clipping Versus Endovascular Treatment

Early recognition and securement of the aneurysm reduces the risk of re-rupture and potential mortality. Securement choice is individualized based on aneurysm and patient characteristics. Post procedure nursing care depends on the choice of securement. Aneurysm clipping requires a surgical craniotomy with the placement of a metal clip at the base of the aneurysm. Nursing care will follow post craniotomy care. Endovascular treatment may include filling the aneurysm with coils or placement of a flow diverting device. Flow diverting devices prevent high-pressure arterial flow into the weakened aneurysm sac. Nursing care for aneurysmal endovascular treatment will follow assessment and monitoring similar to that for ischemic stroke DSA or thrombectomy.[18]

Post Craniotomy or Craniectomy Care

Stroke patients undergoing decompressive cranial surgery require frequent neurological assessments to monitor the procedure's impact on neurological function. Depending on the elevation of ICP pre-procedure, brain tissue may bulge from the

Table 4
Hyperosmolar agents[17]

Agent	Pro	Con	Indication for Use	Conditions to Avoid
Mannitol 20% bag 25% vials (no therapeutic difference in formulations)	Given as rapid IV bolus or IV push	May cause volume depletion leading to hypotension, hypernatremia, and renal insufficiency	Diuresis for increased ICP No central line access	Kidney failure Hypotension
Key Nursing Points	Potential to crystalize – must use a filter set or filter needle			
Hypertonic Saline Sodium Chloride Sodium Acetate	Given as a bolus dose or continuous infusion; improves CPP and a volume expander	Volume overload; flash pulmonary edema; central line, extreme hypernatremia, renal insufficiency	Volume expansion or improve CPP	Decompensated heart failure, baseline hyponatremia (risk of CPM)
Key Nursing Points	• 23.4% sodium chloride may require a central line and be administered by the provider • 3% sodium chloride may require a central line • 2% sodium chloride is generally permitted via a peripheral intravenous line • If running a hypertonic saline infusion, may also administer a bolus dose • Use of sodium acetate with elevated chloride levels to prevent metabolic acidosis • Monitor for rapid changes in sodium levels (6 meq/L in 6 hours or 10 meq/L in 24 hours) due to the risk of CPM.			

Abbreviations: CPM, central pontine myelinolysis; CPP, cerebral perfusion pressure; ICP, intracranial pressure; IV, intravenous; meq/L, milliequivalents per liter.

skull defect after craniectomy, causing compression on adjacent tissue and blood vessels and leading to new neurological deficits. Nurses should monitor the skin turgor over the exposed cranium for evidence of tension and for cerebral spinal leaks. Routine surgical site assessments for bleeding or signs and symptoms of infection should be performed. In patients whose bone flap is removed during surgery and not replaced, the nursing team should avoid turning the patient on the side of the open skin flap to prevent the risk of injury. Positioning devices to prevent pressure may be used for head positioning during the hospital stay. The nursing team should anticipate future skull protection with a helmet once the patient is ready for mobilization.[19]

Nursing interventions to reduce complications within the first 24 hours

Nurses are key to preventing complications and improving patient outcomes through assessment and monitoring, the use of standard protocols, and bedside stroke nursing care (**Table 5**).[20,21]

Glucose monitoring

Hyperglycemia is common in AIS and is associated with worse outcomes because of worsening stroke injury, increased risk of hemorrhagic conversion, and increased mortality risk.[20,22] Research has shown that aggressive blood glucose lowering does not improve outcomes; thus, the guidelines recommend a range of 140 to 180 mg/dL and avoid hypoglycemia (<60 mg/dL).[11,15] Nurses should monitor glucose levels every 6 hours for the first 72 hours, preventing hyperglycemia and hypoglycemia.[4]

There is a lack of randomized clinical trials evaluating hyperglycemia treatment in ICH. However, the Normoglycemia in Intensive Care Evaluation and Surviving Using Glucose Algorithm Regulation trial found intensive glucose control (81–109 mg/dL) versus standard control (<180 mg/dL) was associated with increased all-cause mortality at 90 days. Thus, glucose targets should be less intensive, with a goal of < 180 mg/dL in critically ill patients with ICH.[7]

Hyperglycemia on admission and within the first 72 hours is associated with vasospasm, delayed cerebral ischemia (DCI), and worse outcomes in aneurysmal subarachnoid (aSAH). Yet, there remains a lack of consensus on optimal treatment goals.[23]

Cardiac monitoring

New-onset cardiac conditions are common poststroke (50–70%) and increase the risk of readmission, recurrent ischemic stroke, and mortality.[24,25] Common abnormalities include prolonged QT intervals, abnormal T-waves, tachycardia, heart block, and atrial fibrillation, with at least 40% of patients with ischemic stroke experiencing a myocardial infarction.[24] Continuous cardiac monitoring is recommended for the first 24 hours and may need to be extended to assist with diagnosing atrial fibrillation.[11,15]

Patients experiencing SAH may experience ST elevation and QRS prolongation because of increased catecholamine release. Nurses should anticipate cardiac arrhythmias and notify the provider of potential diagnostic exams such as serial cardiac enzymes, electrocardiograms, or cardiac echocardiograms to guide further treatment plans.[13]

DELAYED CEREBRAL ISCHEMIA

Delayed cerebral ischemia in SAH is a phenomenon producing focal neurologic deterioration during the first 2 weeks after aneurysm rupture. Although the mechanism of

Table 5
Nursing interventions for potential complications[20,21]

Complication	Nursing Intervention
Hypertension or Hypotension	Monitor hemodynamic parameters per individualized needs and orders; administer medications per orders; maintain IVs; administer fluids and oxygen per orders; maintain pain control monitoring for hypotension with pharmacologic pain administration
Seizure	Perform neurological assessment per individualized needs and orders; monitor for changes in alertness, loss of consciousness, nystagmus, facial twitching, uncontrolled movements, blank staring, aphasia, and difficulty breathing; notify the provider of worsening neurological exam and seizure activity; monitor the electroencephalogram and administer prescribed medications
Hyperglycemia or Hypoglycemia	Monitor blood glucose levels per individualized needs and orders; maintain glucose levels per set parameters; and provide nutritional support when clinically possible
Arrhythmia	Maintain continuous cardiac monitoring and individualize telemetry parameters; differentiate rhythm characteristics; and notify the provider of abnormalities
Pyrexia or Hypothermia	Assess body temperature per individualized needs and orders; temperatures falling outside the normal ranges may require more frequent monitoring and management; keep patients dry; follow the institution's shivering protocol
Venous Thromboembolism	Monitor for signs of VTE; apply sequential or intermittent pneumatic compression devices, ensuring proper fit; administer pharmacological prophylaxis as ordered
Dysphagia	Maintain nothing by mouth until bedside swallowing is performed; if the screen failed, continue nothing by mouth and confirm a speech-language pathologist consult has been obtained; provide nutritional support when clinically possible
Cerebral Edema	Monitor intracranial and cerebral perfusion pressure, notifying providers if ICP is outside defined parameters; monitor LOC and pupillary function; maintain BP control; maintain adequate oxygenation; prevent volume overload; maintain HOB at a determined level to promote venous drainage; maintain normal body temperature
Vasospasm	Monitor for neurological decline; monitor BP and maintain prescribed parameters; maintain euvolemic fluid status
Hypernatremia or Hyponatremia	Monitor sodium levels per individualized needs and orders; maintain sodium levels per set parameters via fluid replacement; monitor strict I&Os; maintain IV access

action is unknown, treatment with nimodipine decreases the risk of DCI. Treatment with nimodipine 60 mg every 4 hours, either orally or per gastric tube, should be initiated within 24 hours of admission. Treatment dosing and frequency may be altered dependent on the drugs' effect on the patient's BP. Treatment should be continued for the first 21 days post SAH. Additional DCI prevention strategies include maintaining euvolemia and elevating the patient's BP.[13]

SEIZURE

Approximately, 11% of patients will experience a seizure. Seizures can be early (within the first 24 hours) or late onset (6–12 months) after stroke. Risk for poststroke seizures is associated with stroke size, hemorrhagic stroke, cortical involvement, age less than 65 years, and family history of seizures. The use of a continuous electroencephalogram is beneficial in identifying interictal or ictal abnormalities.[26] The nurse should perform neurological examinations per orders, notifying the medical team of any seizure activity while promoting airway clearance and preventing injury.

TEMPERATURE

Elevated temperature occurs in approximately 60% of patients poststroke, and is associated with worsening infarct size, neurologic deterioration, increased length of stay, morbidity, mortality, and worse outcomes.[21,24] The most common etiology is infection (pneumonia, urinary tract infections), but it can also be neurogenic because of an immune activation response or brain injury effect on the thermoregulatory centers.[24] Guidelines recommend the nurse monitor the temperature every 6 hours and maintain normothermia (targets of 36.5°C to 37.5°C) for the first 72 hours.[20,22] Targeted temperature management may lead to the common side effect of shivering. Shivering can occur in 40% of patients, and nurses should utilize a bedside shiver scale to assess the patient.

DEEP VENOUS THROMBOSIS/VENOUS THROMBOEMBOLISM PROPHYLAXIS

Venous thromboembolism (VTE), which includes deep vein thrombosis and pulmonary embolism, is a common consequence of immobilization because of stroke. There is a 75% risk without VTE prophylaxis. VTE can be prevented with appropriate prophylaxis measures, including intermittent pneumatic compression, low-molecular-weight heparin, anticoagulants, unfractionated heparin, and early mobilization.[15] Nurses should place intermittent pneumatic compression in immobile patients without contraindications[11] and assess for signs of VTE, including extremity tenderness, edema, redness, warmth, and pulmonary embolism, and also signs of anxiety, dyspnea, tachypnea, chest pain, tachycardia, hypoxia, and hypotension.

Patients with ICH are at 4 times the risk for deep venous thrombosis (DVT) versus those with ischemic stroke. DVT prophylaxis should be implemented on the day of admission to prevent this serious complication. Treatment should include, at minimum, the application of intermittent sequential compression devices. In addition, pharmacological prophylaxis with low-dose heparin or low-molecular-weight heparin should be considered for nonambulatory ICH stroke patients to prevent pulmonary embolus.[7] The timing of initiation of pharmacological prophylaxis for DVT prophylaxis in aneurysmal SAH is unclear but should be considered early in the patient's admission.[27]

DYSPHAGIA SCREEN

Patients with stroke are at increased risk of aspiration because of dysphagia, which occurs in up to 67% of patients.[4] Dysphagia increases the risk of malnutrition, which is an independent risk factor for increased morbidity and mortality.[15] A dysphagia screen should be performed as early as possible within 24 hours of admission, utilizing a validated screening tool, prior to any oral intake of medications, food, or liquids. Patients who fail the initial nurse screen should be assessed by a speech-language pathologist.[20]

PATIENT AND FAMILY SUPPORT: NURSING PALLIATIVE CARE

Although stroke survival has improved, there remains a 2.1% ischemic and 9.7% hemorrhagic stroke mortality risk during hospital admission.[28] In addition, stroke is the leading cause of disability. Because of the increased disability and mortality risk, palliative care needs are extensive, and palliative care services should be incorporated into stroke care regardless of prognosis. Palliative care strategies nurses can promote include patient-family-centered values and preferences, establishing goals of care to ensure the patient and family share in decision making, incorporating spiritual needs, addressing symptom management to improve quality of life, and responding to end of life decisions.[29] The use of severity scores (NIHSS, Hunt and Hess score for SAH, ICH score) to predict functional outcomes or mortality may assist the care team in discussions with the patient and family during treatment decisions. In addition, patient frailty and other imaging and clinical factors should be considered in shared decision making during this time.[7]

Case 1: Acute Ischemic Stroke

- NIHSS: 12
- CT: left middle cerebral artery (MCA) hyperdense sign, indicative of a clot
- CTA/CTP: large vessel occlusion in the left MCA and perfusion-core mismatch indicate the patient is a good candidate for mechanical thrombectomy.

Immediate Nursing Interventions

- BP 192/99—Nicardipine infusion initiated to target SBP < 185 mmHg prior to alteplase treatment and mechanical thrombectomy

Key Nursing Care in the First 24 Hours

- Vital signs and neurological assessments are performed every 15 minutes for 2 hours, every 30 minutes for 6 hours, and hourly until 24 hours after treatment
- To promote venous drainage, maintain HOB at 30°
- Nicardipine continued to maintain SBP below 180 mmHg
- Blood glucose maintained around 140 mg/dl
- Acetaminophen to maintain normothermia
- Intermittent pneumatic compression device placed until low-molecular-weight heparin is ordered
- Maintained nothing by mouth after failing swallowing evaluation

Case 2: Intracerebral Hemorrhage

- CT shows left basal ganglia hemorrhage with intraventricular extension

Immediate Nursing Interventions

- BP 194/112—Nicardipine infusion initiated to target SBP between 130-150 mmHg
- Monitor airway and respiratory status
- Administer the DOAC reversal agent as soon as available

Key Nursing Care in the First 24 Hours

- Every 1 hour neurological assessment for early detection of neurological deterioration in a critical care bed with nurses trained to provide stroke care and orders/protocols that adhere to evidence-based care
- Monitor airway and respiratory status
- Continue antihypertensives to control SBP between 130-150 mmHg
- Perform a dysphagia screen or maintain NPO status
- Repeat CT 6 hours and 24 hours after admission to detect hematoma expansion
- Support family and patients in decision making for ongoing treatment

Case 3: Subarachnoid Hemorrhage

- CT shows diffuse SAH with IVH suggestive of an aneurysm and hydrocephalus

Immediate Nursing Interventions

- Intubate for airway protection
- BP 210/96 — Nicardipine infusion initiated to target SBP < 160 mmHg
- Hypertonic saline bolus of 250 mL of 3% sodium chloride for ICP management
- Prepare for EVD placement, maintaining sterility during insertion

Key Nursing Care in the First 24 Hours

- Every 1 hour neurological assessment, including GCS, for early detection of neurological deterioration in a critical care bed with nurses trained to provide stroke care with orders/protocols that adhere to evidence-based care
- Administer antihypertensives to control SBP <160 mmHg or as ordered
- Implement nursing measures to decrease ICP and, if ordered, hyperosmolar therapy
- Monitor sodium and glucose levels
- Insert a gastric tube for nimodipine administration within 24 hours for DCI prevention
- Maintain sterility and implement safety measures for EVD management
- After DSA, aneurysm, and patient characteristic assessments, support the family in shared decision making; anticipate early aneurysm securement

CLINICS CARE POINTS

- Emergency Department triage nurses should be provided ongoing skills training regarding recognizing typical and atypical signs and symptoms of stroke.
- Stroke order sets and pathways standardize the emergent assessment and required diagnostic studies to facilitate and expedite treatment.
- The treatment goal is for eligible patients to receive alteplase as soon as possible and for patients with suspected large vessel occlusions to receive rapid noninvasive neurovascular imaging to determine endovascular intervention eligibility.
- Neurological nursing expertise is important for monitoring, identifying, and managing stroke related complications.

DISCLOSURE

Dr S.E. Wilson and Dr S. Ashcraft have no financial conflicts of interest or funding sources.

REFERENCES

1. Clare C. Role of the nurse in acute stroke care. Nurs Stand 2020;35(4):75–83.
2. Centers for Disease Control and Prevention. Stroke Facts. 2022. Available at: https://www.cdc.gov/stroke/facts.htm. Accessed October 27, 2022.
3. Ashcraft S, Wilson SE, Burrus T, et al. Care of the patient with acute ischemic stroke (prehospital and acute phase of care): update to the 2009 comprehensive nursing care scientific statement: a scientific statement from the American Heart Association. Stroke 2021;52(5):e164–78.
4. Middleton S, Grimley R, Alexandrov A. Triage, treatment and transfer evidence-based clinical practice recommendations and models of nursing care for the first 72 hours of admission to hospital for acute stroke. Stroke 2015;46:e18–25.
5. Hill M, Baumann J, Newcommon N. Nursing care of the acute ischemic stroke endovascular thrombectomy patient. Stroke 2022;53:2958–66.
6. Demeestere J, Wouters A, Christensen S, et al. Review of perfusion imaging in acute ischemic stroke. Stroke 2020;51:1017–24.
7. Greenberg SM, Ziai WC, Cordonnier C, et al. 2022 Guideline for the management of patients with spontaneous intracerebral hemorrhage: a guideline from the American heart association/American stroke association. Stroke 2022;53: 282–361.
8. Babkair LA. Cardioembolic stroke: a case study. Crit Care Nurse 2017;37(1): 27–39.
9. Wilson SE, Ashcraft S. Ischemic stroke: management by the nurse practitioner. J Nurse Pract 2019;15(1):47–53.
10. Naito H, Hosomi N, Kuzume D, et al. Increased blood pressure variability during the subacute phase of ischemic stroke is associated with poor functional outcomes at 3 months. Sci Rep 2020;10(811):1–7.
11. Powers W, Rabinstein A, Ackerson T, et al. Guidelines for the early management of patients with acute ischemic stroke: 2019 update to the 2018 guidelines for the early management of acute ischemic stroke: a guideline for healthcare professionals from the American heart association/American stroke association. Stroke 2019;50:e344–418.
12. Keigher KM. Large vessel occlusion in the acute stroke patient: identification, treatment, and management. Critical Care Nursing Clinics 2020;32:21–36.
13. Wilson SE, Ashcraft S, Troiani L. Aneurysmal subarachnoid hemorrhage: management by the advanced practice provider. J Nurse Pract 2019;15:553–8.
14. Frochlich K, Macha K, Gerner ST, et al. Angioedema in stroke patients with thrombolysis. Stroke 2019;50:1682–7.
15. Rodgers M, Fox E, Abdelhak T, et al. Care of the patient with acute ischemic stroke (endovascular/intensive care unit-postinterventional therapy): update to 2009 comprehensive nursing care scientific statement. Stroke 2021;52:1–13.
16. Sacco TL, Davis JG. Management of intracranial pressure part II. Nonpharmacologic interventions. Dimens Crit Care Nurs 2019;38(2):61–9.
17. Cook AM, Jones GM, Hawryluk G, et al. Guidelines for the acute treatment of cerebral edema in neurocritical care patients. Neurocritical Care 2020;32:647–66.
18. Zhao J, Lin H, Summers R, et al. Current treatment strategies for intracranial aneurysms: an overview. Angiology 2018;69(1):17–30.
19. Livesay S, Moser H. Evidence-based nursing review of craniectomy care. Stroke 2014;45:e217–9.
20. Green T, McNair N, Hinkle J, et al. Care of the patient with acute ischemic stroke (posthyperacute and prehospital discharge): update to the 2009 comprehensive

nursing care scientific statement: a scientific statement from the American heart association. Stroke 2021;52:e179–97.

21. Censullo J, Firikh A, Mulkey M, et al. Nursing care of the patient with aneurysmal subarachnoid hemorrhage: AANN Clinical Practice Guideline Series. American Association of Neuroscience Nurses; 2018. Available at: https://aann.org/uploads/Publications/CPGs/Nursing_Care_Patient_Aneurysmal_CPG_SAH_final2.pdf. Accessed October 27, 2022.

22. Guanci M. Management of the patient with malignant hemispheric stroke. Crit Care Nurs Clin 2020;32:51–66.

23. Santana D, Mosteiro A, Pedrosa L, et al. Clinical relevance of glucose metrics during the early brain injury period after aneurysmal subarachnoid hemorrhage: an opportunity for continuous glucose monitoring. Front Neurol 2022;13:977307.

24. Amatangelo MP, Thomas SB. Priority nursing interventions caring for the stroke patient. Crit Care Nurs Clin 2020;32:67–84.

25. Buckley B, Harrison S, Hill A, et al. Stroke-heart syndrome: Incidence and clinical outcomes of cardiac complications following stroke. Stroke 2022;53:1759–63.

26. Xu M. Poststroke seizure: optimising its management. Stroke and Vascular Neurology 2019;4:48–56.

27. Jakob DA, Lewis M, Benjamin ER, et al. Timing of venous thromboembolic pharmacological prophylaxis in traumatic combined subdural and subarachnoid hemorrhage. Am J Surg 2022;223:194–1199.

28. Neves G, Cole T, Lee J, et al. Demographic and institutional predictors of stroke hospitalization mortality among adults in the United States. eNeurological Science 2022;26:1–6.

29. Holloway R, Arnold R, Creutzfeldt C, et al. Palliative and end-of-life care in stroke: a statement for healthcare professionals from the American heart association/American stroke association. Stroke 2014;45:1887–916.

Evaluation of Wide Complex Tachycardia

Anthony M. Angelow, PhD, ACNPC, ACNP-BC, AGACNP-BC, CEN, FAEN, FAANP[a],*, Jennifer Coates, DNP, MBA, ACNPC, ACNP-BC[b]

KEYWORDS

- Ventricular tachycardia • Supraventricular tachycardia • Aberrant conduction
- Wide QRS complex

KEY POINTS

- Common causes of a wide complex tachycardia (WCT) include ventricular tachycardia, supraventricular tachycardia with aberrant conduction, ventricular pacing, and electrical artifact. Ventricular tachycardia accounts for up to 80% of WCTs.
- One of the most common causes of a wide complex supraventricular tachycardia with aberrant conduction is a bundle branch block.
- Ventricular pacing is an expected WCT and considered a "normal" function of cardiac pacemakers.
- Immediate synchronized cardioversion is first-line therapy for patients experiencing hemodynamic instability with ventricular tachycardia.
- Adenosine is considered first-line pharmacologic therapy for hemodynamically stable patients who have a wide complex supraventricular tachycardia or ventricular tachycardia that is regular and monomorphic.

INTRODUCTION

Wide complex tachycardia (WCT) can be defined as an electrical cardiac rhythm with a rate of more than 100 beats per minute and a QRS complex width greater than 120 milliseconds.[1] There are several reasons why a person may have WCT, ranging from benign to potentially lethal. The bedside nurse should be able to quickly differentiate between the various causes to help deliver rapid and appropriate care to their patient. In this article, we differentiate between the potential causes of WCT and discuss the treatment guidelines for each.

[a] Advanced Practice Nursing, Division of Graduate Nursing, Drexel University, College of Nursing & Health Professions, Philadelphia, PA 19104, USA; [b] Adult-Gerontology Acute Care Nurse Practitioner Program, Drexel University, College of Nursing & Health Professions, Philadelphia, PA 19104, USA
* Corresponding author. 60 North 36th Street, Health Sciences Building, Philadelphia, PA 19104.
E-mail address: ama435@drexel.edu

Nurs Clin N Am 58 (2023) 325–336
https://doi.org/10.1016/j.cnur.2023.05.014
nursing.theclinics.com
0029-6465/23/© 2023 Elsevier Inc. All rights reserved.

NORMAL CARDIAC CONDUCTION

A normal heart rate for adults ranges between 60 and 100 beats per minute.[2] Tachycardia is defined as a heart rate that is greater than 100 beats per minute.[2] Bradycardia is defined as a heart rate of less than 60 beats per minute.[2] For the remainder of this article we will focus on the management of specific WCT.

The cardiac conduction pathway is composed of 5 essential components: the sino-atrial (SA) node, the atrio ventricular (AV) node, the bundle of His, the left and right bundle branches, and the Purkinje fibers.[2] In typical cardiac conduction, the SA node releases electrical stimuli, which creates a conduction cascade to the AV node, down the bundle of His, through the right and left branches to the Purkinje fibers.[2]

When functioning normally, this pathway will produce a cardiac cycle that has a narrow QRS complex, defined as a QRS of 120 milliseconds or less.[2] Abnormal (or aberrant) conduction through the pathway can cause delays or slowing. This slowing can cause a delayed or widened QRS.[2] Common causes of conduction delay that can result in a wide QRS include bundle branch block (BBB) or conduction through an accessory pathway.[2] Retrograde conduction is another possible cause of a wide QRS.[2] When an electrical impulse originates in the ventricles, it can travel backward up the normal pathway, which causes retrograde conduction.[2]

Common Causes of Wide Complex Tachycardia

There are several causes for WCT. Four of the most common causes observed in clinical practice are discussed below.[1]

Ventricular Tachycardia

Ventricular tachycardia, or VT, is defined as a WCT with 3 or more consecutive beats that originate in the ventricles.[3] In VT electrical impulses that originate in the ventricles produce retrograde conduction that ascends the typical pathway.[3] This creates a QRS interval that is prolonged (hence the appearance of a WCT). VT accounts for up to 80% of cases of WCT.[3]

Supraventricular Tachycardia with Aberrant Conduction

A supraventricular tachycardia, or SVT, is defined as a WCT that has an impulse that originates above the ventricles, typically somewhere in the atrium.[3] In SVT, sometimes, the impulse is not conducted through the His Purkinje system in the typical manner. Abnormal (or aberrant) conduction occurs due to one of several reasons. A common reason is when the right or left bundle of His is blocked, causing a BBB.[3] Another common reason occurs if conduction is through an accessory pathway.[3] SVT accounts for approximately 15% to 25% of WCTs.[3]

Ventricular Pacing

Ventricular pacing is an expected WCT produced by the "normal" function of a cardiac pacemaker. Pacemakers produce a WCT on telemetry. Thus, the presence of a pacemaker should be identified when eliciting medical/surgical history and documented in the medical record. Characteristic pacemaker spikes are often visible preceding the cardiac cycle (the QRS wave). Additionally, many commercial telemetry systems have pacemaker detection functions available, which helps differentiate pacemaker spikes from other causes of WCTs.[4]

Electrical Artifact

Electrical artifact is created by external interference with the cardiac monitor by an outside source. These alterations cause baseline waves to be rhythmically distorted and may seem as a WCT. Common causes of artifact include shaking or musculoskeletal movement, cellular phones within 25 cm (about 9.84 in) of the electrocardiogram (ECG) sensor, electrical beds, or surgical and fluorescent lamps.[4] The presence of electrical artifact can be assessed through patient evaluation and removal/cessation of any competing impulses.[4]

The remainder of this article will focus on differentiating between the 2 most impactful causes of WCT: SVT with aberrant conduction and VT, which collectively account for 95% of the cases of WCT.[3]

CLINICAL HISTORY

If the nurse finds a patient in WCT, the first priority is to determine if the patient is hemodynamically stable by assessing patient responsiveness, heart rate, and blood pressure. If the patient is *unstable*, evaluation of the rhythm is deferred to focus on stabilization of the patient. Once the patient is stable, the nurse can shift the focus on evaluation of the cardiac rhythm. Thus, resuscitative care should always be prioritized over diagnostic evaluation of cardiac rhythm.[5]

Assessing a patient's clinical history is helpful in determining the cause of the WCT. For example, if structural heart disease is present, particularly history of myocardial infarction, there is an increased likelihood that the WCT will be VT.[6] Similarly, if a patient has a history of chronic atrial fibrillation, the presence of a regular WCT is likely to be VT. Aberrant conduction during atrial fibrillation would create an irregular rhythm.[5]

Age is another important consideration when evaluating the rhythm. If the patient is aged older than 35 years, a WCT is more likely to be VT, whereas SVT is more common in younger patients. However, VT cannot be ruled out in a younger patient, especially in someone with a family history of arrhythmogenic cardiac disease.[3]

COMMONALITIES AMONG DIFFERENT WIDE COMPLEX TACHYCARDIAS USING ELECTROCARDIOGRAM CRITERIA

Prompt identification and management of the WCT is the goal. However, there is no single criterion that can reliably identify the cause of WCT in all patients. Instead, nurses and other health-care providers can use clues within the 12-lead ECG to help determine cause of the underlying rhythm. Below we discuss key features that are highly correlated with each cause. Understanding these common features will help the bedside nurse correctly identify the rhythm.

Atrio Ventricular Dissociation

The 12-lead ECG must be evaluated for the presence of AV dissociation, a key diagnostic feature of VT.[1] AV dissociation, as the name implies, means that the atrial depolarization and the ventricular depolarization are totally unrelated (asynchronous). When evaluating for AV dissociation, the nurse should look for dissociated P waves, capture beats, or fusion beats.[1] The first feature, P wave dissociation, occurs if the P waves are not consistently coupled with QRS complexes. This can be manifested as either no association between the P and QRS complexes, the presence of P waves on some, but not all, QRS complexes, or variable intervals between the P wave and the QRS complex.[1] A second indicator of AV dissociation is the presence of fusion and/or capture beats. The presence of fusion and/or capture beats in a patient with WCT is considered diagnostic for VT. A capture beat occurs when an electrical impulse originates from the sinus node and then reaches the AV node at the time when the ventricles are able to "accept" the impulse (between the wide complexes). Thus, the "beat" has a normal (narrow) QRS complex.[1] The presence of the capture beat implies that the normal conduction system has temporarily "captured" control of the electrical impulses being produced from the VT foci.[1] Whereas a fusion beat is observed when one impulse is from above the ventricles (from a supraventricular source) and a second impulse is initiated from a ventricular source. The resulting QRS complex morphology will resemble a mix (or fusion) of the foci. Intermittent fusion beats are diagnostic of AV dissociation.[1]

Extreme Axis Deviation

The axis on the 12-lead ECG describes the net (average) direction of the electrical energy that flows through the heart. Typical ventricular activation results in a frontal plane axis between 90° and −30°. This is considered a "normal" QRS axis.[1] Although sources vary in the exact cut points for what is considered normal (ie, some sources indicate a normal axis in adults ranges from between 100° and −30°).

The axis can also be deviated left (between −30° and −90°) or deviated right (between 90° and 180°). Extreme axis deviation (northwest axis) is present when the QRS axis is between −90° and 180°. The presence of extreme axis on ECG in a patient with WCT is strongly associated with VT.[6]

Concordance Throughout the Precordial Leads

Chest lead concordance is another criterion used to evaluate a WCT for the presence of VT. Concordance occurs when all the QRS complexes throughout the 6 precordial (chest) leads (V1-V6) are monophasic, which means all are in the same general direction.[1] For example, positive chest lead concordance occurs when the polarity is positive, resulting in entirely positive (pointing up) QRS complexes throughout the chest leads.[1] Conversely, negative chest lead concordance occurs when the polarity is negative, resulting in entirely negative QRS complexes throughout the chest leads.[1] When either positive or negative chest lead concordance is present, it is highly specific for VT.[6]

Rhythm Regularity

Most WCTs are regular rhythms. However, occasionally a WCT is irregular. The presence of a WCT that is irregular typically represents atrial fibrillation with aberrant conduction because atrial fibrillation is an irregular rhythm.[5]

Morphology Criteria

Typical right bundle branch block (RBBB) morphology on the 12-lead ECG seems as a small "r" wave in lead V1.[1] In other words, the QRS complex starts as larger R wave (points up), followed by an S wave (points down), and ends with another (smaller) R wave (pointing up—verbally called "r prime"). However, in patients with VT, the activation will produce a prominent R wave because it progresses from the left ventricle.[1] Therefore, when a prominent R wave is present in V1, VT is the favored diagnosis.[1] In a typical RBBB pattern the R:S ration in V6 will be greater than 1. In VT, the R:S ratio in V6 is usually less than 1. **Fig. 1**A depicts the common morphology of an RBBB.

Typical left bundle branch block (LBBB) morphology will not have a Q wave (negative deflection) in V6.[1] If a Q wave is present in V6, this favors a VT diagnosis.[1] In addition, the presence of a broad R wave, slurred or notched down stoke of the S wave in V 1 are strong predictors for VT. **Fig. 1**B depicts the common morphology of an LBBB.

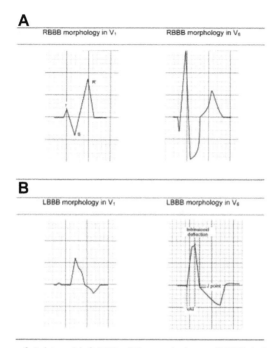

Fig. 1. Morphology of right and left BBBs. (*A*) morphology of RBBB in leads V1 and V6; (*B*) morphology of LBBB in leads V1 and V6. (*Original image from*: Rose L, Kuhn L. ECG interpretation part 2: determination of bundle branch and fascicular blocks. Journal of Emergency Nursing. 2009;35(2):123–126. doi:10.1016/j.jen.2008.03.009.)

AN ALGORITHMIC APPROACH FOR EVALUATING WIDE COMPLEX TACHYCARDIA

There are different clinical algorithms available for using ECG data to help differentiate between VT and SVT with aberrancy.[1] Three of the most frequently used include the Brugada criteria, the Vereckei criteria, and the Ventricular Tachycardia score.[1]

The Brugada Criteria

The Brugada criteria are a stepwise approach for evaluating WCTs using 4 main criteria.[1] If any of the 4 criteria (listed below) are positive, then there is a high chance of VT.[1] The Brugada criteria have a reported accuracy in predicting VT of 98%.[1]

1. Absence of RS complex in the precordial leads

   Determine whether all the QRS complexes in the precordial lead are either completely positive or completely negative (precordial concordance). If precordial concordance exists, then this criterion would be positive, and the diagnosis of VT is likely.[1]

2. Wide R to S interval

   If there is an RS complex present, the nurse should measure the distance between the R and S waves. If the distance between R and the S wave is greater than 100 milliseconds in one precordial lead, then this criterion would be positive and the diagnosis of VT is likely.[1]

3. Atrioventricular dissociation

If AV dissociation is present, then this criterion would be positive, and the diagnosis of VT is likely.[1]

4. Morphology criteria

If morphology criteria discussed above is present for VT in both V1 and V6, this criterion would be positive, and the diagnosis of VT is likely.[1]

The Vereckei Criteria

The Vereckei criteria are used as an algorithm to diagnose VT using a single ECG lead (augmented vector right [aVR]).[3] These criteria are applied in a stepwise fashion, where a VT diagnosis is suggested if any step suggests VT.[3]

1. If an initial dominant R wave in aVR is present, then this criterion would be positive, and the diagnosis of VT is likely.[3]
2. If the width of an initial R or Q wave is greater than 40 milliseconds, then this criterion would be positive, and the diagnosis of VT is likely.[3]
3. If there notching present on the initial downstroke of the QS wave in aVR, then this criterion would be positive, and the diagnosis of VT is likely.[3]
4. If the ventricular activation-velocity ratio (vi/vt) is less than or equal to 1, this criterion is positive and the diagnosis of VT is likely.[3] The ventricular activation-velocity ratio can be measured but calculating the vertical excursion in millivolts during the initial (vi) and the terminal 40 milliseconds (vt) in the QRS complex.

The Ventricular Tachycardia Score

Another scoring tool is the VT score; a scoring system for VT based on 7 ECG features.[7] Each feature is assigned one point when present, except AV dissociation, which was assigned 2 points.[7] The accuracy of VT diagnosis with a score of 1 or more is 83% with a specificity of 63%.[7] Notably, specificity increases as the score increases, reaching 99.6% with a score of 3 or more and 100% with a score of 4 or more.[6]

The 7 criteria are as follows:

1. Initial R wave in V1
2. Initial r > 40 milliseconds in V1/V2
3. Notched S in V1
4. Initial R in aVR
5. Lead II R wave peak time greater than 50 milliseconds
6. No RS in V1 to V6
7. AV dissociation

NURSING ASSESSMENT FOR PATIENTS WITH WIDE COMPLEX TACHYCARDIA

Once a dysrhythmia is identified, the nurse needs to be astute in assessing the patient to ensure that the patient is responsive, if there is an adequate airway, effective breathing, and effective circulation. While performing these assessments, a rapid response or emergency alert system should be activated simultaneously (or as soon as possible).[8,9] Checking for responsiveness can be a visual assessment to determine if the patient is awake and alert. If the patient is not awake and alert, the nurse should shake the patient and shout their name to determine if they are arousable. An airway assessment consists of ensuring the patient's airway is patent and they are able to maintain their own airway. It is important to note that if a patient is not alert or responsive, their airway is at risk. Breathing assessment consists of ensuring that the patient has adequate rise and fall of the chest, in addition to determining if those respirations are adequate. Furthermore, an assessment of respiratory rate is imperative to determine if the patient is at risk for respiratory failure. The circulation assessment consists of looking for adequate signs of circulation and checking for presence and strength of peripheral pulses. However, if the patient is initially unresponsive, the nurse should check for a pulse immediately. In the absence of a pulse, the nurse should begin quality cardiopulmonary resuscitation (CPR) and signal for help until additional help arrives.[9,10] In addition to the emergency assessment of the patient, the nurse should also quickly evaluate the identity of the cardiac dysrhythmia (as discussed earlier).

FIRST-LINE TREATMENT FOR EACH IN HOSPITALIZED PATIENTS

To treat the patient experiencing a narrow or WCT promptly and effectively, the nurse must be prepared to have emergency equipment at the bedside. The following equipment should be readily available.

1. Crash cart with emergency equipment
2. Defibrillator or automated external defibrillator
3. Emergency medications
4. Oxygenation equipment
5. Emergency intubation equipment
6. Rapid sequence intubation medications
7. Suction equipment

The first-line treatment will depend on the type of dysrhythmia present. The nurse also needs to consider factors that influence patient stability such as hemodynamic stability, presence of pulses, and mental status.[11,12] Next, we present the first-line treatment, which is appropriate for both VT and SVT. Each treatment recommendation will follow the current evidence-based practice guidelines for treatment of these dysrhythmias.

Supraventricular Tachycardia

In the event of SVT, the nurse needs to determine if the patient is hemodynamically stable. The presence of hemodynamic stability or instability will influence the first-line treatment options. If the patient is or becomes hemodynamically unstable, more aggressive treatment options would be recommended. In cases where there is a loss of palpable pulses and signs of circulation, CPR must be started immediately.[11,12]

Fig. 2 outlines the process for evaluating and treating a patient with SVT. For the patient who is hemodynamically stable, nonpharmacologic and pharmacologic measures will be instituted. The nurse can assist the patient in performing vagal maneuvers such as the Valsalva maneuver or diving reflex.[11–13] Carotid massage is a historical treatment option but due to the low efficacy of the intervention and associated risks, the practice is debated. There are many contraindications to carotid massage including stroke, carotid artery stenosis, transient ischemic attack, or carotid artery disease.[14,15] Performing carotid artery massage in these circumstances may result in devastating neurologic consequences.[15] Other vagal maneuvers remain safer and more effective.[15]

If vagal maneuvers fail to convert the rhythm, then pharmacotherapy with adenosine (Adeoncard) should be instituted.[12,13] Due to the medication's extremely short half-life, adenosine is administered via rapid intravenous push and followed immediately

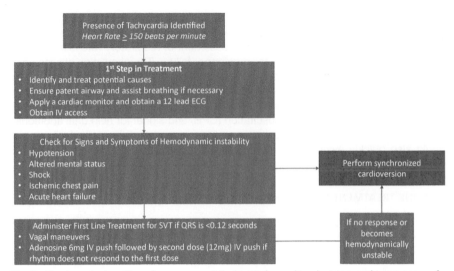

Fig. 2. Treatment algorithm for supraventricular tachycardia. decision-making process for first-line treatment of supraventricular tachycardia. (*Data from* [Adult tachycardiac with a pulse algorithm. American Heart Association. Updated 2020. Accessed November 30, 2022. https://cpr.heart.org/en/resuscitation-science/cpr-and-ecc-guidelines/algorithms].)

by a rapid intravenous push of a saline flush.[16] Keep in mind that continuous ECG monitoring (with a running strip) should be used during administration of adenosine to capture on paper the effectiveness of the treatment, including the first beat after the predicted "pause" caused by the medication. Even if the first (or second) dose of the adenosine does not completely resolve the tachycardia, the first beat gives a clue to the underlying rhythm.

If the patient remains unresponsive to this first-line therapy, a beta-blocker or calcium channel blocker can be administered intravenously.[13] If the patient fails to convert from SVT to a normal rhythm after other treatments or becomes hemodynamically unstable then synchronized cardioversion should be performed.[12,13] A patient who is hemodynamically stable requiring synchronized cardioversion should be sedated appropriately before the procedure and the procedure should be performed in a controlled environment, if possible.[17] Regardless of the treatment options used, the patient should receive a consultation with an expert cardiology professional.[13]

Ventricular Tachycardia

In the event of VT, a WCT, the nurse needs to determine if the patient is hemodynamically stable by first determining if a pulse is present. If no pulse is present, the nurse should begin high-quality CPR immediately and follow the Advanced Cardiac Life Support algorithm for cardiac arrest, which includes high-quality CPR, defibrillation, and pharmacotherapy.[18] The presence of hemodynamic stability or instability will influence the first-line treatment options. If the patient is or becomes hemodynamically unstable, more aggressive treatment options would be recommended.[11,12] **Fig. 3** outlines the process for evaluating and treating a patient with VT.

First-line treatment of VT will depend on the patient's stability. Patients experiencing hemodynamic instability with VT would receive immediate synchronized cardioversion. Patients who are not responsive to initial pharmacotherapy would also receive synchronized cardioversion. Patients who do not respond to initial cardioversion,

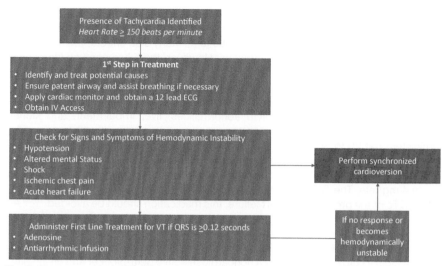

Fig. 3. Treatment algorithm for ventricular tachycardia. Decision-making process for first-line treatment of ventricular tachycardia. (*Data from* [Adult tachycardiac with a pulse algorithm. American Heart Association. Updated 2020. Accessed November 30, 2022. https://cpr.heart.org/en/resuscitation-science/cpr-and-ecc-guidelines/algorithms].)

would receive additional cardioversion at an increased energy level. The energy delivery for synchronized cardioversion will depend on the manufacturer's recommendation for the specific device.[13]

If the patient does not need immediate cardioversion, pharmacotherapy should be the first step in a patient experiencing stable VT. Adenosine may be considered as first-line therapy if the patient's rhythm is regular and monomorphic.[13] However, there are limitations to the use of adenosine in VT (such as irregular or polymorphic WCTs). Hence, other pharmacotherapeutic agents are typically used as first-line therapy.[19] Three main pharmacotherapeutic agents that are used for VT based on evidence-based guidelines include amiodarone (Coradrone), procainamide (Pronestyl), and sotalol (Sotacor). Before administering any pharmacologic agent, the nurse needs to determine if there are any potential drug-to-drug interactions, sensitivities, and/or contraindications to the medication.

Amiodarone is a class III antiarrhythmic medication that has a specific effect on the myocardial depolarization and repolarization by blocking the potassium channels. To a lesser extent, the medication can block sodium and potassium channels as well as beta-adrenergic and alpha-adrenergic receptors. There are side effects of the cardiovascular system, neurological system, and the liver, which should be considered, especially if the patient will be taking this medication on a prolonged basis. However, in an emergency amiodarone is a reasonable choice in most circumstances because side effects tend to present with chronic therapy.[20] The appropriate dosing for amiodarone consists of an initial dose of 150 mg given intravenous push over 10 minutes. This dose can be repeated as necessary if VT tachycardia reoccurs. This is followed by a maintenance infusion of 1 mg/min for the first 6 hours of treatment and then titrated, as necessary. All patients undergoing amiodarone therapy should also be evaluated by a cardiology specialist.[13]

Procainamide is a class IA antiarrhythmic agent. The medication binds to fast sodium channels, which inhibits recovery after repolarization. In addition, this medication prolongs the action potential and reduces the speed on impulse conduction. Altogether, this medication decreases myocardial excitability, slows the conduction velocity, and reduces myocardial contractility. Due to its many side effects, the medication is not used routinely due to safer alternative. However, there has been an increase in procainamide use in recent years. The major side effects include bradycardia, hypotension, and QT corrected (QTc) prolongation, which worsen with increasing level of procainamide. The medication must also be used cautiously in patients with a known diagnosis of heart failure, electrolyte abnormalities, liver impairment, and kidney impairment.[21] The appropriate dosing for procainamide starts with 10 to 17 mg/kg administered at 20 to 50 mg/min. This dose is continued until the dysrhythmia converts, hypotension is present, QRS duration increased by more than 50%, or the maximum dose of 17 mg/kg is achieved. This is followed by a maintenance infusion of 1 to 4 mg/min. The QTc interval should be measured, and if there is a known prolonged QTc or the presence of heart failure, this medication should be avoided.[13,20] As with the other antiarrhythmic agents, patients undergoing procainamide therapy should also be evaluated by a cardiology specialist.[13]

Sotalol is a class I antiarrhythmic agent and is only indicated in the presence of hemodynamically stable VT. Sotalol is a noncardioselective beta-blocker and an inhibitor of the potassium current. Sotalol is effective in prolonging the action potential and the effective refractory period in the atrium, ventricles, nodal tissue, and extranodal tissue. Sotalol has an ability to prolong the QTc interval and should be avoided in patients with a known prolonged QTc interval. Patients receiving IV therapy should be monitored for QTc prolongation every 15 minutes during therapy. Patients with kidney impairment (CrCl <40 mL/min) are also at higher risk of these side effects.[22,23] The appropriate dosing for sotalol starts with 100 mg (1.5 mg/kg) over 5 minutes. This is then transitioned to oral dosing based on the patient's creatinine clearance. Patients undergoing sotalol therapy should also be evaluated by a cardiology specialist. In addition, it is recommended that sotalol is only used by an individual who has experience with treating ventricular dysrhythmias.[13,23]

PATIENT AND FAMILY EDUCATION

Patients undergoing treatment of wide or narrow complex tachycardias need to understand the signs of a reentry tachycardia. The most common signs and symptoms of reentry tachycardia are palpitations, shortness of breath, dizziness, and/or syncope. If left untreated the dysrhythmia can lead to cardiac arrest. If the patient experiences any of these signs, any symptoms, they should immediately report to emergency care.[24,25] The patient and family also need to understand the medical regimen including when to take the medications, possible side effects of the medications, and who to contact should they experience any side effects.[26] Finally, patients should be aware of potential triggers of these dysrhythmias and avoid those triggers if possible. Common triggers may include smoking or nicotine use, increased caffeine intake, excessive alcohol use, over-the-counter cold and flu medications, cocaine use, methamphetamine use, and dehydration.[27]

SUMMARY

Although the focus of this article was on VT, the information presented pertains to SVT as well, especially related to distinguishing between wide and narrow complex tachycardias. Nurses should prioritize making sure the patient with a suspected WCT is hemodynamically stable before taking additional time to determine which specific WCT is present. Nurses need to be familiar with policies and procedures within their own institution(s) when confronted with patients experiencing WCT who are hemodynamically unstable including how to activate the emergency response team and their primary role in the treatment of patients who experience these conditions.

CLINICS CARE POINTS

- When discovering a patient in a WCT, assess the patient for hemodynamic stability versus initially focusing on the reason for the dysrhythmia.

- Once establishing hemodynamic stability, nurses and other health-care providers can use clues within the 12-lead ECG to help determine the cause of the WCT.

- When evaluating a WCT, look for AV dissociation on the 12-lead ECG—where the P waves are not associated with some, but not all, of the QRS complexes often accompanied by fusion and/or capture beats.

- Chest lead concordance, when all the QRS complexes in leads V1 to V6 are in the same general direction, is a clue that the WCT is likely ventricular tachycardia.

- When administering adenosine intravenously, the medication should be followed immediately by a rapid IV push of saline flush simultaneously with continuous ECG monitoring to capture the effectiveness of the treatment.

DISCLOSURE

There are no commercial or financial conflicts of interest and no funding sources to report for either author.

REFERENCES

1. Katritsis DG, Brugada J. Differential Diagnosis of Wide QRS Tachycardias. Arrhythmia Electrophysiol Rev 2020;9(3):155–60.
2. Katritsis DG, Morady F. Clinical cardiac Electrophysiology: a practical Guide. 1st edition. Elsevier; 2021.
3. Vereckei Andras. Current algorithms for the diagnosis of wide QRS complex tachycardias. Current cardiology reviews vol 2014;10(3):262–76.
4. Pérez-Riera AR, Barbosa-Barros R, Daminello-Raimundo R, et al. Main artifacts in electrocardiography. Ann Noninvasive Electrocardiol 2018;23(2):e12494.
5. Al-Khatib SM, Stevenson WG, Ackerman MJ, et al. 2017 AHA/ACC/HRS Guideline for Management of Patients with Ventricular Arrhythmias and the Prevention of Sudden Cardiac Death: Executive Summary: A Report of the American College of Cardiology/American Heart Association Task Force on Clinical Practice Guidelines and the Heart Rhythm Society. Circulation (New York, NY 2018;138(13): e210–71.
6. Abualsuod AM, Miller JM. Removing the complexity from wide complex tachycardia. Trends Cardiovasc Med 2022;32(4):221–5.
7. Jastrzebski M, Sasaki K, Kukla P, et al. The ventricular tachycardia score: a novel approach to electrocardiographic diagnosis of ventricular tachycardia. Europace (London, England) 2016;18(4):578–84.
8. Granitto M, Linenfelser P, Hursey R, et al. Empowering nurses to activate the rapid response team. Nursing 2022;50(6):52–7.
9. Angelow Anthony M, Specht Dawn M. Responding to a rapid response. Essential procedures: Acute care. Philadelphia, PA: Wolters Kluwer; 2022. p. 281–4.

10. Nave J, Smola C. Clinical progress note: AHA ACLS/PALS/NRP updates and cardiac arrest management in the time of COVID-19. J Hosp Med 2022;17(5):364.
11. Merchant RM, Topjian AA, Panchal AR, et al. Part 1: executive summary: 2020 American Heart Association guidelines for cardiopulmonary resuscitation and emergency cardiovascular care, Circulation, 2020;142:(16_Suppl_2):S337–S357.
12. Angelow Anthony M. Review of cardiac dysrhythmia emergency treatment and postcardiac arrest treatment. Exam Review Plus practice Questions: Adult-Gerontology Acute care nurse Practitioner. Philadelphia, PA: FA Davis; 2022. p. 197–202.
13. Adult tachycardiac with a pulse algorithm. American Heart Association. Updated 2020. Accessed November 30, 2022. https://cpr.heart.org/en/resuscitation-science/cpr-and-ecc-guidelines/algorithms.
14. Pasquier M, Clair M, Pruvot E, et al. Carotid Sinus Massage. N Engl J Med 2017; 377(15):e21.
15. Collins NA, Higgins GL. Reconsidering the effectiveness and safety of carotid sinus massage as a therapeutic intervention in patients with supraventricular tachycardia. Am J Em Med 2015;33(6):807–9.
16. Singh S, McKintosh R. Adenosine - statpearls - NCBI bookshelf. Adenosine. https://www.ncbi.nlm.nih.gov/books/NBK519049/Updated September 10, 2022. Accessed November 30, 2022.
17. Al-Zaiti SS, Magdic KS. Paroxysmal supraventricular tachycardia. Crit Care Nurs Clin 2016;28(3):309–16.
18. Adult cardiac arrest algorithm. American Heart Association. Updated 2020. https://cpr.heart.org/en/resuscitation-science/cpr-and-ecc-guidelines/algorithms. Accessed November 30, 2022.
19. Lerman BB. Ventricular tachycardia. Circulation 2015;8(2):483–91.
20. Florek JB, Grizadas D. Amiodarone - StatPearls - NCBI Bookshelf. National Library of Medicine. https://www.ncbi.nlm.nih.gov/books/NBK482154/. Updated July 25, 2022. Accessed November 30, 2022.
21. Pritchard B, Thompson H. Procainamide - StatPearls - NCBI Bookshelf. National Library of Medicine. https://www.ncbi.nlm.nih.gov/books/NBK557788/. May 15, 2022. Accessed November 30, 2022.
22. Mubarik, A., Kerndt, C.C., & Cassagnol, M. Sotalol - StatPearls - NCBI Bookshelf. National Library of Medicine. https://www.ncbi.nlm.nih.gov/books/NBK534832/. Updated June 10, 2022. Accessed November 30, 2022.
23. Sotalol IV. Dosing & administration. Sotalol hydrochloride. https://www.sotaloliv.com/dosing-administration/Published February 18, 2021. Accessed November 30, 2022.
24. Kotadia ID, Williams SE, O'Neill M. Supraventricular tachycardia: An overview of diagnosis and management. Clin Med 2020;20(1):43–7.
25. John's Hopkins Medicine. Ventricular tachycardia. Ventricular Tachycardia | Johns Hopkins Medicine. https://www.hopkinsmedicine.org/health/conditions-and-diseases/ventricular-tachycardia Published February 22, 2021. Accessed November 30, 2022.
26. Talbot B. Improving patient medication education. Nursing 2018;48(5):58–60.
27. American Heart Association. Tachycardia: Fast heart rate. www.heart.org. https://www.heart.org/en/health-topics/arrhythmia/about-arrhythmia/tachycardia–fast-heart-rate Published November 15, 2022. Accessed November 30, 2022.

Updates and Advances in Cardiovascular Nursing
Peripheral Arterial Disease

Debra Kohlman-Trigoboff, RN, MS, ACNP-BC, CVN

KEYWORDS

- Peripheral arterial disease • Claudication • Critical limb ischemia
- Critical limb threatening ischemia • Acute limb ischemia

KEY POINTS

- Peripheral arterial disease (PAD) is a marker for other cardiovascular conditions.
- Early detection can prevent life and limb loss.
- Nurses can play a key role in the detection and management of PAD.

INTRODUCTION

Peripheral arterial disease (PAD) is defined as stenosis or occlusion from atherosclerosis in the aorta or the arteries of the limbs. Because atherosclerosis is a systemic arterial disease process, patients with PAD have an increased risk of ischemic cardiovascular, cerebrovascular, and limb events. Although risk from PAD is often underappreciated compared with coronary artery disease and cerebrovascular disease, PAD may increase the risk of adverse outcomes equal to or greater in magnitude than coronary artery disease or stroke. The 2018 American Heart Association (AHA)/American College of Cardiology (ACC) Cholesterol Guideline categorizes patients with 2 or more major atherosclerotic cardiovascular diseases as very high risk.[1] The focus of this article is on lower extremity PAD. Lower extremity PAD is associated with exertional leg symptoms, functional decline, and poor quality of life.[2]

Registered nurses are in a unique position to monitor and detect lower extremity PAD in both inpatient and outpatient settings. The goal of this article is to review the latest information about the prevalence, symptoms, classification, diagnosis, and treatment of PAD focusing on nursing implications.

PREVALENCE OF PERIPHERAL ARTERIAL DISEASE

PAD affects more than 230 million people worldwide with more than 8 million people in the United States.[2] The prevalence of PAD increases with age. For example,

4415 Grip Drive, Fayetteville, NC 28312, USA
E-mail address: dktrigoboff@yahoo.com

Nurs Clin N Am 58 (2023) 337–356
https://doi.org/10.1016/j.cnur.2023.05.004
0029-6465/23/© 2023 Elsevier Inc. All rights reserved.

percentage of individuals age 40 years and older is about 4.3%, increasing to 14.5% in those 70 years and older, and greater than 20% in those 80 years or older.[3] Prevalence for PAD in Black Americans and Native Americans are about twice that of non-Hispanic Whites at any given age.[4] Whereas, Black and Hispanic women have equal rates of PAD.[5] Notably, these percentages may underestimate the actual prevalence because PAD is often underdiagnosed and undertreated in the general population, especially for Black Americans, resulting in an even greater disparity than reported. Refer to **Box 1**, which displays the risk factors for PAD.

DISPARITIES IN PERIPHERAL ARTERIAL DISEASE

Black Americans are not only more likely to have PAD than other racial and ethnic groups but also tend to present with more severe disease, have more atypical symptoms, and are more likely to suffer worse outcomes.[5] The poorer outcomes seen in Black Americans can be explained by the differences in the prevalence and treatment of cardiovascular risk factors. Studies have shown that Black Americans have a higher prevalence of cardiovascular risk factors such as hypertension, diabetes, chronic kidney disease, and obesity.[7]

Health outcomes can be affected by social determinants of health. Black and Hispanic populations are typically disadvantaged in areas of housing, education level, income, and access to quality health care. Having a low household income and a low education level has been associated with the development of PAD in US adults. Patients with lower socioeconomic status and those on Medicaid insurance have been shown to be more likely to receive amputation for critical limb ischemia.[8]

Black and Hispanic populations are also less likely to have treatment of the atherosclerotic risk factors of tobacco use, hypertension, diabetes mellitus, and dyslipidemia.

Furthermore, socioeconomically disadvantaged adults have high levels of chronic stress and are less likely to attain smoking cessation and afford medications.[5]

SYMPTOMS OF PERIPHERAL ARTERIAL DISEASE

The classic symptom of PAD is intermittent claudication, characterized by exertional fatigue or a cramping pain in the muscles of the lower extremities that is relieved by rest (usually within 10 minutes). Critical limb ischemia or critical limb threatening ischemia is a more advanced level of lower extremity PAD that is chronic associated with a high risk of lower extremity amputation, cardiovascular events, and death, involving more than one area of the lower extremity arterial tree.[8,9]

Box 1
Risk factors for peripheral arterial disease

Age $\geq$ 65 years

Age 50 to 64 years with risk factors for atherosclerosis such as diabetes mellitus, history of smoking, dyslipidemia, hypertension, or family history of PAD

Age less than 50 years with diabetes mellitus and one additional atherosclerotic risk factor

Individuals with known atherosclerotic disease in another vascular bed (ie, coronary artery disease, cerebrovascular disease, renal, mesenteric artery stenosis, and abdominal aortic aneurysm).

Data source: Gerhard-Herman, 2017.[6]

Approximately 20% to 34% of individuals with (a diagnostic test for PAD to be discussed later in the article) ankle-brachial index (ABI) less than 0.9 are asymptomatic for PAD.[9,10] In patients with PAD, 70% to 80% will have stable claudication and 10% to 20% will have worsening claudication, with only a fraction requiring revascularization.[11] However, 20% will have a myocardial infarction (MI) or stroke and 15% to 30% will die (most of them from cardiovascular causes), all within 5 years after the diagnosis of PAD.[12,13] In the Euclid trial (n = 13,885 subjects) there was a 9.1% death rate in the median 30-month follow-up period, of which 706 patients (55.9%) died of a cardiovascular cause.[14] The most common cause of cardiovascular death was sudden cardiac death (20.1%), whereas MI (5.2%) and ischemic stroke (3.2%) were less common.[14] Variables that were associated with higher rates of cardiovascular death in the study were older age, lower ABI values, and prior amputation.[14] Whether a patient has asymptomatic or symptomatic PAD, patients in both groups are functionally impaired, have a more rapid physical decline, and carry the same cardiovascular risk as compared with patients without PAD.[15]

Because many patients with PAD are asymptomatic or they attribute their leg symptoms to aging or arthritis, it is important for a nurse to know what questions to ask patients to determine if they have PAD. The muscles of the legs need more blood flow when active, thus PAD symptoms (cramping or fatigue) typically occur with exertion and resolve with rest. Another common finding is that pain in the feet occurs when supine when the nerves of the feet do not get enough blood supply at rest. Patients often find that if they dangle their feet off the side of the bed, the foot pain at night (rest pain) resolves when in a dependent position, allowing gravity to increase blood flow to the feet. Whereas tissue loss that does not heal and/or presence of the gangrene are signs of more advanced PAD or critical limb ischemia. Refer to **Box 2**, which displays

---

Box 2
History taking in patients with suspected peripheral arterial disease

1. Ask patients if they have:
   - Exertional leg pain at a set distance that resolves within 10 minutes of rest
   - Pain in feet at night when legs are level with the body
   - Any skin lesion that does not heal
   - Any foot or toe gangrene
   - Impotence (in men)

2. Presence of other cardiovascular risk factors:
   - Diabetes
   - Dyslipidemia
   - Smoking/tobacco use
   - Hypertension

3. Presence of associated comorbidities:
   - Coronary artery disease
   - Carotid stenosis
   - Renal/mesenteric artery stenosis
   - Chronic kidney disease

4. Prior procedures:
   - Lower extremity procedures (arteriograms, cardiac catheterization, intraaortic balloon pump)
   - Pelvic radiation
   - Prior lower extremity revascularization

5. Family history of cardiovascular disease

Data from Gerhard-Herman,[6] Gul[16] & Swenty.[17,18]

questions that nurses can ask patients with suspected PAD. Another helpful resource for obtaining a vascular history and for patients, available through the AHA, is the PAD Symptom Checklist: https://www.heart.org/-/media/Files/Health-Topics/Peripheral-Artery-Disease/PAD-Symptom-Checker.pdf.

PHYSICAL EXAMINATION

The physical examination provides an opportunity to detect asymptomatic vascular disease. The 4 elements of a physical examination are observation, palpitation, percussion, and auscultation. For the lower extremity physical examination percussion is not typically a part of the examination. Equipment needed for the lower extremity vascular examination include a stethoscope and a Doppler, if needed.[19] Nurses should notify the physician or other provider of any abnormal findings from the physical examination.

Observation

Over time, patients who lack blood supply to their lower extremities develop changes to the skin and tissue. Thus, it is important for the nurse to instruct patients to take off their shoes and socks in order to fully evaluate them for PAD. When there is lack of blood to the skin, hair loss can be seen and the skin may seem shiny. Chronic arterial ischemia can cause thickened toenails as well as atrophy to the normal fat pad on the toes/heels (creating a hollowness to these areas, making them more prone to pressure sores). Lastly, nurses should evaluate the patient's skin for slow healing ulcers, cracks between the toes, or gangrene (all signs of critical limb ischemia). Refer to **Box 3**, which displays clinical signs of PAD.

Palpation and Auscultation

When conducting a vascular physical examination, it is important to for the nurse to compare color and temperature of the feet and palpate pulses. In addition, nurses should check for bruits by placing the stethoscope over the iliac and femoral arteries. If the patient has a known aortic abdominal aneurysm, then the nurse should palpate for femoral or popliteal aneurysms. **Box 4** displays information about doing a pulse examination.

If a pedal pulse is not palpable, nurses should use a handheld Doppler to assess perfusion (refer to **Fig. 4**). To do so, the nurse should first add conduction gel to the skin and then place the Doppler probe over the area where the pulse should be located. It is important to angle the Doppler probe toward the patient's head.

A normal arterial waveform has triphasic flow (**Fig. 5**). Arterial stenosis can dampen the arterial signal on a Doppler to biphasic or monophasic (typically indicating multilevel arterial disease).

Box 3
Clinical signs of peripheral arterial disease

- Decreased hair growth
- Trophic nail changes (refer to **Fig. 1**)
- Tissue loss or gangrene (refer to **Fig. 2**)
- Loss of fat pad on toes or heels

Data source: Gogalniceanu.[20]

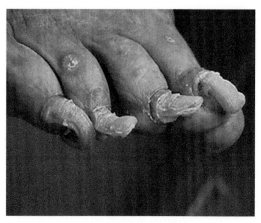

Fig. 1. Trophic nails from chronic arterial ischemia. (Image courtesy of Kohlman-Trigoboff.)

CLASSIFICATION OF PERIPHERAL ARTERIAL DISEASE

Based on reporting standards, PAD is classified into stages, ranging from stage 0 (asymptomatic) to stage 6 (critical limb ischemic with the presence of gangrene noted). Refer to **Box 5**, which displays the stages of PAD.

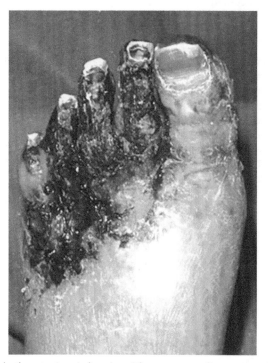

Fig. 2. Critical limb threatening ischemia with gangrene. (Image courtesy of Kohlman-Trigoboff.)

> **Box 4**
> **Conducting a pulse examination on a vascular patient (refer to Fig. 3)**
>
> Pulses to palpate:
> - Femoral
> - Popliteal
> - Anterior tibial
> - Dorsalis pedis
> - Posterior tibial
>
> Pulse rating:
> - 0 = Absent
> - 1 = Diminished
> - 2 = Normal
> - 3 = Bounding
>
> *Data from* Gogalniceanu[20] and Gerhard-Herman.[6]

Claudication

The origin of claudication is Latin meaning "to limp" and is defined as non–joint-related cramping, discomfort, or fatigue in the leg muscles that occurs a consistent distance of activity due to insufficient arterial supply to meet the demands of exertion. Claudication is generally relieved within 10 minutes of rest. Arterial stenosis usually occurs at an arterial bifurcation due to the turbulence of blood flow. The muscle group involved in claudication generally occurs below the area of arterial stenosis. For example, the calf muscle is a common area of claudication due to superficial femoral artery stenosis. Only a small percentage (<10%–15%) of patients with claudication progress to ischemia.[6,22]

Critical Limb Ischemia/Critical Limb Threatening Ischemia

Critical limb ischemia (CLI) or critical limb threatening ischemia (CLTI) is a chronic progression of PAD and refers to lack of blood supply that can lead to tissue or limb loss if untreated. Three levels of CLI or CLTI include rest pain, tissue loss, and gangrene. Rest pain (foot pain at rest) occurs in patients with CLI due to lack of blood to the nerves. Tissue loss occurs due to skin trauma in the setting of arterial insufficiency, resulting in a sore or ulcer on the foot that fails to heal. Gangrene is tissue death due to inadequate arterial perfusion.[6] Patients with CLI have high mortality rates exceeding those of symptomatic coronary artery disease, reflecting the systemic atherosclerotic burden of CLI.[23]

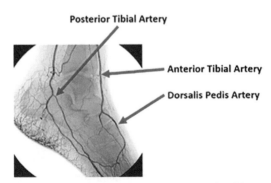

Fig. 3. Location for pedal pulse palpation. (Image courtesy of Kohlman-Trigoboff.)

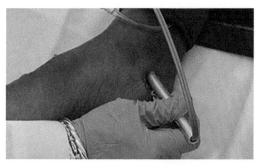

Fig. 4. Assessing the posterior tibial pulse with a handheld Doppler. (Image courtesy of Dr. Keith Horton.)

CONSEQUENCES OF CRITICAL LIMB ISCHEMIA/CRITICAL LIMB THREATENING ISCHEMIA
Risk of Lower Extremity Amputation

Approximately 10% to 40% of patients with CLI have a major amputation within 6 months of diagnosis.[9] There is a higher risk of amputation in Black patients with claudication, diabetes, and kidney disease as compared with white patients with CLI.[7] Furthermore, nearly half of all patients age 65 years and older with PAD die within 1 year of major lower extremity amputation.[24,25]

Acute Limb Ischemia

Acute limb ischemia (ALI) differs from CLI or CLTI in that it involves a sudden reduction in limb perfusion that results in a potential threat to limb viability. Symptom onset is less than 2 weeks duration. Globally, the incidence of ALI is 1 to 1.5 individuals per 10,000 individuals per year.[26] Those at risk for ALI include persons who smoke tobacco, have diabetes, or have a history of revascularization. However, ALI may be the first indicator in a patient with previously asymptomatic PAD.[27]

The mortality, morbidity, and limb loss rates from acute lower extremity limb ischemia remain high; limb loss rates are as high as 30%, whereas in-hospital mortality rates of ALI are 20%.[27] ALI is a medical emergency; thus, early diagnosis and rapid revascularization are essential in this patient population.[27–29] Because of the time-sensitive nature of ALI, nurses can be instrumental in detecting ALI in patients with

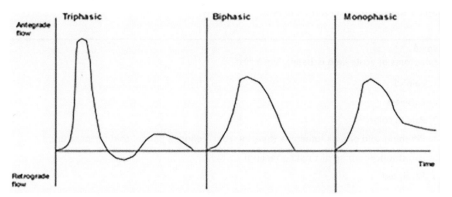

Fig. 5. Use of hand-held Doppler. (Image courtesy of Kohlman-Trigoboff.)

Box 5
Stages of peripheral arterial disease

Stage 0: Asymptomatic

Stage 1: Mild Claudication

Stage 2: Moderate Claudication (200 m)

Stage 3: Severe Claudication

Stage 4: Critical Limb Ischemia: Rest Pain

Stage 5: Critical Limb Ischemia: Ulceration/Tissue Loss

Stage 6: Critical Limb Ischemia: Gangrene

Data from Stoner.[21]

---

known or suspected vascular disease. Refer to **Box 6**, which displays the symptoms of ALI.

Limb viability in the setting of ALI is based on the Rutherford Classification of ALI. This classification is based on assessment of symptoms (sensory) changes, motor changes, and arterial and venous Doppler signaling results. Refer to **Table 1**, which displays the 3 categories of limb viability.

DIAGNOSTIC TESTING

When PAD is suspected, diagnostic testing helps to establish the diagnosis of PAD. Nurses should be familiar with vascular diagnostic testing and have a general understanding of how to interpret the results.

Ankle-Brachial Index

The ABI is a simple, cost-effective screening tool to diagnose lower extremity PAD and can be done on patients in the inpatient or outpatient setting. Typically, blood pressures in the ankles are equal to (or greater than) the blood pressures in the arms. The ABI is a ratio of the higher ankle systolic pressure to the higher arm systolic pressure, both taken with a Doppler. The sensitivity of an ABI for detecting PAD ranges 68% to 84%, whereas the specificity ranges from 84% to 99%. However, in patients with diabetes, chronic kidney disease, and the elderly, ABIs may be falsely elevated due to noncompressibility from medial artery calcification.[6] Refer to **Box 7**, which display the interpretation of the ABI.

Box 6
Symptoms of acute limb ischemia: the 6 "Ps"

1. Painful

2. Pulseless

3. Pale in color

4. Perishing cold or poikilothermia (freezing cold feeling; a painful cold temperature).

5. Paresthetic (burning or tingling feeling)

6. Paralyzed

Data from: Olinic.[29]

Table 1 Categories of limb viability in acute limb ischemia				
Category	Sensory Change	Motor Change	Arterial Doppler Signal	Venous Doppler Signal
VIABLE	None	None	Audible	Audible
THREATENED	Rest pain	Moderate	Inaudible	Audible
IRREVERSIBLE	Anesthetic	Paralysis	Inaudible	Inaudible

Data from Olinic.[29]

In addition, the Society for Vascular Nursing provides a helpful worksheet for calculating the ABI (**Fig. 6**).

Toe-Brachial Index

The toe-brachial index (TBI) is a helpful diagnostic test that is used to diagnose patients with suspected PAD when the ABI is noncompressible (>1.40) (**Fig. 7**). Because the digital arteries in the toe are rarely calcified, the diagnosis of PAD can be made using TBI. To obtain the TBI place a blood pressure cuff on the first toe on each foot. The TBI is then calculated by dividing the toe pressure by the higher of the 2 arm blood pressures taken by Doppler. A TBI of less than 0.6 or a toe pressure less than 30 to 50 mm Hg indicates CLI and suggests a limited ability for wound healing.[6]

Rest and Exercise Ankle-Brachial Indices

ABIs measured at rest can be normal in patients who have lower extremity claudication. When the vascular history suggests claudication, rest and exercise ABIs can help diagnose PAD and are typically done in the outpatient setting. During exercise, the arterial dilation lowers the blood pressure in the legs, and if arterial stenosis exists, the ABI drops. An exercise ABI drop of greater than 20% as compared with the resting ABI indicates PAD. In addition to being diagnostic, an exercise ABI can be used as an objective measure of functional improvement in response to claudication treatment (such as structured exercise program or revascularization).[6,30]

Pulse Volume Recording

Pulse volume recording (PVR), also known as plethysmography, is a vascular test done in the outpatient setting. PVR is a noninvasive imaging test that evaluates the lower extremity blood flow using the same principles as the ABI (**Fig. 8**). PVRs involve applying 2 blood pressure cuffs on both the thigh and calf to help determine the origin of arterial stenosis, as PAD is diagnosed if there is a drop of more than 20 to 30 mm Hg

Box 7 Interpretation of ankle-brachial index results
Abnormal ABI ($\leq$0.90)
Borderline ABI (0.91–0.9)
Normal ABI (1.0–1.4)
Noncompressible ABI (>1.4)
Data from Gerhard-Herman.[6]

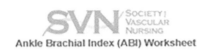

Ankle Brachial Index (ABI) Worksheet

Ankle Brachial Index (ABI): A non-invasive measurement of the ratio of the systolic blood pressure of arm to the systolic blood pressure of the leg
- Place patient supine for 5—10 min
- Apply the appropriately sized blood pressure cuff on the extremity at the arm
- Apply Doppler gel to skin surface
- Place the probe in the area of the pulse at a 45—60degree angle to the surface of the skin
- Inflate the cuff to 20mm Hg above the point where systolic sound is no longer heard
- Gradually deflate until the arterial signal returns. Record the systolic pressure reading.
- Repeat for all extremities

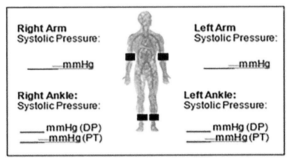

Right Arm Systolic Pressure:	Left Arm Systolic Pressure:
_____mmHg	_____mmHg
Right Ankle: Systolic Pressure:	Left Ankle: Systolic Pressure:
_____ mmHg (DP) _____ mmHg (PT)	_____ mmHg (DP) _____ mmHg (PT)

Calculating the ABI:

Right Leg ABI

= Higher right ankle pressure (DP or PT pulse) / Higher Arm Pressure (of either arm)

Left Leg ABI

= Higher left ankle pressure (DP or PT pulse) / Higher Arm Pressure (of either arm)

☐ = _____   ☐ = _____

ABI Values

<0.90 or less: Abnormal
1.0–1.40: Normal
>1.40: Poorly compressible/calcified vessels
0.91 — 0.99: Borderline further investigation
    may be indicated

When to Refer

Rest pain or tissue loss
Lifestyle-limiting claudication
Normal ABI with high suspicion of PAD
Poorly compressible/calcified vessels

Fig. 6. ABI worksheet.

between cuff pressures. The PVR can confirm the anatomic location of lower extremity PAD and is useful in determining the course of treatment.[31]

Arterial Duplex Ultrasound

An arterial duplex is a noninvasive ultrasound of the lower extremity arteries using color flow imaging and Doppler waveforms to identify blood flow in the arteries (**Fig. 9**). This diagnostic test determines the anatomic location and degree of stenosis in the arteries. Findings are helpful in planning for therapeutic intervention and are valuable in monitoring the patency of a revascularization procedure.[6]

Other Diagnostic Tests

Other modes of diagnostic testing for lower extremity PAD include computed tomography angiography (CTA), magnetic resonance angiography (MRA), and angiography.

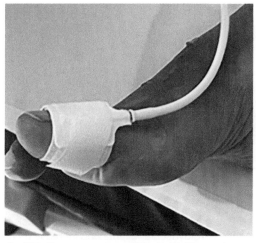

Fig. 7. Toe pressure for TBI. (Image courtesy of Dr. Keith Horton.)

These invasive diagnostic studies carry an increased risk for the patient (potential for contrast-induced nephropathy, allergy to contrast, radiation exposure, and arterial injury) and are typically ordered by the vascular specialist. Nurses should monitor patients' vital signs, peripheral pulses, and kidney function and observe the access sites after diagnostic testing.

CTA may be done with or without intravenous contrast to identify the lower extremity arterial anatomy and areas of stenosis. CTA can be useful in planning lower extremity revascularization (**Fig. 10**).[32]

MRA uses radio waves and magnetic fields to create detailed images showing arterial blood flow. Gadolinium, a noniodinated contrast media, may be used to improve the test's accuracy by making the arteries more visible (**Fig. 11**). Gadolinium is not without consequence, as it can trigger nephrogenic systemic fibrosis in patients with kidney disease. However, an advantage of MRA is that it can precisely define arterial stenosis as well as identify the structure of atherosclerotic plaque.[33]

A lower extremity arteriogram uses standard digital subtraction arteriography to define and treat arterial stenoses. Intravenous contrast is injected into the lower extremity arterial tree to locate and revascularize areas of stenoses (**Fig. 12**). The typical access site is the common femoral artery on the nontreatment leg. Once arterial access is obtained on the contralateral femoral artery, the arterial catheter is passed up and over the iliac bifurcation into the treatment leg.[34]

TREATMENT OF PERIPHERAL ARTERIAL DISEASE

Once PAD is diagnosed, guideline-directed medical therapy (GDMT) including exercise training, cardioprotective medications (antiplatelet agents, anticoagulants,

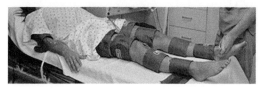

Fig. 8. Obtaining a pulse volume recording. (Image courtesy of Dr. Keith Horton.)

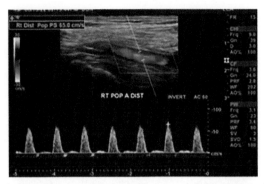

Fig. 9. An arterial duplex ultrasound. (Image courtesy of Kohlman-Trigoboff.)

statins, and antihypertensives), lifestyle modifications, and risk factor modification should be used to reduce cardiovascular events and increase functional status. However, studies have shown that patients with PAD are less likely to receive GDMT as compared with patients with coronary artery disease.[6,35]

Cardiovascular Risk Factor Modification

Cigarette smoking, hypertension, type 2 diabetes, hypertension, and dyslipidemia account for 75% of risk associated with the development of PAD.[10] Thus controlling these risk factors is essential to preventing and improving patient outcomes.

Tobacco use

One of the leading preventable causes of death is tobacco use. Cigarette smoking is a stronger risk factor for PAD than for coronary artery disease and is the single greatest modifiable risk factor for PAD. Smoking increases risk of PAD by 2.3-fold.[36] Observational studies have shown that MI, death, and amputations are higher in patients who smoke cigarettes, with or without lower extremity revascularization.[37,38] Nurses should advise patients with PAD who use tobacco (smoke or use other forms of tobacco) to quit smoking at every visit, whether in the inpatient or outpatient setting. Nurses can help patients develop a plan for smoking cessation by discussing non-pharmacologic techniques, pharmacotherapy (ie, varenicline, bupropion, and/or nicotine replacement therapy), or assisting with a referral to a smoking cessation program. Patients with PAD should also be advised to avoid exposure to secondhand smoke at home, work, and in public places.[6,39]

Hypertension

Several large studies found a significant association of hypertension with PAD.[3] Hypertension (defined as blood pressure $\geq$ 130/80 mm Hg)[40] increases the odds of developing PAD by 50%; each 20 mm Hg increase in systolic blood pressure increases

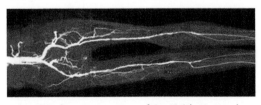

Fig. 10. Lower extremity CTA. (Image courtesy of Dr. Keith Horton.)

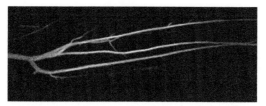

Fig. 11. Lower extremity MRA. (Image courtesy of Dr. Keith Horton.)

the association of hypertension with PAD.[10] Furthermore, there is a 60.2% lifetime risk for cardiovascular disease at age 60 years in patients with hypertension.[10] Patients with hypertension and PAD should be on an angiotensin-converting enzyme inhibitor or angiotensin receptor blocker to reduce the incidence of MI, stroke, heart failure, or cardiovascular death by 25%.[6]

Diabetes

There is a higher risk for major lower extremity amputation in patients with PAD and diabetes as compared with patients with PAD who do not have diabetes.[25] The reduction of the hemoglobin A1c to less than 7.0% through GDMT for diabetes with PAD can reduce microvascular complications and improve cardiovascular outcomes and reduce limb-related outcomes.[41] Glucose control and cardiovascular risk reduction can also be achieved by using sodium-glucose cotransporter-2 inhibitors (SGLT2) and glucagon-like peptide-1 receptor agonist (GLP-1).[41] Nurses can help reinforce the importance of glucose control and adherence to GDMT toward ideal A1C goal.

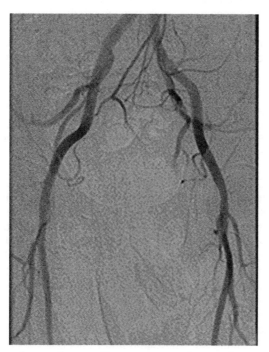

Fig. 12. Lower extremity arteriogram. (Image courtesy of Dr. Keith Horton.)

Dyslipidemia

Dyslipidemia is an elevation in the total cholesterol, triglycerides, or low-density lipoprotein cholesterol (LDL-C) and/or a low level of high-density lipoprotein (HDL). In patients with symptomatic PAD, the target LDL-C is less than 70.[1] All patients with known PAD (whether symptomatic or asymptomatic) should be on a statin to reduce cardiovascular outcomes and to improve walking distance.[1,6] Research has shown that statin use reduced adverse limb-related events (ie, worsening claudication, new CLI, new lower extremity revascularization, new ischemic amputation) and the relative risk of peripheral vascular events (including noncoronary revascularization, aneurysm repair, major amputation, or PAD death) compared with placebo.[6]

Medications for Peripheral Arterial Disease

Antiplatelet agents

Antiplatelet medications are recommended in patients with PAD to reduce the incidence of MI, stroke, or cardiovascular death.[6] All patients with symptomatic PAD (lower extremity claudication or prior lower extremity revascularization) should be on an antiplatelet such as aspirin alone (75–325 mg/d) or clopidogrel alone (75 mg/d) to reduce (22% odds reduction) cardiovascular events.[6] Dual antiplatelet therapy with aspirin and clopidogrel has been shown to reduce the risk of limb-related events in patients with symptomatic PAD after lower extremity revascularization for a duration of up to 6 months.[6] Among patients with symptomatic PAD, compared with clopidogrel, ticagrelor did not reduce primary endpoints of cardiovascular mortality, MI, or ischemic stroke.[42,43]

Phosphodiesterase inhibitor/antiplatelet agents

Cilostazol is a phosphodiesterase type 3 inhibitor that increases the flexibility of red blood cells (RBCs), decreases platelet aggregation, and may cause vasodilation, which allows RBCs to pass more easily through arterial stenosis.[6,44] Cilostazol (50-100mg 2 times per day) is effective in improving claudication symptoms and increasing walking distance by 40% to 60% after 3 to 6 months of therapy.[6] Cilostazol should *not* be prescribed to patients with heart failure, as it can cause fluid retention, act as a negative inotrope, and may increase ventricular arrhythmias.[6,45]

Anticoagulants

The Cardiovascular Outcomes for People Using Anticoagulation Strategies (COMPASS) trial showed that a combination of an anticoagulant (rivaroxaban, 2.5 mg, twice daily) and aspirin (81 mg/d) reduced major adverse cardiovascular events and major adverse limb events.[46,47]

Foot Care

Diabetic foot ulcers are one of the most common complications of diabetes mellitus.[48] It is estimated that between 19% and 34% of persons with diabetes will develop foot ulcers in their lifetime.[49] PAD increases the risk of foot ulcers, foot infection, and amputation.[50] In patients with PAD who have diabetes, there is a 40% rate of death at 5 years after foot ulcer development.[48] Risk factors for foot ulcer development include prior amputation, foot deformity, prior history of foot ulcers, peripheral neuropathy, PAD, visual impairment, poor glycemic control, and tobacco use. Foot surveillance and foot care can prevent foot ulcers that may lead to amputations and death.[50] Nurses can play a key role in educating patients and their families regarding foot care, which consists of nail and skin care, washing and drying the feet daily, doing foot exercises, and wearing socks and appropriately fitting shoes to prevent foot problems.[51] Please refer to **Box 8** for resources on Foot Care.

> **Box 8**
> **Peripheral arterial disease resources**
>
> *2016 AHA/ACC PAD Guidelines-* https://www.ahajournals.org/doi/10.1161/CIR.0000000000000470
>
> It is anticipated that the updated AHA/ACC PAD guidelines will be published in mid-2023.
>
> *European Society of Cardiology (ESC) PAD Guidelines*—https://www.escardio.org/Guidelines/Clinical-Practice-Guidelines/Peripheral-Artery-Diseases-Diagnosis-and-Treatment-of
>
> *Guidelines for Risk Factor Management*—https://www.ahajournals.org/doi/10.1161/CIR.0000000000000678
>
> *PAD National Action Plan-* https://professional.heart.org/-/media/PHD-Files-2/Science-News/p/PAD-National-Action-Plan.pdf
>
> *PAD Tool Kit for Healthcare Professionals*—https://lsc-pagepro.mydigitalpublication.com/publication/?i=705127
>
> *PAD Webinars*—https://www.heart.org/en/health-topics/peripheral-artery-disease/peripheral-artery-disease-webinars
>
> *PAD Fact Sheet for Patients*—https://www.heart.org/-/media/Files/Health-Topics/Peripheral-Artery-Disease/PVD-vs-PAD.pdf
>
> *Talking to your Patients About PAD*—https://www.heart.org/-/media/Files/Health-Topics/Peripheral-Artery-Disease/Talking-About-PAD.pdf
>
> *PAD Symptom Checklist for Patients*—https://www.heart.org/-/media/Files/Health-Topics/Peripheral-Artery-Disease/PAD-Symptom-Checklist.pdf
>
> *Society for Vascular Nursing Patient Education Booklets/Handouts*—https://svnnet.org/resources/patient-education-resources/
>
> *Ankle-Brachial Index Worksheet (Society for Vascular Nursing)*—https://svnnet.org/resources/clinician-education-resources-2/
>
> *Preventative Cardiovascular Nurses Association (PCNA) PAD Resources*—https://pcna.net/clinical-resources/provider-tools/peripheral-artery-disease-provider-tools/
>
> *Society for Vascular Surgery PAD Resources*—https://vascular.org/news-advocacy/articles-press-releases/peripheral-arterial-disease-resources
>
> *Vascular Cures PAD Patient Education*—https://vascularcures.org/patients/peripheral-artery-disease/
>
> *Society for Vascular Medicine Provider and Patient PAD Resources*—https://myperipheralarterydisease.com/
>
> *Diabetes and Foot Care*—https://www.niddk.nih.gov/health-information/diabetes/overview/preventing-problems/foot-problems Diabetes & Foot Problems | NIDDK (nih.gov)
>
> *Diabetes Foot Complications*—https://diabetes.org/diabetes/foot-complications Foot Complications | ADA (diabetes.org)
>
> *Diabetes and Your Feet*—https://www.cdc.gov/diabetes/library/features/healthy-feet.html Diabetes and Your Feet | CDC

Supervised Exercise Therapy

Structured exercise therapy (SET) is an important component of care for patients with stable symptomatic PAD and helps to build collateral blood flow to improve distance to claudication. Thus, SET can improve walking performance, functional capacity, and quality of life. SET is performed for a 60-minute session, 3 times per week for 12 weeks.[52]

Patients who do not improve with comprehensive medical therapy (pharmaco-therapy and structured exercise) or who have CLI (ischemic rest pain, nonhealing wounds, or gangrene) or ALI should be immediately referred to a vascular specialist. Patients with CLI and tissue loss should be evaluated by the interdisciplinary care team to provide comprehensive care to achieve complete wound healing and functional outcomes.[6,53]

REVASCULARIZATION

Endovascular procedures are a form of catheter-based revascularization done at the time of an arteriogram. Endovascular revascularization can be achieved by the use of covered stents, cutting balloon, drug-coated balloons, and/or stents.[6] Use of endovascular treatment of PAD (atherectomy, angioplasty with or without stenting) is more common than surgical revascularization and has lower complication rates.[54] However, endovascular treatments for PAD are less durable than surgical revascularization, often requiring repeat interventions. Revascularization should be offered for lifestyle-limiting lower extremity claudication that does not respond to GDMT to improve quality of life and functional status.[55]

During surgical revascularization of patients with CLTI, surgical bypass to the popliteal or infrapopliteal arteries (ie, tibial, pedal) should be constructed with autogenous vein. This procedure has superior patency rates over prosthetic graft material, especially below the knee.[6]

Another revascularization treatment option is with hybrid procedures; this is when physicians perform a combination of endovascular and surgical revascularization therapies. Hybrid procedures are ideal for patients with CLI with complicated arterial lesions such as combining a common femoral artery endarterectomy with endovascular treatment of the superficial femoral artery.[56]

TEAM-BASED APPROACH TO CARE

A key component of patient-centered health care for patients with PAD is shared decision-making whereby clinicians and patients work together to make decisions about treatments and develop a plan of care based on clinical evidence that balances risks and expected outcomes with patient preferences and values.[57] Because patients with PAD are complex, it is helpful to have a multispecialty team to coordinate efforts for medical management, revascularization, risk factor reduction, and wound healing.[58] Multispecialty care teams include experts in revascularization, foot ware (to offload pressure on feet), infection control, wound care, risk factor reduction, and patient education.[58]

Nursing care is an integral part of this multispecialty care team. Whether working in an inpatient or outpatient setting, it is important to recognize the association between PAD and other cardiovascular conditions. Nurses should know the risk factors and signs and symptoms of PAD. Simple assessments such as having the patient take off their socks during a physical examination could yield important findings. Nurses should be comfortable doing a vascular pulse examination and using a handheld Doppler when needed. When recovering patients from diagnostic or revascularization procedures, nurses can monitor for complications. Nurses can educate patients with PAD about signs and symptoms to report to their continuing care providers, such as rest pain, nonhealing foot or leg wounds, disabling lower extremity claudication, hematoma or wound dehiscence following revascularization, or any symptoms of ALI (sudden onset of foot pain, pallor, coldness, paralysis, or paresthetic feeling).

SUMMARY

PAD can be associated with exertional leg symptoms, functional decline, and poor quality of life. More than 200 million people have PAD around the world. The prevalence of PAD increases with age and affects men and women equally. Black Americans have a higher incidence of PAD than non-Hispanic whites. There is a higher incidence of MI, stroke, and cardiovascular death, resulting in higher rates of all-cause mortality compared with patients without PAD. Thus, the presence of PAD is a marker for systemic atherosclerotic disease and can lead to the early detection and treatment of coronary artery or cerebrovascular disease. The diagnosis of PAD is often ignored and once diagnosed is undertreated. Goals of care include early detection of lower extremity PAD to facilitate guideline-based treatment that ultimately can improve cardiovascular outcomes, walking fitness, and quality of life of patients. Nurses are key members of the multispecialty team needed to care for patients with PAD.

CLINICS CARE POINTS

- Patients diagnosed with PAD should be evaluated for other cardiovascular conditions such as coronary artery or cerebrovascular disease.
- When PAD is detected early, both life and limb loss can be prevented and quality of life can be improved.
- Nurses are key members of the multispecialty team that are needed in the detection and management of patients with PAD through guideline-based treatment.

DISCLOSURE

No disclosures.

REFERENCES

1. Grundy SM, Stone NJ, Bailey AL, et al. 2018 AHA/ACC/AACVPR/AAPA/ABC/ACPM/ADA/AGS/APhA/ASPC/NLA/PCNA Guideline on the Management of Blood Cholesterol: A Report of the American College of Cardiology/American Heart Association Task Force on Clinical Practice Guidelines. Circulation 2019;139(25): e1082–143.
2. Aday AW, Matsushita K. Epidemiology of Peripheral Artery Disease and Polyvascular Disease. Circ Res 2021;128(12):1818–32.
3. Criqui MH, Aboyans V. Epidemiology of peripheral artery disease. Circ Res 2015; 116(9):1509–26.
4. Shu J, Santulli G. Update on peripheral artery disease: Epidemiology and evidence-based facts. Atherosclerosis 2018;275:379–81.
5. Hackler EL 3rd, Hamburg NM, White Solaru KT. Racial and Ethnic Disparities in Peripheral Artery Disease. Circ Res 2021;128(12):1913–26.
6. Gerhard-Herman MD, Gornik HL, Barrett C, et al. 2016 AHA/ACC Guideline on the Management of Patients with Lower Extremity Peripheral Artery Disease: Executive Summary: A Report of the American College of Cardiology/American Heart Association Task Force on Clinical Practice Guidelines. Circulation 2017; 135(12):e686–725.
7. Arya S, Binney Z, Khakharia A, et al. Race and Socioeconomic Status Independently Affect Risk of Major Amputation in Peripheral Artery Disease. J Am Heart Assoc 2018;7(2):e007425.

8. Demsas F, Joiner MM, Telma K, et al. Disparities in peripheral artery disease care: A review and call for action. Semin Vasc Surg 2022;35(2):141–54.

9. Uccioli L, Meloni M, Izzo V, et al. Critical limb ischemia: current challenges and future prospects. Vasc Health Risk Manag 2018;14:63–74.

10. Tsao CW, Aday AW, Almarzooq ZI, et al. Heart Disease and Stroke Statistics-2022 Update: A Report From the American Heart Association. Circulation 2022; 145(8):e153–639.

11. Mizzi A, Cassar K, Bowen C, et al. The progression rate of peripheral arterial disease in patients with intermittent claudication: a systematic review. J Foot Ankle Res 2019;12:40.

12. Pérez Mejias EL, Faxas SM, Taveras NT, et al. Peripheral Artery Disease as a Risk Factor for Myocardial Infarction. Cureus 2021;13(6):e15655.

13. Kolls BJ, Sapp S, Rockhold FW, et al. Stroke in Patients With Peripheral Artery Disease. Stroke 2019;50(6):1356–63.

14. Kochar A, Mulder H, Rockhold FW, et al. Cause of Death Among Patients With Peripheral Artery Disease: Insights From the EUCLID Trial. Circ Cardiovasc Qual Outcomes 2020;13(11):e006550.

15. Drachman DE, Beckman JA. The Exercise Ankle-Brachial Index: A Leap Forward in Noninvasive Diagnosis and Prognosis. JACC Cardiovasc Interv 2015;8(9): 1245–7.

16. Gul F, Janzer SF. In: Peripheral Vascular Disease. In: StatPearls [Internet]. Treasure Island (FL). StatPearls Publishing; 2023.

17. Swenty CF, Hall M. Peripheral vascular disease. Home Healthc Now 2020;38(6): 294–301.

18. Bickley L, Bates B. Bates' Guide to physical Examination and history taking. 13th edition. Philadelphia: Lippincott Williams &Wilkins; 2020.

19. Gogalniceanu P, Lancaster RT, Patel VI. Clinical Assessment of Peripheral Arterial Disease of the Lower Limbs. N Engl J Med 2018;378(18):e24.

20. Islam SN, Deka N, Hussain Z. Role of Doppler Ultrasound in Assessing the Severity of Peripheral Arterial Diseases of the Lower Limb. J Med Ultrasound 2021;29(4):277–80.

21. Stoner MC, Calligaro KD, Chaer RA, et al, Society for Vascular Surgery. Reporting standards of the Society for Vascular Surgery for endovascular treatment of chronic lower extremity peripheral artery disease: Executive summary. J Vasc Surg 2016;64(1):227–8.

22. Society for Vascular Surgery Lower Extremity Guidelines Writing Group, Conte MS, Pomposelli FB, Clair DG, et al, Society for Vascular Surgery. Society for Vascular Surgery practice guidelines for atherosclerotic occlusive disease of the lower extremities: management of asymptomatic disease and claudication. J Vasc Surg 2015;61(3 Suppl):2S–41S.

23. Mustapha JA, Katzen BT, Neville RF, et al. Disease Burden and Clinical Outcomes Following Initial Diagnosis of Critical Limb Ischemia in the Medicare Population. JACC Cardiovasc Interv 2018;11(10):1011–2.

24. Jones WS, Patel MR, Dai D, et al. High mortality risks after major lower extremity amputation in Medicare patients with peripheral artery disease. Am Heart J 2013; 165(5):809–15.e1.

25. Teraa M, Conte MS, Moll FL, et al. Critical Limb Ischemia: Current Trends and Future Directions. J Am Heart Assoc 2016;5(2):e002938.

26. Howard DP, Banerjee A, Fairhead JF, et al, Oxford Vascular Study. Population-Based Study of Incidence, Risk Factors, Outcome, and Prognosis of Ischemic

Peripheral Arterial Events: Implications for Prevention. Circulation 2015;132(19): 1805–15.

27. Björck M, Earnshaw JJ, Acosta S, et al, Esvs Guidelines Committee. Editor's Choice - European Society for Vascular Surgery (ESVS) 2020 Clinical Practice Guidelines on the Management of Acute Limb Ischaemia. Eur J Vasc Endovasc Surg 2020;59(2):173–218.

28. Hess CN, Huang Z, Patel MR, et al. Acute Limb Ischemia in Peripheral Artery Disease. Circulation 2019;140(7):556–65.

29. Olinic DM, Stanek A, Tătaru DA, et al. Acute Limb Ischemia: An Update on Diagnosis and Management. J Clin Med 2019;8(8):1215.

30. Alqahtani KM, Bhangoo M, Vaida F, et al. Predictors of Change in the Ankle Brachial Index with Exercise. Eur J Vasc Endovasc Surg 2018;55(3):399–404.

31. Hashimoto T, Ichihashi S, Iwakoshi S, et al. Combination of pulse volume recording (PVR) parameters and ankle-brachial index (ABI) improves diagnostic accuracy for peripheral arterial disease compared with ABI alone. Hypertens Res 2016;39(6):430–4.

32. Mishra A, Jain N, Bhagwat A. CT Angiography of Peripheral Arterial Disease by 256-Slice Scanner: Accuracy, Advantages and Disadvantages Compared to Digital Subtraction Angiography. Vasc Endovasc Surg 2017;51(5):247–54.

33. Roy TL, Chen HJ, Dueck AD, et al. Magnetic resonance imaging characteristics of lesions relate to the difficulty of peripheral arterial endovascular procedures. J Vasc Surg 2018;67(6):1844–54.e2.

34. Chung J, Modrall JG, Knowles M, et al. Arteriographic Patterns of Atherosclerosis and the Association between Diabetes Mellitus and Ethnicity in Chronic Critical Limb Ischemia. Ann Vasc Surg 2017;40:198–205.

35. Krishnamurthy V, Munir K, Rectenwald JE, et al. Contemporary outcomes with percutaneous vascular interventions for peripheral critical limb ischemia in those with and without poly-vascular disease. Vasc Med 2014;19(6):491–9.

36. Bevan GH, White Solaru KT. Evidence-Based Medical Management of Peripheral Artery Disease. Arterioscler Thromb Vasc Biol 2020;40(3):541–53.

37. Barua RS, Rigotti NA, Benowitz NL, et al. 2018 ACC Expert Consensus Decision Pathway on Tobacco Cessation Treatment: A Report of the American College of Cardiology Task Force on Clinical Expert Consensus Documents. J Am Coll Cardiol 2018;72(25):3332–65.

38. Ratchford EV, Evans NS. Smoking cessation. Vasc Med 2016;21(5):477–9.

39. Lu L, Mackay DF, Pell JP. Secondhand smoke exposure and risk of incident peripheral arterial disease and mortality: a Scotland-wide retrospective cohort study of 4045 non-smokers with cotinine measurement. BMC Publ Health 2018; 18(1):348.

40. Whelton PK, Carey RM, Aronow WS, et al. 2017 ACC/AHA/AAPA/ABC/ACPM/ AGS/APhA/ASH/ASPC/NMA/PCNA Guideline for the Prevention, Detection, Evaluation, and Management of High Blood Pressure in Adults: A Report of the American College of Cardiology/American Heart Association Task Force on Clinical Practice Guidelines. Hypertension 2018;71(6):e13–115.

41. American Diabetes Association Professional Practice Committee. 9. Pharmacologic Approaches to Glycemic Treatment: Standards of Medical Care in Diabetes-2022. Diabetes Care 2022;45(Suppl 1):S125–43.

42. Jones WS, Baumgartner I, Hiatt WR, et al, International Steering Committee and Investigators of the EUCLID Trial. Ticagrelor Compared With Clopidogrel in Patients With Prior Lower Extremity Revascularization for Peripheral Artery Disease. Circulation 2017;135(3):241–50.

43. Berger JS, Abramson BL, Lopes RD, et al. Ticagrelor versus clopidogrel in patients with symptomatic peripheral artery disease and prior coronary artery disease: Insights from the EUCLID trial. Vasc Med 2018;23(6):523–30.

44. Desai K, Han B, Kuziez L, et al. Literature review and meta-analysis of the efficacy of cilostazol on limb salvage rates after infrainguinal endovascular and open revascularization. J Vasc Surg 2021;73(2):711–21.e3.

45. Balinski AM, Preuss CV. Cilostazol. Updated 2022 Sep 21. In: StatPearls Internet. Treasure Island (FL): StatPearls Publishing; 2022. Available at: https://www.ncbi. nlm.nih.gov/books/NBK544363/.

46. Eikelboom JW, Connolly SJ, Bosch J, et al. Rivaroxaban with or without Aspirin in Stable Cardiovascular Disease. N Engl J Med 2017;377(14):1319–30.

47. Anand SS, Bosch J, Eikelboom JW, et al, COMPASS Investigators. Rivaroxaban with or without aspirin in patients with stable peripheral or carotid artery disease: an international, randomized, double-blind, placebo-controlled trial. Lancet (London, England) 2018;391(10117):219–29.

48. Jupiter DC, Thorud JC, Buckley CJ, et al. The impact of foot ulceration and amputation on mortality in diabetic patients. I: From ulceration to death, a systematic review. Int Wound J 2016;13(5):892–903.

49. Everett E, Mathioudakis N. Update on management of diabetic foot ulcers. Ann N Y Acad Sci 2018;1411(1):153–65.

50. Armstrong DG, Boulton AJM, Bus SA. Diabetic Foot Ulcers and Their Recurrence. N Engl J Med 2017;376(24):2367–75.

51. Miikkola M, Lantta T, Suhonen R, et al. Challenges of foot self-care in older people: a qualitative focus-group study. J Foot Ankle Res 2019;12:5.

52. Treat-Jacobson D, McDermott MM, Bronas UG, et al, American Heart Association Council on Peripheral Vascular Disease; Council on Quality of Care and Outcomes Research; and Council on Cardiovascular and Stroke Nursing. Optimal Exercise Programs for Patients With Peripheral Artery Disease: A Scientific Statement From the American Heart Association. Circulation 2019;139(4):e10–33.

53. Conte MS, Bradbury AW, Kolh P, et al, GVG Writing Group. Global vascular guidelines on the management of chronic limb-threatening ischemia. J Vasc Surg 2019;69(6S):3S–125S, e40.

54. Wong KHF, Zucker BE, Wardle BG, et al. Systematic review and narrative synthesis of surveillance practices after endovascular intervention for lower limb peripheral arterial disease. J Vasc Surg 2022;75(1):372–80.e15.

55. Pereira K. Treatment Strategies for the Claudicant. Semin Intervent Radiol 2018; 35(5):435–42.

56. Takayama T, Matsumura JS. Complete Lower Extremity Revascularization via a Hybrid Procedure for Patients with Critical Limb Ischemia. Vasc Endovasc Surg 2018;52(4):255–61.

57. Resnicow K, Catley D, Goggin K, et al. Shared Decision Making in Health Care: Theoretical Perspectives for Why It Works and For Whom. Med Decis Making 2022;42(6):755–64.

58. Dhand S. Multidisciplinary Approach to PAD: Who's on Your Team? Semin Intervent Radiol 2018;35(5):378–83. Eur Heart J. 2004;25:17–24. doi: 10.1016/j.ehj.2003. 10.033.

Update on Valvular Heart Disease for Registered Nurses

Janet F. Wyman, DNP, ACNS-BC*, Crystal Cusin, DNP, AG-ACNP-BC,
Dayna Gjurovski, DNP, AG-ACNP-BC

KEYWORDS

- Valvular heart disease • Aortic valve • Mitral valve • Tricuspid valve
- Transcatheter valve therapy • Heart failure

KEY POINTS

- A dramatic increase in the older adult population has resulted in an increased prevalence of valvular heart disease (VHD) and the associated heart failure when untreated.
- Definitive treatment of VHD is shifting from predominantly surgical procedures in an operating suite to minimally invasive procedures in the cardiac catheterization laboratory.
- Patients with VHD should be referred to a valve center with a multidisciplinary heart team, comprised of cardiologists, surgeons, cardiac imaging specialists, heart failure specialists, cardiac anesthesiologists, nurse practitioners, and nurses.

INTRODUCTION

Valvular heart disease (VHD) significantly impacts health, quality of life, and longevity.

A dramatic global increase in the aging population has caused an increasing burden of VHD. Rheumatic heart disease, the most common form, is predominantly found in developing countries; functional and degenerative diseases are more common in higher income countries. In America life expectancy has increased over the decades with improved health care. Between 2009 and 2019, the number of Americans over the age of 60 years increased from 55.7 million to 74.6 million.[1] Population studies show an increase in prevalence of VHD with age, rising from 0.7% in the 18 to 45 year old group to 13.3% for those greater than 75 years of age.[2–4] These increases have intensified the focus on the management and treatment of VHD and its primary manifestation: heart failure (HF).

Historically, recommendations for treatment of VHD centered on surgeries that repaired or replaced diseased valves. Over the last 2 decades, advances in minimally

Henry Ford Hospital, Structural Heart Disease, Henry Ford Health, Heart and Vascular Service Line, 2799 West Grand Boulevard, Clara Ford Pavilion 439, Detroit, MI 48202, USA
* Corresponding author. Henry Ford Health, 2799 West Grand Boulevard, CFP 439, Detroit, MI 48202.
E-mail address: jwyman1@hfhs.org

Nurs Clin N Am 58 (2023) 357–378
https://doi.org/10.1016/j.cnur.2023.05.012
0029-6465/23/© 2023 Elsevier Inc. All rights reserved.

invasive procedures have upended the approach to valve repair and replacement. Catheter-based procedures driven by assessment of symptom status, disease severity, comorbidities, and cardiac and vascular anatomy also require advanced imaging interpretation. Because of the complexity, recommendations now advocate referral of patients with VHD to valve centers with multidisciplinary heart teams (MDTs) able to provide the comprehensive testing, evaluation, and patient engagement to determine the treatment best suited to their goals.[5] In **Box 1** the minimal requirements for the MDTs are displayed. In this paper, we will focus discussion on the major valve diseases and current guideline treatment options.

AORTIC VALVE DISEASE: STENOSIS

Aortic stenosis (AoS) is a progressive narrowing of the aortic valve (AoV) due to an inflammatory process caused by endothelial damage from mechanical stress, lipid invasion, leaflet thickening, and ultimately calcification of the valve.[6] The most common causes of AoS are related to calcific disease, rheumatic disease, or as a congenitally or acquired bicuspid valve.[7] Rheumatic disease is the primary cause of stenosis around the world. However, calcification of a bileaflet or trileaflet AoV is the most frequently occurring form in developed nations. AoV sclerosis that develops prior to any significant stenosis can be identified by echocardiogram and/or computed tomography.[8]

The prevalence of AoS increases with age, found in approximately 1% to 2% of patients aged 65 years, increasing to over 12% of those aged over 75 years.[9,10] The overall prognosis and long-term survival with untreated severe symptomatic AoS are extremely poor. Approximately 50% of those with severe AoS die within 2 years and at 5 years, the survival rate is approximately 20%.[6,7]

Box 1
The multidisciplinary team: minimum requirements

- Interventional cardiologist
- Cardiac surgeon
- Imaging specialist: echocardiographic and radiographic[a]
- Clinical cardiology valve expert[a]
- Heart failure (HF) specialist (for HF due to LV systolic dysfunction and secondary MR)
- Cardiovascular anesthesiologist
- Nurse practitioner/physician assistant for pre- and peri-procedural care and MDT consults
- Valve coordinator/program navigator
- Institutionally supported data manager for National Registry
- Hospital administration representative as necessary

Abbreviations: LV, left ventricle; MDT, multidisciplinary team; MR, mitral regurgitation.[a] A single individual may provide clinical and imaging expertise.

From Nishimura RA, O'Gara PT, Bavaria JE, Brindis RG, Carroll JD, Kavinsky CJ, Lindman BR, Linderbaum JA, Little SH, Mack MJ, Mauri L, Miranda WR, Shahian DM, Sundt TM 3rd. 2019 AATS/ACC/ASE/SCAI/STS expert consensus systems of care document: a proposal to optimize care for patients with valvular heart disease: a joint report of the American Association for Thoracic Surgery, American College of Cardiology, American Society of Echocardiography, Society for Cardiovascular Angiography and Interventions, and Society of Thoracic Surgeons. J Am Coll Cardiol 2019;72:xxx-xx.

AoS is divided into 4 general stages, with each stage described by patient symptoms, valve anatomy, valve hemodynamics, and changes in the left ventricle (LV) and vasculature.[11] Diagnostic testing with echocardiogram, electrocardiogram (ECG), and a history and physical examination are essential for determining severity, disease burden, symptomatology, and presence of HF. Accurate identification of stage with appropriate symptomatology guides treatment and ongoing surveillance.[11]

CLINICAL PRESENTATION

The cardinal symptoms associated with AoS are shortness of breath, angina, and syncope. Fatigue and dyspnea on exertion with a gradual progression are the most common presenting symptoms while in later stages and severity of disease patients often endorse orthopnea, paroxysmal nocturnal dyspnea, and edema. These symptoms are often associated with LV hypertrophy and diastolic dysfunction. Symptom burden is an important clinical component when determining definitive treatment.

PHYSICAL EXAMINATION

Evaluation of the carotid upstroke, auscultation of a systolic murmur, and signs and symptoms of HF are important clinical findings in AoS. Normally palpating the carotid artery and simultaneously listening to the heart sounds produces a synchronized heartbeat and pulse. A delayed and weak upstroke is called *pulsus parvus e tardus* and is specific for *severe* AoS (SAS). Auscultation of a heart sounds is often the first finding directing the diagnosis of AoS. Located at the right sternal border second intercostal space a high-pitched, crescendo-decrescendo, midsystolic murmur is revealed that radiates to the carotids. Cautious auscultation may reveal a paradoxical split S2, over time the loss of the A2 component may occur with SAS. **Fig. 1** displays murmurs with VHD.

RISK AND FRAILTY ASSESSMENT

Frailty evaluations are an essential component when evaluating patients with AoS for intervention.[11] The Society of Thoracic Surgeons (STS) use the STS score to determine risk of morbidity and mortality in patients undergoing surgical intervention; however, the impact of frailty on surgical risk and recovery is not included. Frailty scores are included in the current guidelines for treatment assessments.[11]

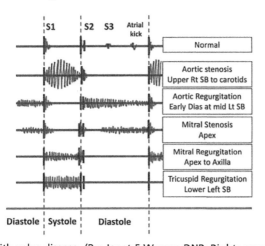

Fig. 1. Murmurs with valve disease. (By: Janet F Wyman DNP; Rights reserved.)

DIAGNOSTIC TESTING

Transthoracic echocardiogram (TTE) is the standard diagnostic test for the evaluation of VHD[11] providing assessment of morphology and severity of disease, chamber size and function, and pulmonary status. TTE metrics quantify disease as mild, moderate, and severe that are the basis for recommendations for treatment.[11] Refer to **Table 1** that displays the echo metrics for AoS.

There are no ECG changes that define AoS, it is used to establish rhythm, and signs of LV hypertrophy. For patients with *asymptomatic* SAS, low level stress testing may be helpful for defining symptom burden. During stress testing exercise intolerance, an abnormal blood pressure response, and other symptoms may reveal SAS when patients have adjusted their lifestyle to symptom progression.[11] Gated computed tomography (CT) scans have become the gold standard to evaluate feasibility for transcatheter procedures. CT is used to assess valve sizing, calcium distribution, disease severity and valve morphology, coronary calcifications, and measurements of the arterial vessels for surgical and minimally invasive valve replacement planning.[11]

TREATMENT

Current research is exploring the underlying progressive fibrocalcific remodeling that occurs with calcific AoS. However, no pharmacotherapy has yet been developed to prevent this process.[10] Aortic valve replacement (AVR) has been shown in randomized controlled trials to be superior to medical management. AVR either surgically or minimally invasive with transcatheter aortic valve replacement (TAVR) is the recommended treatment for symptomatic AoS.[11,12] Bioprosthetic valve placement via TAVR has been shown to be noninferior to surgical procedures and is now recommended for AVR regardless of level of surgical risk.[11] There are select populations in which surgical AVR should be considered: age less than 65 years, anatomy not amenable to TAVR, multivalve, coronary, or aortic disease that also require treatment.

The TAVR procedure is a catheter-based procedure in which a bioprosthetic valve is collapsed on a catheter tip. A major artery, most often a femoral, is used as access to the aorta. The catheter is threaded up, around the aortic arch, down the ascending aorta, and through the diseased valve. The valve is deployed either by self-expansion or balloon inflation in the diseased valve. Catheters are then removed. Although initially performed under TEE guidance and general anesthesia, with improved and radiographic detectable devices and smaller catheter sizes nurse-led conscious sedation has been shown to be safe and effective.[13]

Balloon aortic valvuloplasty (BAV) is a temporizing palliative treatment for severe symptomatic AoS. It is often used as a bridge to definitive treatment (SAVR or

Table 1
Echo metrics for aortic stenosis

Aortic Metric	Aortic Sclerosis	Mild	Moderate	Severe	Very Severe
Jet velocity (m/s)	≤ 2.5	2.6–2.9	3.0–4.0	>4.0	≥ 5
Mean gradient (mm Hg)		<20	20–40	>40	≥ 60
AoVA (cm²)		>1.5	1.0–1.5	<1.0	≤ 0.6
AoVA index (cm²/m²)		>0.85	0.60–0.85	<0.6	

From Ring L, Shah BN, Bhattacharyya S, Harkness A, Belham M, Oxborough D, Pearce K, Rana BS, Augustine DX, Robinson S, Tribouilloy C. Echocardiographic assessment of aortic stenosis: a practical guideline from the British Society of Echocardiography. Echo Res Pract. 2021 Apr 28;8(1):G19-G59. https://doi.org/10.1530/ERP-20-0035. PMID: 33709955; PMCID: PMC8115410.

TAVR) or as a palliative treatment option when there is a concern that patients will not have a significant benefit from TAVR. BAV may provide a symptomatic benefit for a range of 6 to 12 months; however, patients have the same high mortality risk as those who are untreated.[9]

AORTIC VALVE DISEASE: REGURGITATION

Aortic regurgitation, also known as aortic insufficiency (AI), is the backflow of blood from the aorta into the LV during diastole. Approximately 2% of the US population over the age of 75 years have moderate to severe AI.[14] AI is divided into diseases that affect the AoV and leaflets and those that affect the aortic root and/or ascending aorta. For patients undergoing AVR for isolated AI, diseases of the aortic root are now considered to be the most common cause of AI.[15] In those less than 65 year age, the most common cause of AI remains congenital bicuspid AoV.[14] Other causes of AI are endocarditis, rheumatic disease, calcific disease, aortic dilation, arteriosclerosis, Marfan's syndrome, and syphilis.[15]

AI is categorized as acute or chronic. Untreated acute severe AI leads to LV volume overload, decreased cardiac output, and ultimately cardiogenic shock. Severe acute AI is a medical emergency and requires urgent intervention. Its primary causes are endocarditis, aortic dissection, or trauma.

Chronic AI is also categorized in 4 stages. Stage A is for those at risk of AI. Stage B is progressive AI showing mild to moderate AI on imaging (from a TTE). Stage C is asymptomatic severe AI, in this stage stress testing may be used to assess for symptomatology. Lastly, stage D is symptomatic severe AI, with symptoms ranging from mild to severe symptoms.[11]

CLINICAL PRESENTATION

Patients with acute severe aortic insufficiency (ASAI) appear severely ill, presenting with rapid progression of symptoms or sudden cardiovascular collapse. The initial presenting symptoms of ASAI may vary based on the etiology of the disease. For example, a patient with an aortic dissection may present with severe back and chest pain with normal pulse pressure. However, a patient with infective endocarditis may have night sweats, fever, weight loss, and hypotension. The importance of identifying etiology of the clinical presentation is essential for accurate, timely treatment, and support.[14] Unlike ASAI, patients with chronic severe AI remain grossly asymptomatic, until LV dilatation becomes significant.[15] The first symptoms may be dyspnea on exertion, orthopnea, and paroxysmal nocturnal dyspnea, and these tend to develop gradually as the disease progresses and LV enlarges. Late symptoms include nocturnal angina and signs of left-sided HF such as fatigue and shortness of breath. In both decompensated and compensated AI, a wide pulse pressure is present.[12]

PHYSICAL EXAMINATION

The heart sounds associated with ASAI are a low pitched, short duration, early diastolic murmur, and a soft or absent S1 which can be heard best at the left third or fourth intercostal space with the patient leaning forward.[12] The Austin-Flint murmur is frequently found with chronic AI, a low pitched, mid diastolic murmur best heard at the cardiac apex with the patient leaning forward.[12] The importance of a timely and accurate diagnosis for AI, whether acute or chronic, is important for optimal outcomes. Some unique physical examination findings associated with AI are the Corrigan sign: a "water hammer" radial or brachial pulse, a rapidly rising and falling pulse with a wide pulse pressure, and the Duroziez sign: a systolic and diastolic bruit heard when the femoral artery is partially compressed.

DIAGNOSTIC TESTING

The TTE is necessary for evaluation of severity of AI disease, LV function and volume, and AV assessment (leaflets, vegetation, and morphology).[15] Transesophageal echocardiogram (TEE), cardiac MRI, or cardiac catheterization may be used to determine LV size and function, degree of AI, and assessment of the aortic root to assess for enlargement, dissection, and/or congenital abnormality.

TREATMENT

Indications for treatment of AI are based on the clinical presentation, severity of disease, chronicity, and symptomatology. Currently, surgical replacement/repair for acute and chronic severe native valve AI is the mainstay of treatment.[11] The timing of intervention is critical for optimal outcomes. In the setting of pulmonary edema, hypotension, or signs of low cardiac output emergent intervention with surgical AVR is indicated. ASAI from infective endocarditis and aortic dissection require initial stabilization before surgery with aims to decrease LV afterload. Beta-blockers, often used in the setting of aortic dissection, should be avoided in almost all causes of acute ASAI as frequent compensatory mechanism is tachycardia and attempts to decrease heart rate (HR) may cause further hypotension.[11]

At this time, there are no commercially approved percutaneous transcatheter AVRs for patients with symptomatic severe AI. However, investigational trials are underway for native AI. TAVR: valve-in-valve is approved for patients with surgical bioprosthetic AV failure requiring replacement.

MITRAL VALVE DISEASE: STENOSIS

Mitral stenosis (MS) occurs when blood flow from the left atrium (LA) through the mitral valve (MV) to the LV is obstructed, resulting in increased LA pressure and ultimately pulmonary vascular congestion. These increases in LA pressure and pulmonary congestion may also result in pulmonary hypertension, hemoptysis due to pulmonary vein rupture, right ventricular (RV) strain, and tricuspid regurgitation (TR). MS is predominately caused by untreated streptococcus, an infection resulting in rheumatic fever and VD; this etiology accounts for approximately 50% to 70% of patients with symptomatic MS.[16] Additional causes may include mitral leaflet calcification, vegetations associated with infective endocarditis that obstruct the valve orifice, and congenital stenosis.[16]

The incidence of MS is low in high income countries and has been declining in low- and middle-income countries. The prevalence in the United States is now estimated to be approximately 1 in 100,000 and 35 cases per 100,000 persons in developing nations. MS is also found more commonly in women, with approximately 80% of cases in this population.[11]

CLINICAL PRESENTATION

Progression of MS causes symptoms of congestion and HF prompting patients to seek evaluation.[17] Presentation with MV disease is similar regardless of pathophysiology (stenosis vs regurgitation). Classic symptoms include fatigue, decreased exercise tolerance, shortness of breath, dyspnea on exertion, orthopnea, and paroxysmal nocturnal dyspnea. Additionally, patients may complain of chest discomfort, lower extremity edema, and dizziness or lightheadedness. Symptom onset is gradual and progressive over time. Conditions or activities that augment the HR and cardiac output may exacerbate symptoms. This includes fever, anemia, hyperthyroidism, pregnancy, rapid arrythmias, emotional stress, or sexual intercourse.[3] **Table 2** displays symptoms and etiologies of MV disease.

PHYSICAL EXAMINATION

The classic MS murmur is a low-frequency decrescendo diastolic murmur caused by turbulent flow of blood across the stenotic valve as it passes from the atria to the ventricle during diastole, best heard in the left lateral position. It begins after the opening snap of the MV, with the duration of the murmur correlating with the severity of the stenosis (refer to **Fig. 1**). On palpation, the chest may reveal an RV "tap" in patients with an increased RV pressure.

DIAGNOSTIC TESTING

The primary diagnostic tool for identifying MS is the TTE. It is used to evaluate stenosis severity, generally revealing thickened mitral leaflets with abnormal fusion at the commissures and restricted separation during diastole.[3] Disease severity is classified as mild, moderate, or severe. A TEE is helpful to view the valve and the LA when a TTE has limited quality. See **Table 3** for echo metrics for MS severity.

Cardiac catheterization and/or an exercise stress test may also be useful for better evaluation of MS when physical examination or symptomology do not correlate with TTE findings.

TREATMENT

Treatment for MS largely depends on the etiology of the disease. For patients with rheumatic MS, which is clinically determined by appearance of the mitral valve leaflets on TTE coupled with a past medical history of rheumatic fever, recommendations are for percutaneous mitral balloon valvuloplasty.[11] Percutaneous valvuloplasty is performed via the femoral vein with a balloon tipped catheter. The catheter is advanced into the RA, across the atrial septal wall into the LA then down into the MV annulus. Positioned across the MV, the balloon is inflated, "stretching" or "cracking" the valve to allow improved leaflet mobility. This treatment is first-line therapy for rheumatic MS and may be used to provide relief while undergoing further workup for definitive replacement. In rheumatic MS it may provide several years of symptomatic relief for

Table 2 Mitral disease symptoms and etiologies	
Symptom	**Pathophysiology**
Shortness of breath	Pulmonary venous congestion due to high left ventricular end diastolic pressures (LVEDP)
Chest discomfort	Pulmonary hypertension
Fatigue	Liver congestion
Early satiety or a sense of heaviness in the abdomen	Abdominal wall edema
Lower extremity edema	Volume overload
Orthopnea	Pulmonary venous congestion
Paroxysmal nocturnal dyspnea	Pulmonary venous congestion

Table 3
Echo metrics for mitral stenosis: AEA/ASE recommendations

Mitral Metric	Mild	Moderate	Severe
MV area (cm^2)	>1.5	1.0–1.5	<1.0
Supportive findings			
Mean gradient (mm Hg)[a]	<5	5–10	>10
Pulmonary artery (PA) pressure (mm Hg)	<30	30–50	>50

Abbreviations: American Society of Echocardiography; European Association of Echocardiography
 [a] At heart rates 60–80 bpm and sinus rhythm.
 From Baumgartner H, Hung J, Bermejo J, Chambers JB, Evangelista A, Griffin BP, et al. Echocar[1] diographic assessment of valve stenosis: EAE/ASE recommendations for clinical practice. J Am Soc Echocardiogr 2009; 22 (1):1-23.

some patients.[11] At the current time, open surgical replacement remains the gold standard therapy for other forms of MS.

MITRAL VALVE DISEASE: MITRAL REGURGITATION

Mitral regurgitation (MR) is the third most common VHD in the world, affecting 24.2 million people[18] and the most common form of VHD in the United States.[19] It is primarily found in the elderly, with an overall prevalence of 1.7%, but an increasing prevalence with age, ranging from 0.5% in those aged 18 to 44 years to 9.3% in those aged greater than or equal to 75 years.[20]

MR is the reversal of blood flow from the LV through the MV into the LA during the systolic phase of the cardiac cycle. MR is classified by duration (acute vs chronic). Chronic MR is further differentiated by etiology: primary/degenerative, secondary/functional, or mixed (a combination of both). Acute MR may occur in the setting of infectious endocarditis leading to leaflet perforation, spontaneous chordal rupture, or as the result of a myocardial infarction (MI).[11] Acute MR can lead to rapid decompensation, need for intensive care, and possibly mechanical circulatory support until curative treatment of the valve is performed.

Chronic MR is differentiated into 2 categories based on the cause of the malfunction. Primary/degenerative MR (dMR) occurs when there is a structural abnormality of the valve apparatus (leaflets, chordae, papillary muscles, annulus).[16] Acute causes include endocarditis, trauma, and chordal rupture but are largely due to genetic predispositions.[18] Structural abnormalities prevent the valve from closing, allowing backflow of blood into the LA at the location of the defect. Secondary/functional MR (fMR) accounts for 65% of MR cases and arises when annular dilatation prevents coaptation of the leaflets.[18] Secondary MR originates from dilated atria or ventricles.

CLINICAL PRESENTATION

MR regardless of type presents with the similar complaints: fatigue, decreased exercise tolerance, shortness of breath, dyspnea on exertion, orthopnea, and paroxysmal nocturnal dyspnea. A differentiating component is the timing and development of the symptom burden. Acute MR shows relatively rapid symptom progression: sudden MV chordal rupture causing acute MR presents with abruptly developing symptoms and rapid progression of severity, versus the gradual progression found with chronic MR or MS. With chronic MR, patients may be asymptomatic for years, showing progressive decline in activity tolerance with shortness of breath that evolves due to decreasing cardiac output. Patients with chronic severe MR may also present with symptoms of right-sided HF including abdominal fullness and peripheral edema.

PHYSICAL EXAMINATION

Patients with MR may be asymptomatic or have florid pulmonary edema depending on progression of HF. The prototypical murmur of MR is a holosystolic (pansystolic) murmur, heard best at the apex with the patient in the left lateral decubitus position in chronic MR; the murmur may radiate to the axilla. The apical impulse may be more laterally displaced due to LV enlargement. In MR due to mitral valve prolapse the murmur may also radiate to the anterior or posterior chest depending on the eccentricity of the jet. Having the patient change positions, such as leaning forward or lying on their left side, may help you appreciate a mitral murmur better. A narrow pulse pressure is often seen in severe MR. Signs of left-sided HF, including pulmonary rales, may be present, along with indications of right HF, including distended jugular veins and pitting edema of the lower extremities.

DIAGNOSTIC TESTING

Diagnostic testing of MR consists of echocardiogram, either TTE or TEE. TTE provides assessment of LV function, pulmonary artery pressure, and importantly the severity and mechanism of MR regardless of etiology or chronicity.[11] Whereas TEE is helpful in determining etiology of MR (functional vs degenerative), as well as detection of papillary muscle, chordal rupture, valvular vegetations, or annular abscesses that may be present.[11]

Although not the primary modality for diagnosing MR, hemodynamic assessments performed during cardiac catheterization also provide evidence for MR. A prominent systolic *c-v* wave is seen in pulmonary capillary wedge pressure tracings during ventricular systole with MR. Ventriculograms (done during cardiac catheterization) are also be used to quantify the severity of MR.

TREATMENT

Acute MR from chordal or papillary muscle rupture or infective endocarditis almost always requires surgical treatment. The patient may require stabilization prior to the procedure with vasodilator therapy to reduce arterial systemic resistance and augment forward flow. This may temporarily relieve symptoms of pulmonary vascular congestion by reducing regurgitant volume.[3] For some patients with acute MR who are deemed prohibitive risk for surgical intervention, transcatheter therapies (such as mitral valve edge-to-edge repair also referred to as MV TEER) may be considered as lifesaving standalone procedure or used as a stabilizing measure as a bridge to surgery.[21]

Medical therapy for chronic MR is based on the etiology. fMR requires a different treatment pathway from dMR. The first-line treatment for fMR with LV HF with reduced ejection fraction (HFrEF) is optimizing guideline-directed medical therapy (GDMT). The goal of GDMT is recovery of LV systolic function that facilitates restoration of the annulus to its original size and shape, thereby reducing the severity of MR. GDMT involves reducing afterload and excess volume. The first-line therapy for afterload reduction is initiation of angiotensin-converting enzyme inhibitors (ACE-Is) or angiotensin receptor blockers (ARBs) and beta-blockers.[3] Initiation of loop diuretics and/or mineralocorticoid receptor antagonists (MRAs) to manage excess fluid volume are additional components of GDMT for fMR.[11] See **Table 4** for review of GDMT for fMR with LV HFrEF.

Table 4
Guideline directed medical therapy for HFrEF

Class	Examples	Max (Target) Dosage	Mechanism of Action in HF	LOE
SGLT2i	Empagliflozin/ Dapagliflozin	10 mg daily/ 10 mg daily	Reduces glucose/sodium reabsorption and increases urinary glucose exertion and sodium delivery to tubules	1, A
ARNi	Sacubitril/ valsartan Entresto	97/103 mg/ twice daily	Decreases BNP, selectively antagonizes angiotensin II AT1 receptors, reduces cardiovascular death and hospitalization by 20%	1, A
ACEi (unable to tolerate ARNi)	Lisinopril/ Enalapril/ Ramipril/ Benazepril	40 mg/daily 40 mg/daily 10 mg/daily 20 mg/daily	Inhibits angiotensin converting enzyme interfering with conversion of angiotensin I to II, reduces morbidity and mortality	1, A
ARB (unable to tolerate ARNi/ACEi)	Losartan/ Valsartan	150 mg daily/ 320 mg daily	Selectively antagonizes angiotensin II AT1 receptors, reduces morbidity and mortality	1, A
MRA	Spironolactone/ Eplerenone	50 mg daily/ 50 mg daily	Antagonizes aldosterone-specific mineralocorticoid receptors decreasing Na and water reabsorption, improves all cause mortality and hospitalization	1, A
BB	Bisoprolol/ Metoprolol succinate/ Carvedilol	10 mg daily/ 200 mg daily/ 25-50 mg/ twice daily	Selectively antagonizes beta 1 adrenergic receptors, reduces risk of death and/or hospitalization, can improves LVEF, lessen symptoms of HF, improves clinical status	1, A
LOOP diuretic	Bumetanide/ Furosemide/ Torsemide	10 mg daily/ 600 mg daily/ 200 mg daily	Inhibits loop of Henle and prox and distal convoluted tubule sodium and chloride resorption, decreases physical signs of fluid retention, and improves symptoms, QOL, and exercise tolerance	1, B
Thiazide (not responsive to LOOP diuretics)	Chlorothiazide/ Chlorthalidone/Hydro-chlorothiazide/Indapamide/ Metolazone	1000 mg daily/ 100 mg daily/ 200 mg daily/ 5 mg daily/ 20 mg daily	Inhibits cortical diluting site and proximal convoluted tubule sodium resorption, decreases physical signs of fluid retention, and improves symptoms, QOL, and exercise tolerance	1, B

Abbreviations: COR, class of recommendation; LOE, level of evidence; QOL, quality of life.

There is no evidence that use of vasodilator therapy is helpful with dMR.[9] However, GDMT should be pursued when systolic dysfunction or hypertension is present.[11] **Table 5** reviews GDMT for dMR.

With chronic MR, open surgical repair is stilled reserved as the most appropriate treatment for those who are surgical candidates. Advances in transcatheter therapies have allowed for the treatment of MR in patients at high or prohibitive risk for standard surgical treatment. Transcatheter edge-to-edge repair (MV TEER) is commercially

Table 5
Guidelines directed medical therapy for HFpEF

Medication Type	Examples	Max (Target) Dosage	Mechanism of Action in HF	COR/LOE
SGLT2i	Empagliflozin	10 mg/daily	Reduces glucose/sodium reabsorption and increases urinary glucose exertion and sodium delivery to tubules	2a, B
	Dapagliflozin	10 mg/daily		
MRA (aldosterone antagonist)	Spironolactone	50 mg/daily	Antagonizes aldosterone-specific mineralocorticoid receptors decreasing Na and water reabsorption, improves all-cause mortality and hospitalization	2b, B
ARNi	Sacubitril/valsartan	97/103 mg twice/daily	Decreases BNP, selectively antagonizes angiotensin II AT1 receptors, reduces cardiovascular death and hospitalization by 20%	2b, B
LOOP diuretic	Bumetanide/ Furosemide/ Torsemide	10 mg/daily 600 mg/daily 200 mg daily	Inhibits loop of Henle and prox and distal convoluted tubule sodium and chloride resorption, decreases physical signs of fluid retention, and improves symptoms, QOL, and exercise tolerance	1, B-NR
Thiazide diuretic (not responsive to LOOP diuretic)	Chlorothiazide Chlorthalidone Hydrochlorothiazide Indapamide Metolazone	1000 mg/daily 100 mg/daily 200 mg/daily 5 mg/daily 20 mg/daily	Inhibits cortical diluting site and proximal convoluted tubule sodium resorption, decreases physical signs of fluid retention, and improves symptoms, QOL, and exercise tolerance	1, B-NR
ARB	Candesartan Losartan Valsartan	32 mg/daily 150 mg/daily 160 twice/daily	Selectively antagonizes angiotensin II AT1 receptors, reduces hospitalization for heart failure and cardiovascular death	2b, B

Abbreviations: COR, class of recommendation, LOE, level of evidence; NR, nonrandomized.

available for severe MR. The procedure is performed in the cardiac catheterization laboratory with TEE guidance under general anesthesia. "Clips" are used to capture the anterior and posterior mitral valve leaflets, creating a double or triple orifice valve, effectively reducing the mitral valve opening. Up to 3 clip devices may be placed during the MV TEER procedure. Studies have shown that patients undergoing MV TEER can have a significant reduction in severity of MR and an improvement in quality of life.

TRICUSPID VALVE

The tricuspid valve has recently emerged as a major focus in cardiology innovation and research. Tricuspid regurgitation (TR) has high prevalence in the general population[22] with progression to severe disease associated with high morbidity and mortality.[23,24] Incidence has increased in recent years due to the rise in use of pacemakers.[18] Although a common finding on TTEs, TR was thought benign unless associated with pulmonary hypertension, RV failure, or LV failure.

TR is distinguished by backflow of blood into the RA, the volume or load varying based on pre-load and structural changes. With disease progression, backflow extends into the superior and inferior vena cava. TR is categorized into 3 types: primary, secondary, and isolated. Primary TR accounts for ~8% to 10% of all cases and involves etiologies in which the valve is structurally abnormal, either congenital or acquired causes. Congenital abnormalities include Ebstein's disease in which the origin of the leaflets is shifted toward the apex and there are no chordae. Acquired abnormalities include iatrogenic damage (biopsies, pacer leads), leaflet damage (endocarditis, rheumatic or systemic disease, drug induced), leaflet displacement (pacemaker or defibrillator leads, tumors, carcinoid disease, commissural fusion, chordal tethering, or rupture).[25] Pacemaker wire induced TR is the most common acquired cause.

Secondary TR is the more commonly found form, most often caused by RV dilatation and dysfunction resulting in the tethered leaflets, annular dilatation, and malcoaptation of leaflets. Secondary TR is highly associated with other left-sided valvular and myocardial disease; up to half of patients with severe MR and 25% with SAS also show TR.[23]

A third form of TR, called "isolated" TR, is morphologically different from the first 2. Isolated TR is commonly found in the elderly with atrial fibrillation which causes right atrial dilatation, annular dilatation, and malcoaptation of the leaflets. See **Fig. 2** for a schematic representation of types of TR.

CLINICAL PRESENTATION

Patients with severe TR generally present with complaints of right-sided HF or low cardiac output symptoms. Symptoms of fatigue, weakness, shortness of breath, and exercise intolerance may build over for years due to the slow progression of the disease process.

PHYSICAL EXAMINATION

During inspection, severe TR may show prominent, distended, or pulsatile jugular veins from the regurgitant flow into the superior vena cava. Over time, persistent regurgitation into the inferior vena cava results in lower extremity edema and abdominal distention with ascites.

Palpation of the chest may show a dynamic RV heave from RV dilatation. The liver may be enlarged, tender, and pulsatile in association with the TR murmur. The abdomen enlarged, becoming taunt with increasing fluid buildup.

CENTRAL ILLUSTRATION: Schematic Drawing of the Different Morphologic Types of Tricuspid Regurgitation

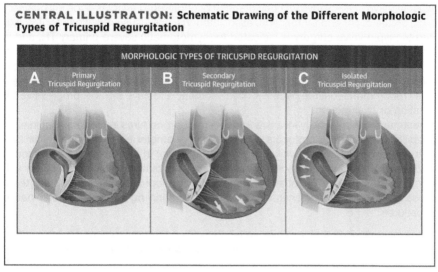

MORPHOLOGIC TYPES OF TRICUSPID REGURGITATION

A   Primary Tricuspid Regurgitation

B   Secondary Tricuspid Regurgitation

C   Isolated Tricuspid Regurgitation

Fig. 2. Types of tricuspid regurgitation: Primary (*A*); Secondary (*B*); Isolated (*C*). (*From* Prihadi E, Delgado V, Leon M, et al. Morphologic Types of Tricuspid Regurgitation. J Am Coll Cardiol Img. 2019 Mar, 12 (3) 491–499. https://doi.org/10.1016/j.jcmg.2018.09.027.[25])

Classic TR is associated with a holosystolic murmur found at the right lower and mid sternal border with little radiation. A visual display of murmurs with VHD is shown in **Fig. 1**.

DIAGNOSTIC TESTING

TTE and TEE are used to assess severity of regurgitation, leaflet motion, dimensions, interventricular septal motion, RA and RV size, and evidence of superior and inferior vena cava reflux. These echocardiogram findings provide prognostic indicators and direction for treatment.

There are no ECG changes associated with TR. However, there may be changes associated with the primary process causing TR. For example, RV hypertrophy with severe pulmonary hypertension or Q-waves in right-sided precordial (chest) leads with RV infarction may be seen on the 12-lead ECG.

Right heart catheterization pulmonary pressures and vascular resistance can help clarify severity of TR when there is inconsistent echocardiographic data. Cardiac MRI may be useful in defining RV anatomy and wall motion.

TREATMENT

Medical therapy focusing on HF management is the primary strategy with TR. Diuretic therapy for fluid and volume management is the first line of treatment. In secondary TR, addressing the cause of the TR is recommended, such as pursuing GDMT with LV-HF or vasodilators with pulmonary hypertension.[11] As previously shown, **Tables 4** and **5** display GDMT for Heart Failure with reduced ejection fraction (HFrEF) and Heart Failure with preserved ejection fraction (HFpEF). Neurohormonal antagonists can be included to improve diuretic therapy by reducing the body's attempts to compensate for volume loss or treatments for pulmonary hypertension.

Surgical repair has been the gold standard for the treatment of severe symptomatic TR when left-sided valve surgery is indicated. Recent recommendations regarding tricuspid valve surgery involve consideration of numerous variables: type and severity of TR, status of RV and LV function, associated VD, and cause of secondary TR. Isolated tricuspid valve surgery is indicated for symptomatic severe primary TR, and in asymptomatic or mildly symptomatic TR when there is evidence of RV enlargement of deteriorating function.[11] For patients with previous left-sided valve surgery who develop severe TR, early surgery is recommended when symptomatic.[9] Early surgery is also recommended if the patient is asymptomatic and have signs of progressive RV dilatation or dysfunction.[11]

Treatment with minimally invasive transcatheter procedures is predominant in early feasibility and research protocols. There are transcatheter edge-to-edge repair systems approved in Europe, while commercial approval in United States expected is pending. The complex tricuspid valve anatomy, surrounding electrical system and structures that require negotiation have made development of transcatheter techniques challenging. Two general approaches are being pursued as catheter-based procedures.[23]

- Repair: devices that improve leaflet coaptation through an edge-to-edge suture or clip; annuloplasty systems that use a cinching or suturing system to reduce the size of the TC annulus.
- Replacement: orthotopic valves delivered into the tricuspid valve via the venous route and heterotopic valves placed in either bi-caval or inferior vena cava position. Caval-atrial valve junction implantation is thought to reduce backflow into the vena-cava, reducing venous system congestion but does not treat the TR.

POSTPROCEDURE NURSING CARE

Nursing care following transcatheter valve procedures begins in the cardiac catheterization laboratory and extends to hospital discharge. Initial postprocedure nursing care focuses on sedation/anesthesia recovery, hemostasis with access site management, hemodynamic stability, cardiac rhythm and perfusion monitoring, neurologic monitoring, and eventual mobilization. Variations in care are determined by which valve was treated, the type of intervention performed, and individual patient needs—all affecting recovery. Refer to **Table 6** that displays priorities for postprocedure nursing care.

Access Site Management

Access site management is one of the most important areas of postprocedure care. The most common access sites are the femoral arteries and veins, unilateral or bilateral, often both. When peripheral disease is present alternate access sites (carotid, subclavian, axillary, caval) may be engaged. Catheter sizes range from 6 French to 24 French. French size identifies the outer diameter of the catheter and is calculated to millimeters by dividing the French size by 3 (eg, 14 French/3 = 4.7 mm). A smaller French size indicates a smaller puncture to the vessel. Vascular closure devices are frequently used with large French catheters to assist in site management. Identification of catheter size, site of deployment, arterial versus venous placement, and use of closure device are key elements of postprocedure and ongoing clinical care. In the event of any disruption in hemostasis or hemodynamic stability quick recognition and knowledge of access characteristics are essential for effective management. Refer to **Table 7** for access site management recommendations.[26]

Cardiac Rhythm Monitoring

The anatomic proximity of the conduction system to the various heart valves impacts the risk of conduction defects postvalve procedures. Conduction defects are primarily

Table 6	
Potential protocol for postprocedure clinical care	
General Guidelines	**Parameters**
1. Assess vital signs (BP, HR, RR, SatO$_2$) and cardiac rhythm 2. Assess access site for bleeding, hematoma formation and swelling 3. Assess perfusion: peripheral pulses distal to access site 4. Assess neurovascular status: mentation, recovery from sedation	q15 min x4, q30 min x2, q1 h x 4, then q4 h until discharge
5. Assess pain status	Administer analgesics as indicated
6. Diet	Resume preprocedure diet
7. Medications	Resume preprocedure regimen, adjust HF regimen based on hemodynamics Note: addition of antiplatelet therapy

8. Notification parameters:
  a. Decrease/absence of peripheral pulses.
  b. Development of access site hematoma/ uncontrolled bleeding
  c. Increase in pain at access site or extremity
  d. Development of chest pain or shortness of breath	

Femoral access (arterial or venous) 1. Activity: bedrest for 4–6 h based on access catheter size. Head of bed elevation up to 30° 2. Avoid flexion of hip on access side for duration of bedrest. 3. Compression device based on institutional protocol	
Brachial or radial access 1. Activity: may sit up in bed, progress to ambulation based on recovery from sedation 2. Site: apply sequential pressure dressing to access site. Pressure reduction per device protocol 3. Instruct patient to avoid prolonged periods of arm flexion, hyperextension, or lying on access arm or wrist	

associated with AoV procedures and rarely seen with mitral procedures. Transcatheter tricuspid valve procedures are primarily in research protocols with incidence yet to be determined. Telemetry monitoring for a minimum of 24 hours is recommended for all patients post TAVR to ensure no development of high grade atrioventricular (AV) block occurs. Patients at the highest risk are those with a pre-existing right bundle branch block or second-degree heart block Mobitz type I.[27] If there are new, progressive or preexisting conduction disturbances that change postprocedure, electrophysiology studies should be considered and continued monitoring for ≥48 hours is recommended.[27] Patients with new conduction delays that do not progress to high grade AV block while hospitalized may be discharged home with mobile cardiac telemetry device to monitor for late onset conduction disturbances for a minimum of 14 days.[27]

Pericardial Effusion

Risk for pericardial effusion can be seen with any transcatheter valve procedure. Catheters and wires present a risk of perforation leading to the risk of bleeding into the pericardial sac, restricting movement of the heart. Observant clinical care is essential for early detection and treatment of this rare but life-threating condition. Signs of

Table 7
Access site management: guidelines[24]

Access site	Monitoring: access and hemodynamics	Initial manual pressure	Management: late access site bleeding	Management: hemostasis achieved
Venous access	q15 min x4, q30 min x2, q1 h x 4, q4h	*Distal* to access site	Apply direct pressure distal to access site uninterrupted for 15 min, if continues to bleed/ooze continue to apply pressure and notify provider (MD/APP)	Apply clean, dry dressing; restart hemodynamic, access site monitoring
Arterial access	q15 min x4, q30 min x2, q1 h x 4, q4h	*Proximal* to access site	Apply direct pressure proximal to access site uninterrupted for 15 min, continue to apply pressure and notify provider	Apply clean, dry dressing; restart hemodynamic, access site monitoring

Developed by: C Cusin DNP;

Abbreviations: APP, advanced practice provider; MD, medical doctor.

Table 8	
Patient education: preparing for procedure, discharge and recovery	
Preprocedure	
Patient goals	• Establish purpose for procedure • Identify patient goals and preferences
Procedure description	• Include description: surgical, minimally invasive, transcatheter; replacement, repair, or palliative • Describe procedure, access, devices used, forms of anesthesia, anticipated duration of procedure, expected duration in recovery area • Teaching aides: models, diagrams, illustrations assist in visualization • Education materials and resources for patient and family: booklets and websites
Risks	• Describe potential risks and risk reduction strategies
Medication instruction	• Review medication regimen: with same day admissions identify medications to hold or take prior to arriving to hospital • In presence of renal dysfunction and anticipated use of contrast, nephrotoxic agents may be held
Allergies	• Review allergies • For contrast allergies provide instruction for prophylaxis preparation • Identify antibiotic allergies
Diet	• Preprocedure: hold intake after midnight or specified duration • Postprocedure: resuming heart healthy diet
Activities	• Expectations re: postprocedure monitoring and testing, telemetry monitoring, frequent access site monitoring and neurovascular checks, bedrest, electrocardiograms, chest X-ray, TTE, blood work • Expectations for post procedure bedrest (BR), activity progression following BR, and ambulation thereafter • Post procedure activity limitations expected based on procedure type. Weight limitations, stair climbing, driving • Cardiac rehabilitation postprocedure for recovery
Length of stay	• Anticipated hospital stay duration. • Next day discharge for majority of procedures. Identify discharge and home resources
Postprocedure through discharge	
Activity: initial, progression, restrictions	• Bedrest duration • Reinforce limitations in flexion of hip, arm, and wrist based on access sites • Activity progression following bed rest • Restrictions following discharge

(continued on next page)

Table 8 (continued)	
Medications	• Review resumption of previous medications. • Addition of anti-platelet or anticoagulation therapy. • Adjustments in heart failure regimens. • Pain regimen: strategies to reduce/limit; medications
Heart Failure	• Reinforce HF teaching. • Daily weights. Recognizing significant weight changes. • Dietary directions. • Medications: diuretics, BB, ACEi/ARB/ARNis, SGLT2i, MRA's etc.
Discharge Instructions	
Follow up	• Appointment types and frequency. • Clinic evaluations. • Dental prophylaxis: life long • Diagnostic evaluations: blood tests, imaging: TTE, TEE, CT etc.
Activity	• Bathing: no soaking access sites in water until healed. • Progression. • Cardiac Rehabilitation enrollment
Complications	• Specific complications to be aware of bleeding, breathing, pain, HF, procedure specific
Emergency	• When to call: unexpected outcomes, • Who to call: phone number • When to call for Emergency Support (911)

pericardial effusion include decreasing systolic blood pressure with an increasing HR. The rising HR is a compensatory mechanism to increase cardiac output as the LV becomes compressed from an effusion resulting in decreased stroke volume. Symptoms include complaints of pain or shortness of breath. The pain maybe localized to the chest or reported in the back, neck, or upper abdomen. Shortness of breath may be gradual or abrupt in onset. These signs and symptoms in a postprocedure setting indicate rapid assessment with TTE and escalation of care.

Medical Therapy—Heart Failure

Patients with VHD generally present with HF. Although transcatheter procedures treat a valve lesion, the existing HF remains and requires ongoing treatment. Adjustments to preprocedural regimens may be indicated due to changes resulting from valve treatment. Optimal GDMT as outlined in guidelines is recommended based on underlying preserved or reduced ejection fraction.[28] As discussed (and displayed in **Table 4**) GDMT for HFrEF includes SGLT2is, ARNis (ACE-Is or ARBs if ARNi's are not appropriate), MRAs, and beta-blockers (only the ones approved for HF). Generally, loop diuretics are used for fluid management primarily due to comorbid kidney disease, adding thiazide diuretics when unresponsive to loop diuretics.[28]

Medical therapy for HFpEF (LVEF ≥50%) focuses on afterload reduction and volume management. As discussed earlier (and displayed in **Table 5**) recent 2022 guidelines added sodium-glucose cotransporter-2 inhibitors (SGLT2i), ARNis (ACE-Is or ARBs, if ARNis are not appropriate), and MRAs for the management of HFpEF.[28]

Recommendations remain the same for treatment of hypertension, atrial fibrillation, use of ARBs, and avoidance of nitrates or phosphodiesterase-5 inhibitors.[28] As with HFrEF, loop diuretics can be used with fluid retention in addition to thiazide diuretics (when unresponsive to loop diuretics alone).[28]

Medical Therapy—Antiplatelet and Anticoagulation Therapy

Antiplatelet therapy following transcatheter procedures has been based on their use in the initial research protocols. Early TAVR protocols used dual antiplatelet therapy (DAPT) with clopidogrel and aspirin to reduce the risk of thrombus formation on leaflets or devices thought to increase the risk for stroke. Currently DAPT is recommended in the TAVR expert consensus decision pathway.[29] However, a more recent meta-analysis found that following TAVR single antiplatelet therapy is associated with a lower bleeding risk with no increase in ischemic events.[30]

PATIENT EDUCATION

For any procedure, whether surgical or a minimally invasive, pre- and postprocedure education is essential for the patient, family, or/and significant others. Providing education for patients and their support systems regarding procedures, expected hospital events, and the postdischarge period helps prepare for optimal outcomes, obtaining resources for success and avoidance of both real and perceived barriers. **Table 8** provides key topics to address in patient education and content to include.

SUMMARY

Over the last few decades, the treatment of VHD has rapidly transitioned from a surgical to a transcatheter approach. Transcatheter treatments are less invasive and associated with lower complication rates, allowing therapies to be offered to complex patients traditionally considered at increased risk for surgery. This paradigm shift has elevated the need for multidisciplinary teams to provide patient care. Teams in which nursing plays the integral role of coordinating patients with their families through a maze of testing and intricate procedures manage HF, providing support, guidance, and education for success. As the aging population continues to increase and the innovation in the treatment of VHD continues there will be a simultaneous demand for nursing to actively engage in creating safe, effective, efficient, and patient centric care pathways.

CLINICS CARE POINTS

- Patients with valve disease are often first identified by the presence of a heart murmur, exploration of symptoms, and then confirmed by echocardiogram. Echocardiogram is the primary diagnostic test for assessing for valve disease and cardiac function.

- Symptoms of valve disease are nonspecific. Patients present with dyspnea on exertion, reduced exercise capacity, and complaints associate with HF: shortness of breath, orthopnea, and paroxysmal nocturnal dyspnea. Although lower extremity edema is associated with right HF and severe tricuspid regurgitation, it is also associated with noncardiac sources such as lymph, liver, and kidney disease.

- When assessing for symptoms explore timing and progression, symptoms often develop slowly and are not recognized. Explore with time comparison questions:
  - When was the last time you were able to (cut the lawn, walk around the block)?
  - How does your activity this summer compare to your activity last summer?

- The echocardiogram assessment is not just about the valve but also about assessing cardiac function. It is essential for evaluating impact of valve disease on overall cardiac function as well as the contribution of cardiac damage on valve function. Assess left and right ventricular size and function as well as left and right atrial size and function.
- Valve disease often occurs secondary to another condition. For example, left ventricular chamber enlargement from long standing untreated hypertension can cause "stretching" of the mitral annulus resulting in secondary/functional MR; atrial arrhythmias cause atrial enlargement that stretches the tricuspid annulus creating tricuspid regurgitation.
- Although the transthoracic echocardiogram may be the primary diagnostic tool for identifying valve disease, a meticulous history and physical examination, chest X-ray, electrocardiogram, and lab tests are essential to fully explore when assessing valve disease.
- Primary valve disease is a mechanical problem of the valve and requires the valve to be "fixed." Secondary valve disease occurs due to another issue that requires treatment in order to improve the valve disease.

DISCLOSURE

The authors have no disclosures relevant to this publication.

REFERENCES

1. 2020 Profile of Older Americans. In: United States Department of Health and Human Services editor: Administration for Community Living; 2021.
2. Nkomo VT, Gardin JM, Skelton TN, et al. Burden of valvular heart diseases: a population-based study. Lancet 2006;368(9540):1005–11.
3. d'Arcy JL, Prendergast BD, Chambers JB, et al. Valvular heart disease: the next cardiac epidemic. Heart 2011;97(2):91–3.
4. Baumgartner H, Falk V, Bax JJ, et al. ESC/EACTS Guidelines for the management of valvular heart disease. Eur Heart J 2017;38(36):2739–91.
5. Nishimura RA, O'Gara PT, Bavaria JE, et al. AATS/ACC/ASE/SCAI/STS Expert Consensus Systems of Care Document: A Proposal to Optimize Care for Patients With Valvular Heart Disease: A Joint Report of the American Association for Thoracic Surgery, American College of Cardiology, American Society of Echocardiography, Society for Cardiovascular Angiography and Interventions, and Society of Thoracic Surgeons. J Am Coll Cardiol 2019;73(20):2609–35.
6. Joseph J, Naqvi SY, Giri J, et al. Aortic Stenosis: Pathophysiology, Diagnosis, and Therapy. Am J Med 2017;130(3):253–63.
7. Osnabrugge RL, Mylotte D, Head SJ, et al. Aortic stenosis in the elderly: disease prevalence and number of candidates for transcatheter aortic valve replacement: a meta-analysis and modeling study. J Am Coll Cardiol 2013;62(11):1002–12.
8. Lindman BR, Bonow RO, Otto CM. Aortic valve stenosis. In: Libby P, Bonow RO, Mann DL, editors. Braunwald's Heart Disease; A Textbook of Cardiovascular Medicine. Philadelphia, PA: W. B. Saunders Company; 2022. p. 1399–418.
9. Lindman BR, Clavel MA, Mathieu P, et al. Calcific aortic stenosis. Nat Rev Dis Primers 2016;2:16006.
10. Goody PR, Hosen MR, Christmann D, et al. Aortic Valve Stenosis: From Basic Mechanisms to Novel Therapeutic Targets. Arterioscler Thromb Vasc Biol 2020; 40(4):885–900.
11. Otto CM, Nishimura RA, Bonow RO, et al. 2020 ACC/AHA Guideline for the Management of Patients With Valvular Heart Disease: A Report of the American

College of Cardiology/American Heart Association Joint Committee on Clinical Practice Guidelines. Circulation 2021;143(5):e72–227.

12. Evangilista A, Tornas P, Bonow RO. Aortic Regurgitation: Clinical Presentation, Disease Stages and Management. In: Otto CM, Bonow RO, editors. Valvular heart disease: a Companion to Braunwald's heart disease. Philadelphia, PA: Elsevier; 2021. p. 179–96.

13. Keegan P, Lisko JC, Kamioka N, et al. Nurse Led Sedation: The Clinical and Echocardiographic Outcomes of the 5-Year Emory Experience. Structural Heart 2020;4(4):302–9.

14. Chambers JB. Epidemiology of Valvular Heart Disease. In: Otto CM, Bonow RO, editors. Valvular heart disease: a Companion to Braunwald's heart disease. Philadelphia, PA: Elsevier; 2021. p. 3–17.

15. Bonow RO, Nishimura RA. Aortic Regurgitation. In: Libby P, Bonow RO, Mann DL, et al, editors. Braunwald's heart disease: a Textbook of cardiovascular medicine. Philadelphia, PA: Elsevier; 2022. p. 1419–29.

16. Lilly LS, Harvard Medical School. Pathophysiology of heart disease : a collaborative project of medical students and faculty. Philadelphia: Wolters Kluwer; 2016.

17. Nguyen T, Hu D, Chen SL, et al. Management of complex cardiovascular problems. Chichester, West Sussex, UK ; Hoboken, NJ: John Wiley & Sons Inc.; 2016. p. 1, online resource.

18. Aluru JS, Barsouk A, Saginala K, et al. Valvular Heart Disease Epidemiology. Med Sci 2022;10(2).

19. Peters AS, Duggan JP, Trachiotis GD, et al. Epidemiology of Valvular Heart Disease. Surg Clin North Am 2022;102(3):517–28.

20. Cahill TJ, Prothero A, Wilson J, et al. Community prevalence, mechanisms and outcome of mitral or tricuspid regurgitation. Heart (British Cardiac Society), heartjnl-2020-318482 2021. https://doi.org/10.1136/heartjnl-2020-318482.

21. Haberman D, Dahan S, Poles L, et al. Transcatheter edge-to-edge repair in acute mitral regurgitation following acute myocardial infarction: Recent advances. Kardiol Pol 2022;80(12):1190–9.

22. Fender EA, Zack CJ, Nishimura RA. Isolated tricuspid regurgitation: outcomes and therapeutic interventions. Heart 2018;104(10):798–806.

23. Condello F, Gitto M, Stefanini GG. Etiology, epidemiology, pathophysiology and management of tricuspid regurgitation: an overview. Rev Cardiovasc Med 2021;22(4):1115–42.

24. Nath J, Foster E, Heidenreich PA. Impact of tricuspid regurgitation on long-term survival. J Am Coll Cardiol 2004;43(3):405–9.

25. Prihadi EA, Delgado V, Leon MB, et al. Morphologic Types of Tricuspid Regurgitation: Characteristics and Prognostic Implications. JACC Cardiovascular imaging 2019;12(3):491–9.

26. Julien M. Cardiac Catheterization. In: Perpetua E, Keegan P, editors. Cadiac nursing. Philadelphia: Wolters Kluwer; 2021. p. 428–60.

27. Lilly SM, Deshmukh AJ, Epstein AE, et al. 2020 ACC Expert Consensus Decision Pathway on Management of Conduction Disturbances in Patients Undergoing Transcatheter Aortic Valve Replacement: A Report of the American College of Cardiology Solution Set Oversight Committee. J Am Coll Cardiol 2020;76(20):2391–411.

28. Heidenreich PA, Bozkurt B, Aguilar D, et al. AHA/ACC/HFSA Guideline for the Management of Heart Failure: A Report of the American College of Cardiology/ American Heart Association Joint Committee on Clinical Practice Guidelines. J Am Coll Cardiol 2022;79(17):e263–421.

29. Otto CM, Kumbhani DJ, Alexander KP, et al. ACC Expert Consensus Decision Pathway for Transcatheter Aortic Valve Replacement in the Management of Adults With Aortic Stenosis: A Report of the American College of Cardiology Task Force on Clinical Expert Consensus Documents. J Am Coll Cardiol 2017; 69(10):1313–46.
30. Guedeney P, Sorrentino S, Mesnier J, et al. Single Versus Dual Antiplatelet Therapy Following TAVR: A Systematic Review and Meta-Analysis of Randomized Controlled Trials. JACC Cardiovasc Interv 2021;14(2):234–6.

Focus on Treatment (Drug and Device Updates)

Anticoagulation for Stroke Prevention in Atrial Fibrillation

Carrie Palmer, DNP, RN, ANP-BC

KEYWORDS

- Atrial fibrillation • Stroke • Oral anticoagulant

KEY POINTS

- Anticoagulation for stroke prevention is a cornerstone of atrial fibrillation management.
- Patients should be carefully assessed for stroke and bleeding risk before initiating anticoagulation therapy.
- Many oral anticoagulant options are available to allow for individualization of therapy.
- Major bleeding while on oral anticoagulation is rare and reversal agents are widely available.
- Non-life-threatening bleeding can generally be managed through withholding anticoagulants and supportive measures.

INTRODUCTION

Cardiovascular disease is a leading cause of death in the United States, and one in six of these deaths is attributed to stroke.[1] Nearly 90% of strokes are ischemic, in which a thrombus, either atherosclerotic or cardioembolic, disrupts blood flow to cerebral parenchyma, eventually causing cell death.[1] Atrial fibrillation (AF) is a leading cause of cardioembolic stroke and causes considerable morbidity and mortality with high recurrence rates. Strokes due to AF are expected to increase due to the aging of the population and prevalence of other risk factors such as obesity, diabetes, hypertension, and coronary artery disease.[2,3] Nurses care for patients with stroke across the continuum, and early management of stroke risk can contribute to improved outcomes.

One of the keystones of AF management is stroke prevention. AF causes uncoordinated atrial contractions, allowing blood to become stagnant in the atria. A common complication of AF is the formation of a clot in the left atrial appendage which can embolize to peripheral tissues, causing a venous thromboembolism, or to the brain, causing cerebral arterial occlusions, or ischemic stroke.[3] Stroke prevention commonly includes

The University of North Carolina at Chapel Hill School of Nursing, 7460 Carrington Hall, Chapel Hill, NC 27599, USA
E-mail address: carrie_palmer@unc.edu

Nurs Clin N Am 58 (2023) 379–387
https://doi.org/10.1016/j.cnur.2023.05.005
0029-6465/23/© 2023 Elsevier Inc. All rights reserved.

anticoagulation with direct oral anticoagulants (DOACs) and vitamin K antagonists (VKA) or procedures like a left atrial appendage closure.[2,3] This article describes medication-based prevention of AF-related strokes, including important information for nurses and caregivers.

PATIENT SELECTION

Patient selection is a distinct aspect of anticoagulation therapy and influences the choice of anticoagulant. An initial distinction is determining if the AF is related to valvular heart disease. Valvular AF generally refers to coexisting AF and mitral stenosis or mechanical mitral valve prosthesis. Nonvalvular AF occurs absent significant mitral valve disease.[4] Patients with valvular heart disease are currently limited to VKA (eg, warfarin) for antico-agulation, whereas those with nonvalvular AF are generally treated with a DOAC.

Further classification of AF includes determining whether it is persistent or self-limiting. Paroxysmal AF usually resolves within seven days while persistent lasts more than 7 days and often becomes chronic or permanent.[4] Despite this distinction, stroke risk and anticoagulation recommendations are based on a calculation of patient-specific risk factors.[4]

A risk assessment to determine stroke risk in patients with AF is crucial. One such risk assessment is the CHA_2DS_2-VASc score, a validated tool to determine stroke risk in patients with AF.[5] The CHA_2DS_2-VASc tool gives greater weight to factors that pose greater risk, particularly previous stroke or systemic embolism.[5] Possible scores range from 0 to 9, with stroke risk increasing exponentially for each point; a score of 0 offers no added stroke risk, whereas a score of 9 indicates over 15% risk for stroke (**Table 1**). A score of 1 or more in men and 2 or more in women indicates a need for stroke pre-vention through anticoagulation.[4]

Finally, consideration of each patient's bleeding risk is crucial when considering anticoagulation. The most commonly used tool is HAS-BLED, which provides a score based on risk factors for bleeding.[6] A score of 3 or more indicates high risk for bleeding warranting cautious use of anticoagulation. These patients are more closely monitored for bleeding, modifiable risk factors (eg, uncontrolled blood pressure) are potentially corrected, and in some cases, alternative treatment options to anticoagulation are considered. Of note, the risk of stroke is generally higher than the risk of bleeding so stroke prevention remains the priority and should be considered during shared decision-making with patients[6] (**Table 2**).

Table 1 CHA_2DS_2-VASc risk scoring schema	
Criterion	**Possible Score**
Congestive heart failure	1
Hypertension	1
Age:	
65–74 y	1
≥75 y	2
Diabetes	1
Prior Stroke or systemic embolism	2
VAscular disease	1
Female Sex Category	1

Adapted from Jame & Barnes, 2020 and Gažová, et al, 2019.

Table 2
HAS-BLED scoring schema

Risk Factors for Bleeding	Points (Maximum Score: 9)
Hypertension (systolic BP > 160 mm Hg)	1
Abnormal Kidney and/or liver function	1 point for each
Stroke	1
Bleeding (history of major bleeding or tendency to bleed)	1
Labile INR or anticoagulation	1
Elderly (age >65 years) or extreme frailty	1
Drugs or substances that promote bleeding (use of non-steroidal antiinflammatory drugs [NSAIDs], aspirin, or alcohol)	1 point for each

Adapted from Methavigul, 2022.

ORAL ANTICOAGULANT MEDICATIONS

Anticoagulation is a primary strategy to prevent death and disability from stroke in patients with AF. Anticoagulants prevent formation or extension of thrombi by interfering with the clotting cascade. Until 2009, VKAs (warfarin) were the only option for stroke prevention in AF. Since that year, several direct, or target-specific, agents have been developed, which provide protection with a more favorable side effect profile and substantially less burden from monitoring.[3]

Warfarin is a VKA that inhibits the production vitamin K-dependent clotting factors II, VII, IX, and X.[7] Warfarin is indicated for stroke prophylaxis in patients with valvular or nonvalvular AF. Warfarin is a narrow therapeutic index drug that requires frequent dose adjustment and laboratory monitoring and has numerous significant drug–drug and drug–food interactions. Its metabolism can be altered by factors such as inflammation, kidney or liver disease, or fever. Anticoagulation with warfarin is monitored by the international normalized ratio (INR). An INR of 2 to 3 is considered therapeutic, balancing the risks of bleeding and embolism. An INR below 2 indicates inadequate stroke protection, whereas an INR above 3 leads to increased bleeding risks.[7–9] Monitoring the INR occurs every few days initially, gradually increasing to monthly INR readings based on the time therapeutic range (TTR).[10] Given these factors, warfarin is primarily recommended for stroke prevention in patients with prosthetic heart valves and valvular AF.[9]

DOACs consist of two classes of target-specific anticoagulants: factor Xa inhibitors and direct thrombin inhibitors. DOACs are approved to prevent stroke in nonvalvular AF. Dabigatran is the only direct thrombin inhibitor currently available. Apixaban, edoxaban, and rivaroxaban are currently available factor Xa inhibitors[11] (**Table 3**). By targeting specific clotting factors later in the cascade, these agents have much more predictable anticoagulation effects, necessitating less monitoring and have fewer interactions while providing adequate stroke protection. In addition, DOACs are fixed dose drugs, requiring no dose adjustments based on coagulation markers such as INR. DOACs have become the favored medication therapy for nonvalvular AF and other thromboembolic conditions primarily based on superiority or noninferiority to warfarin in terms of thrombus prevention. DOACs also have lower bleedings risks, require less monitoring, and are more convenient for patients as they do not require frequent clinic visits and have less potential drug and food interactions.[9,11]

Table 3
Direct oral anticoagulant use in patients with nonvalvular atrial fibrillation

Class and Drug	Dose and Administration	Considerations
Direct Thrombin Inhibitor		
Dabigatran	150 mg twice daily 75 mg twice daily if CrCl 15–30 mL/min or CrCl 30–50 mL/min in those taking concomitant P-gp inhibitors (eg, dronedarone or systemic ketoconazole)	Not recommended in patients with CrCl <15 mL/min or on dialysis Avoid use in patients with CrCl 15–30 mL/min taking concomitant P-gp inhibitors Avoid in patients with BMI ≥ 40kgm²
Factor Xa Inhibitors		
Apixaban	5 mg twice daily 2.5 mg twice daily in adults with 2 or more of the following: Age ≥80 y, weight ≤60 kg, serum creatinine ≥1.5 mg/dL	5 mg twice daily for pts with ESRD on dialysis Avoid in patients with severe liver impairment
Edoxaban	60 mg once daily in patients with CrCl >50 mL/min and CrCl ≤95 mL/min 30 mg once daily in patients with CrCl 15–50 mL/min	Avoid in patients with CrCl < 15 mL/min or Cr Cl > 95 mL/min Avoid in patients with moderate–severe liver impairment Avoid in patients with BMI ≥40 kg/m²
Rivaroxaban	20 mg once daily with the evening meal if CrCl > 50 mL/min 15 mg once daily in patients with CrCl 15–50 mL/min	Avoid in patients with CrCl < 15 mL/min and/or patients on dialysis Avoid in patients with moderate–severe liver impairment

Abbreviations: BMI, body mass index; CrCl, creatinine clearance; ESRD, end-stage renal disease; P-gp, P-glycoprotein.
Adapted from Chen, Stecker, & Warden (2020).

SPECIAL CONSIDERATIONS FOR DIRECT ORAL ANTICOAGULANT SELECTION

Several considerations for selection of DOAC have become apparent since their approvals, particularly chronic kidney disease (CKD), advanced age, and extremes of body weight.[11] Patients with CKD have higher rates of thromboembolic disease yet are at high risk of both bleeding and adverse drug reactions, warranting caution.[11,12] All DOACs are at least partially cleared by kidneys and require dose adjustments based on factors such as creatinine clearance, age, and weight. In patients with AF and moderate CKD, DOACs with appropriate dose adjustments are recommended over warfarin; however, in patients with more severe CKD, dose-adjusted factor Xa inhibitors or warfarin are recommended.[9]

Older adult patients comprise the majority of people with AF, and age above 75 years contributes to a higher CHA_2DS_2-VASc score.[4,5,13] In fact, age above 75 years alone warrants anticoagulation based on current guidelines.[4,5] Anticoagulation for stroke prophylaxis is foundational to AF care in this population, and a careful assessment of patient goals and falls risk is paramount; however, failure to offer anticoagulation when indicated can lead to further death and disability. Studies have failed to show an increased rate of intracranial hemorrhage due to falls in patients on anticoagulants and that the risk of stroke far outweighs bleeding risk in this population.[13] For older adults, major bleeds are more common in warfarin as compared with DOACs, and apixaban has lower rates of gastrointestinal (GI) bleeds in this population.[13]

Although a clear advantage of DOACs is their fixed dosing, the impact of extremes in body weight is unclear. For example, patients with obesity may have subtherapeutic anticoagulation and patients who are underweight may experience higher levels of drug action.[11] A systematic review found that no statistically significant differences in stroke in patients with weight over 120 kg compared with those weighing 60 to 120 kg in terms of stroke, major bleed, and other outcomes, concluding apixaban, dabigatran, and rivaroxaban were all safe and effective treatment options.[14]

COMPLICATIONS AND REVERSAL

Whether anticoagulation is achieved with a DOAC or VKA, one of the most serious complications is bleeding. Although relatively uncommon, major bleeding may occur in up 5% of patients on anticoagulation for stroke prevention.[15] However, not all bleeding events require reversal of anticoagulation. Some bleeding, included some types of major bleeding, can be managed through holding the anticoagulant, hemostatic interventions, circulatory support, and watchful waiting. Decisions about anticoagulation reversal are based on bleeding severity, the specific anticoagulant and timing of the last dose, and the patient's kidney function.

Major or life-threatening bleeding may require the use of reversal agents.[16] Major bleeding includes a rapid drop in hemoglobin of 2 g or more or bleeding into a critical area (eg, intracranial hemorrhage).[17] Other forms of severe bleeding that may warrant reversal include significant bleeding from acute trauma, bleeding that causes imminent death, and bleeding in a patient that needs a life-saving invasive procedure.[16]

Emergent warfarin reversal is typically achieved through administration of oral or intravenous vitamin K 2.5 to 10 mg and four-factor prothrombin complex concentrate (4F-PCC).[17] The reversal of the direct-thrombin inhibitor dabigatran for life-threatening bleeding is achieved with idarucizumab, a monoclonal antibody with an affinity for dabigatran, freeing thrombin from its binding.[17] Factor Xa inhibitor reversal for life-threatening bleeding includes 4F-PCC (andexanet alfa) a recombinant form of inactivated factor Xa that binds with the anticoagulant, freeing factor Xa[17] (**Table 4**). Both of

Table 4
Reversal agents

Agent	Mechanism of Action	Dose	Administration	Cautions
Vitamin K	Increases production of vitamin K-dependent clotting factors	2.5–10 mg for INR >10 or life-threatening bleeding/need for urgent invasive procedure regardless of INR	Oral administration is preferred IV infusion over 10–20 min for life-threatening bleeding or urgent invasive procedure	Anaphylactic responses with rapid IV administration Resumption of embolic risk
4 Factor-PCC	Increases vitamin K-dependent clotting factors and proteins C and S	*For VKA:* INR 2 to 2.5–22.5 to 32.5 units/kg INR 2.5 to 3–32.5 to 40 units/kg INR 3 to 3.5–40 to 47.5 units/kg INR >3.5: IV: >47.5 units/kg Maximum dose 3000 units	IV infusion at rate of 0.12 mL/min	Do not allow blood to enter syringe or tubing to prevent formation of a fibrin clot Resumption of thromboembolic risk
Andexanet alfa	Binds to factor Xa inhibitors and increases thrombin generation	Low-dose factor Xa inhibitor: 400 mg followed by 4 mg/min High-dose factor Xa inhibitor: 800 mg followed by 8 mg/min	Initial IV bolus delivered at 30 mg/min followed by IV infusion of 4–8 mg/min for up to 120 min	Inline protein binding filter required Resumption of embolic risk
Idarucizumab	Binds to dabigatran and its metabolites to diminish anticoagulant activity	2.5 mg twice	IV bolus; second dose delivered within 15 min of first	Administer immediately on preparation Resumption of thromboembolic risk

Adapted from Lexicomp, 2022.

these agents have limited shelf life and once reconstituted must be used within a pre-specified time period.

Non-life-threatening bleeding and preparation for elective invasive procedures can generally be treated without reversal.[18] Non-life-threatening bleeding is bleeding that occurs outside of critical organs and does not otherwise meet the criteria for major bleeding. Holding future doses of the anticoagulant until hemostasis is achieved is often adequate. Providing local hemostatic interventions and circulatory support through intravenous fluids or blood product transfusion can also limit the need to reverse anticoagulation.[18] It is important to remember that once anticoagulation is reversed the patient is at risk for thromboembolic events.

Patient Education

Perhaps the most important role of nurses in the safe use of oral anticoagulation is in providing practical patient education. Primary targets for patient education are rationale for treatment, dosing and administration, lifelong nature of treatment, monitoring for bleeding or embolism, medication adherence, requirements for drug monitoring (primarily for warfarin), potential drug interactions, and when to contact their primary care providers.[19] Because safety in anticoagulation is crucial, The Joint Commission includes patient education as a practice standard for organizations that administer and prescribe these therapies, including DOACs and VKAs. Specifically, patient education should be individualized to the patient and drug.[20] Similarly, the American College of Chest Physicians cite the need for additional education for patients with evidence of nonadherence (eg, persistently subtherapeutic INRs).[9]

Patient education for VKAs should include information about drug–drug and drug–food interactions. Many commonly used medications, foods, and supplements can interact to enhance or diminish VKA effectiveness or increase bleeding risk. These interactions should be reviewed at the time of prescribing warfarin; however, patient education should include recommendations to avoid starting any new medication or supplement without discussion with a provider and for patients to remind any prescriber they are on a VKA. Consistency in the intake of high vitamin K foods, such as dark green leafy vegetables, is also warranted. DOACs do not have the same drug–food interaction considerations and can be taken with or without food. However, for those prescribed dabigatran education should also include the proper storage of capsules in the original package (blister package or bottle) not in any other container (eg, pill boxes or organizers) and that the capsules should not be crushed or chewed. In addition, taking with food may reduce stomach upset.

Regardless of which anticoagulant, patients and caregivers should be taught to monitor for bleeding (eg, blood in their urine or stool; unusual bleeding or bruising) and for emboli (eg, new lower extremity edema, particularly unilaterally, neurologic changes, and signs of hypovolemia such as weakness and rapid heart rate).

CLINICS CARE POINTS

- Anticoagulation for stroke prevention is a key aspect of AF management.
- Patient selection for anticoagulation includes using evidence-based tools such as CHA_2DS_2-VASc and HAS-BLED to calculate patient-specific stroke and bleeding risk scores.
- Most nonmajor and non-life-threatening bleeding can be managed through withholding the anticoagulant, treating the cause of bleeding, and circulatory support.

- Major bleeding while on oral anticoagulation is rare and reversal agents are widely available for all types of oral anticoagulants.
- Patient education should include information on signs and symptoms of bleeding and embolism, potential for drug–drug and drug-food interactions, and monitoring requirements

SUMMARY

Strokes related to AF cause substantial morbidity and mortality in the United States. Oral anticoagulants are the mainstay of stroke prevention. Despite bleeding risks, reduction of death and disability from stroke is important considerations for patients, nurses, and all clinicians. Nurses play an essential role in prevention of bad outcomes through safe administration of anticoagulants, observing for complications, and providing individualized patient education.

DISCLOSURES

The author has no commercial or financial disclosures or conflicts of interest.

REFERENCES

1. Centers for Disease Control and Prevention. Stroke Facts. October 14, 2022. Available at: https://www.cdc.gov/stroke/facts.htm#:~:text=Every%203.5% 20minutes%2C%20someone%20dies%20of%20stroke.&text=Every%20year% 2C%20more%20than%20795%2C000,are%20first%20or%20new%20strokes. &text=About%20185%2C000%20strokes%E2%80%94nearly%201,have%20had %20a%20previous%20stroke. Accessed November 18, 2022.
2. Katsanos AH, Kamel H, Healey JS, et al. Stroke prevention in atrial fibrillation: looking forward. Circulation 2020;142(24):2371–88.
3. Jame S, Barnes G. Stroke and thromboembolism prevention in atrial fibrillation. Heart 2020;106(1):10. https://doi.org/10.1136/heartjnl-2019-314898. Available at: http://libproxy.lib.unc.edu/login?url=https://www.proquest.com/scholarly-journals/ stroke-thromboembolism-prevention-atrial/docview/2348225223/se-2.
4. Gažová A, Leddy JJ, Rexová M, et al. Predictive value of CHA2DS2-VASc scores regarding the risk of stroke and all-cause mortality in patients with atrial fibrillation (CONSORT compliant). Medicine (Baltim) 2019;98(31):e16560.
5. Steffel J, Verhamme P, Potpara TS, et al. The 2018 European Heart Rhythm Association Practical Guide on the use of non-vitamin K antagonist oral anticoagulants in patients with atrial fibrillation. Eur Heart J 2018;39(16):1330–93.
6. Methavigul K. Revised HAS-BLED score for bleeding prediction in atrial fibrillation patients with oral anticoagulants. J Arrhythm 2022;38(3):380–5.
7. Drugs for atrial fibrillation. Med Lett Drugs Ther 2019;61(1580):137–44.
8. Agnieszka K, Michał M, Zbigniew K, et al. Stroke prevention strategies in high-risk patients with atrial fibrillation. Nat Rev Cardiol 2021;18(4):276–90. Available at: http://libproxy.lib.unc.edu/login?url=https://www.proquest.com/scholarly-journals/ stroke-prevention-strategies-high-risk-patients/docview/2502556157/se-2.
9. Lip GYH, Banerjee A, Boriani G, et al. Antithrombotic therapy for atrial fibrillation: CHEST Guideline and Expert Panel Report. Chest 2018;154(5):1121–201. https:// doi.org/10.1016/j.chest.2018.07.040.
10. Patel S., Singh R., Preuss C.V., et al., Warfarin, In: StatPearls [Internet], 2022, StatPearls Publishing; Treasure Island (FL), 1-18. Available at: https://www.ncbi. nlm.nih.gov/books/NBK470313/. Accessed December 28, 2022.

11. Chen A, Stecker E, A Warden B. Direct oral anticoagulant use: a practical guide to common clinical challenges. J Am Heart Assoc 2020;9(13):e017559.
12. Aursulesei V, Costache II. Anticoagulation in chronic kidney disease: from guidelines to clinical practice. Clin Cardiol 2019;42(8):774–82.
13. Salih M, Abdel-Hafez O, Ibrahim R, et al. Atrial fibrillation in the elderly population: challenges and management considerations. J Arrhythm 2021;37(4):912–21.
14. Wiethorn EE, Bell CM, Wiggins BS. Effectiveness and safety of direct oral anticoagulants in patients with nonvalvular atrial Ffbrillation and weighing ≥ 120 kilograms versus 60–120 kilograms. Am J Cardiovasc Drugs 2021;21:545–51.
15. Milling TJ, Pollack CV. A review of guidelines on anticoagulation reversal across different clinical scenarios - is there a general consensus? Am J Emerg Med 2020;38(9):1890–903.
16. Chaudhary R, Sharma T, Garg J, et al. Direct oral anticoagulants: a review on the current role and scope of reversal agents. J Thromb Thrombolysis 2020;49: 271–86. https://doi-org.libproxy.lib.unc.edu/10.1007/s11239-019-01954-2.
17. Milling TJ, Zeibell CM. A review of oral anticoagulants, old and new, in major bleeding and the need for urgent surgery. Trends Cardiovasc Med 2020;30(2): 86–90.
18. Mujer MTP, Rai MP, Atti V, et al. An update on the reversal of non-vitamin K antagonist oral anticoagulants. Adv Hematol 2020;2020:7636104.
19. Hawes EM. Patient education on oral anticoagulation. Pharmacy 2018;6(2):34.
20. Morris L. Life support comes in various forms: Anticoagulation therapy in the ambulatory care setting. AAACN Viewpoint 2022;44(3):1–11. Available at: https://search-ebscohost-com.libproxy.lib.unc.edu/login.aspx?direct=true&db=rzh&AN=1574 69750&site=ehost-live&scope=site. Accessed December 30, 2022.

A Pharmacologic Update
New Treatments for Patients with Cardiovascular Disease

Elizabeth Radchik, PharmD[a], Leslie L. Davis, PhD, NP-BC[b],
Ciantel A. Blyler, PharmD[a],*

KEYWORDS

- Cardiovascular disease • Pharmacotherapy • Hypertrophic cardiomyopathy
- Heart failure • Familial hypercholesterolemia

KEY POINTS

- Pharmacologic therapies are a key part of the medical armamentarium aimed at reducing the significant morbidity and mortality caused by cardiovascular disease (CVD).
- The landscape of CVD treatment is ever evolving with the development of new medication classes and the repurposing of existing medications for new indications.
- Mavacamten is a first-in-class cardiac myosin inhibitor, approved by the FDA in April 2022, for the treatment of obstructive hypertrophic cardiomyopathy.
- Inclisiran is a first-in-class antilipemic small interfering ribonucleic acid agent approved by the FDA in December 2021 for the treatment of familial hypercholesterolemia.
- Dapagliflozin and empagliflozin are sodium-glucose co-transporter-2 inhibitors initially approved by the FDA for the treatment of type 2 diabetes. More recently, the FDA has approved expanded indications for both medications to reduce the risk of cardiovascular death and hospitalization in heart failure patients.

INTRODUCTION

Cardiovascular disease (CVD) remains the leading cause of death in both the United States (US) and worldwide.[1] Nearly half of adults aged > 20 years in the US have one or more types of CVD[1] and the prevalence increases with age. Although lifestyle and surgical interventions play important roles in the management of CVD, pharmacologic treatment is the cornerstone of therapy for most patients. Here, the authors provide an update on pharmacologic therapies for three types of CVD—hypertrophic cardiomyopathy (HCM), familial hypercholesterolemia (FH), and heart failure (HF).

---

[a] Smidt Heart Institute at Cedars-Sinai Medical Center, 127 S. San Vicente Boulevard, Suite A3600, Los Angeles, CA 90048, USA; [b] University of North Carolina at Chapel Hill, School of Nursing, 4007 Carrington Hall, CB # 7460, Chapel Hill, NC 27599-7460, USA
* Corresponding author.
E-mail address: Ciantel.Blyler@cshs.org

Nurs Clin N Am 58 (2023) 389–403
https://doi.org/10.1016/j.cnur.2023.05.006
0029-6465/23/© 2023 Elsevier Inc. All rights reserved.

The authors review clinical indications, pharmacology, practical considerations for the safe and appropriate use of these medications, and implications for nurses.

HYPERTROPHIC CARDIOMYOPATHY

HCM is one of the most common forms of inherited CVD, affecting at least one in 500 individuals.[2,3] The disease rarely presents before the third decade of life, but may occur at any age. HCM is defined by nondilated left ventricular (LV) hypertrophy (LVH) in the absence of other cardiac or systemic causes of LVH.[4] Clinically in adults, an LV wall thickness of greater than 15 mm by echocardiography or by cardiac MRI indicates HCM.[4] For children, HCM is defined as increased LV wall thickness ≥2 standard deviations from the mean for that age or body mass index.[4]

HCM is an autosomal dominant genetic condition, caused by pathogenic variants in at least one of the genes which encode proteins of the cardiac sarcomere. To date, over 1500 individual pathogenic variants have been implicated making HCM both genetically and clinically diverse in its presentation.[5] The mechanism by which different pathogenic variants cause specific clinical phenotypes is not fully understood. It is hypothesized that HCM mutations cause cardiac hypercontractility and activation of signaling pathways that cause both hypertrophy of the heart and fibrosis[6] consequentially leading to a small, stiff ventricle with impaired systolic and diastolic function despite normal LV ejection fraction (LVEF). In two-thirds of patients, this hypertrophy causes a narrowing of the LV outflow tract (LVOT) and obstruction of blood outflow from the LV into the ascending aorta. The narrowing or obstruction of the outflow tract leads to the development of a systolic pressure gradient that further limits ejection from the LV. The LVOT gradient is quantified in millimeters of mercury and is an important predictor of prognosis.[4,7]

For most patients, HCM has a benign disease course with a normal life expectancy. However, those with more severe obstructive disease or diastolic dysfunction, symptoms can be quite limiting and include fatigue, dyspnea, angina, palpitations, and syncope. For a small subset of patients, the development of life-threatening symptoms such as progressive HF, atrial fibrillation with thromboembolism, and sudden cardiac death can occur.[8]

Conventional Approach to Hypertrophic Cardiomyopathy Treatment

Traditionally, pharmacologic treatment of HCM has focused on providing symptom relief.[4] Non-vasodilating beta-blockers, such as metoprolol and propranolol, have been the cornerstone of therapy and were the first medications studied, albeit in small or non-randomized trials, for the treatment of outflow tract obstruction. Non-vasodilating beta-blockers are also effective at relieving ischemic chest discomfort and obstruction-related dyspnea.[4,7] Non-dihydropyridine calcium channel blockers, such as diltiazem and verapamil, are effective alternatives for patients unable to tolerate beta-blockers.[4,7] Disopyramide, a negative inotrope, can further improve symptoms associated with LVOT obstruction when paired with a beta-blocker or non-dihydropyridine calcium channel blocker.[4,7] Diuretics may also be beneficial for patients with HCM, especially those with nonobstructive HCM, with pulmonary edema or in frank HF though minimum effective doses should be used and great care taken to avoid hypovolemia, hypotension, and exacerbation of LVOT obstruction.[4] Ultimately, although these therapies provide a measure of symptomatic relief, they do not directly address underlying disease mechanisms or modify its natural course; necessitating the development of new medicines that directly target HCM disease pathophysiology.

A New Frontier in Hypertrophic Cardiomyopathy Treatment

Mavacamten (Camzyos) is a first-in-class cardiac myosin inhibitor, indicated for adults with symptomatic (New York Heart Association [NYHA] class II to III) obstructive HCM to improve functional capacity and symptoms.[9] A reversible inhibitor selective for cardiac myosin, mavacamten attenuates formation of actin-myosin cross-bridges within the cardiac sarcomere during both systole and diastole. Reducing cardiac contractility and LVOT obstruction, promoting a relaxed energy sparing state and improving cardiac filling pressures.[9]

In early studies, mavacamten improved LV filling and showed promise in reducing LVOT gradients.[10,11] Phase II studies[12] affirmed these results and paved the way for the phase III EXPLORER-HCM study, which enrolled 251 adults aged 18 years or older with obstructive HCM and an LVEF of at least 55% and randomly assigned them to receive either mavacamten or placebo.[13] The primary endpoint was a 1.5 mL/kg/min or greater increase in peak O_2 consumption (a marker of cardiovascular fitness) and improvement of NYHA classification (one category reduction or more), or a 3.0 mL/kg/min or greater improvement in peak O_2 consumption without NYHA class worsening.[13] At 30 weeks, 37% of patients randomized to mavacamten achieved the primary endpoint compared with 17% of patients in the control group ($P = 0.0005$). Mavacamten treatment also led to improvements in both resting and postexercise LVOT gradients when compared with placebo.[13] In an extension phase of the study (median follow-up of 62 weeks), mavacamten showed sustained improvements in functional capacity, LVOT gradients and NYHA classification. Importantly, no significant long-term treatment-related adverse effects were observed.[14]

Mavacamten was subsequently approved by the US Food & Drug Administration (FDA) in April 2022 (**Table 1**).[9] The orally administered medication is currently available through a restricted program under a Risk Evaluation and Mitigation Strategy (REMS) due to its tendency to reduce LVEF potentially causing systolic HF. This requires that prescribers enroll in the REMS program, review complete prescribing information, and successfully complete a knowledge assessment to become eligible to prescribe. Of note, nurses can act as a "physician designee" — performing REMS activities such as counseling patients on the risk of HF, the need for regular cardiac monitoring during treatment, the risk of drug–drug interactions, and the need to inform their health care providers of all the prescription and nonprescription medications they take. Patients must also enroll into the REMS program and comply with monitoring requirements.

Initiation of mavacamten at the recommended dose of 5 mg once daily by mouth (PO) should only be undertaken in patients with LVEF $\geq$55%.[9] Medication titration by the prescriber is guided by the reassessment of echocardiogram at 4, 8, and 12 weeks, then every 3 months with special attention given to LVEF and LVOT gradients (**Fig. 1**). Therapy is discontinued if at any point the LVEF falls below 50% or if the patient experiences HF symptoms or worsening clinical status.[9]

Mavacamten is extensively metabolized in the liver, primarily through cytochrome P450 (CYP) 2C19 (74%), CYP3A4 (18%), and CYP2C9 (8%) making clinically relevant drug–drug interactions commonplace. As a result, concomitant use of moderate to strong CYP2C19 inhibitors/inducers and moderate to strong CYP3A4 inhibitors/inducers are contraindicated.[9] No dosage adjustments are required for either kidney or hepatic impairment.

Mavacamten is relatively well-tolerated with dizziness (27%) and syncope (6%) being the only adverse effects reported more frequently than in placebo-treated patients.[12,13] Decreased LVEF, which occurs in about 6% of patients, is dose-related with an intermediate onset of ~4 weeks post-initiation.[9,15] Risk factors that increase

Table 1
Cardiac myosin inhibitors for treatment of hypertrophic cardiomyopathy

Drug	Route	FDA-Labeled Indications	How Supplied	Time to Peak	Half-Life Elimination	Clinical Pearls
Mavacamten (Camzyos)	PO	Hypertrophic cardiomyopathy with left ventricular outflow tract obstruction	2.5 mg 5 mg* 10 mg 15 mg	1 h; however, T_{max} increases to 4 h when taken with high-fat meal	Normal CYP2C19 metabolizers: 6 to 9 d Poor CYP2C19 metabolizers: 23 d Of note, steady state expected ~6 wk	Swallow capsule whole with or without food No dose adjustments for kidney/liver impairment Contraindicated with moderate to strong CYP2C19 and CYP3A4 inhibitors/inducers May interfere with hormonal contraception; use back-up method REMS program

* Recommended starting dose.
Source: Camzyos (mavacamten) [prescribing information]. Brisbane, CA: MyoKardia Inc; May 2022.

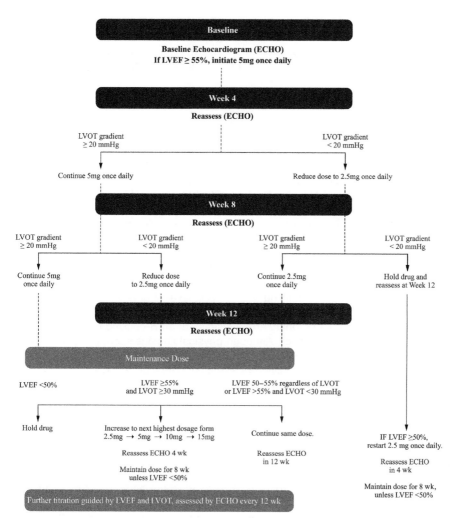

Fig. 1. Mavacamten dose titration algorithm. LVEF, left ventricular ejection fraction; LVOT, left ventricular outflow tract. (*Adapted from*: Camzyos (mavacamten) [package insert]. Brisbane, CA: MyoKardia Inc; May 2022.)

probability of decreased LVEF include concomitant use of CYP450 inhibitors, concomitant illness, uncontrolled tachyarrthymias, and concomitant use of disopyramide with either verapamil or diltiazem.[13,15]

As the first available therapy to directly target the underlying pathophysiology of HCM, mavacamten represents a significant advancement in the management of this condition. The medication is also being evaluated as a treatment option for patients with nonobstructive HCM and high symptom burden, with the proof-of-concept MAVERICK-HCM study[15] paving the way for larger trials currently underway. The FDA has also accepted a supplemental drug application for an expanded indication to reduce the need for septal reduction therapies in patients with obstructive HCM and NYHA class IV symptoms based on the VALOR-HCM studies.[16]

Despite its successes, the limitations of mavacamten (long half-life and drug-drug interactions) have led to the development of aficamten, a novel second-generation cardiac myosin inhibitor.[17] Phase II studies (REDWOOD-HCM) have already shown aficamten to be effective in reducing LVOT gradients and relieving HF symptoms in those with obstructive disease.[18] FDA-approval will likely hinge of the results of the phase III SEQUOIA-HCM trial, which is currently enrolling patients.[18]

FAMILIAL HYPERCHOLESTEROLEMIA

FH is a commonly inherited disorder of impaired lipid metabolism affecting one in 250 people in the United States[19] and one in 200 worldwide.[20] FH is characterized by markedly elevated blood levels of low-density lipoprotein (LDL) cholesterol and premature development of coronary heart disease. FH is an autosomal dominant genetic condition, caused by at least one pathogenic mutation in the LDL-R, apolipoprotein B (ApoB), or proprotein convertase subtilisin/kexin type 9 (PCSK9) genes, which mediate LDL clearance from the circulation.[21,22] Inheritance of two pathogenic variants (homozygotes), as opposed to just one (heterozygotes), confers more severe disease, though this is significantly less common with a prevalence of approximately one in 200,000 to 300,000.[22]

Several diagnostic systems are available to diagnose FH,[23–25] but their clinical criteria vary and there is little consensus on superiority. In 2015, the American Heart Association (AHA) proposed simplified criterion to diagnose heterozygous FH in the absence of genetic testing; defining it as an LDL level of greater than 190 mg/dL in adults or greater than 160 mg/dL in children, with a similarly affected first-degree relative with either premature coronary artery disease or a FH-causing mutation.[26,27]

FH is largely a "silent disease." Although physical findings such as xanthelasmas, tendon xanthomas, and corneal arcus may be present and aid the diagnosis of FH.[21] Left untreated affected individuals experience fatal or nonfatal cardiac events at a rate of 50% in men and 30% of women by the ages of 50 and 60 years, respectively,[22] making early detection and treatment very important.

Conventional Approach to Familial Hypercholesterolemia Treatment

As both the duration and degree of LDL elevation are the primary determinants of poor cardiovascular (CV) outcomes, treatment largely focuses on prompt LDL lowering to improve prognosis. Guidelines support LDL targets of less than 100 mg/dL (<2.6 mmol/L) for adults with FH (or at least 50% reduction), and an even more aggressive goal of less than 70 mg/dL (<1.8 mmol/L) for those with atherosclerotic CVD or diabetes.[28] In children greater than 10 years of age, an LDL target of less than 135 mg/dL (<3.5 mmol/L) is recommended.[28]

Although dietary and lifestyle modifications (ie, smoking cessation) play an essential role in FH management, multidrug treatment is often necessary to achieve LDL targets in most patients.[21] Statins have long been the cornerstone of therapy and are considered first line for all patients with FH. High-dose, high-intensity statins, such as rosuvastatin and atorvastatin, are capable of lowering LDL by 50% to 60% and should be prescribed. If not tolerated, moderate-intensity statin therapy should be substituted.[21,28] For those unable to reach LDL goals on statin therapy alone, ezetimibe, which inhibits cholesterol absorptions from the intestine, is a well-tolerated second-line therapy.[28] Niacin and bile acid sequestrants were previously used as third-line adjuncts but have been replaced with PCSK9 inhibitors (evolocomab and alirocumab) as a more effective option for additional LDL reduction. However, PCSK9 inhibition use is often limited by high cost.[21,28]

A New Option for Treatment of Familial Hypercholesterolemia

Inclisiran (Leqvio), a first-in-class antilipemic synthetic small interfering ribonucleic acid, presents yet another option. Indicated for the treatment of heterozygous FH in adults, inclisiran selectively targets PCSK9 mRNA for breakdown resulting decreased PCSK9 levels, increased LDL receptor recycling and expression on the surface of hepatocytes leading to increased LDL uptake, and decreased LDL in circulation.[29]

Early clinical studies of inclisiran revealed sustained reduction in LDL cholesterol levels following a single dose.[30] These results were confirmed in phase II studies where patients saw dose-dependent decreases in LDL and PCSK9 levels, with multiple doses providing the most profound reductions.[31] Larger phase III trials (ORION10 and ORION11) enrolled 1561 and 1617 patients, respectively, to assess the safety and efficacy of inclisiran in patients with suboptimal LDL cholesterol levels despite maximally tolerated doses of statins plus or minus conventional add-on therapy.[32] Patients were randomly assigned to either inclisiran (dosed on day 1, day 90, and every 6 months thereafter) or placebo and followed for an 18-month period. The primary endpoint was the percentage change in LDL from baseline. At day 510, inclisiran decreased LDL cholesterol levels by 52.3% in the ORION10 trial and by 49.9% in the ORION11 trial ($P < 0.001$). Inclisiran also lowered triglyceride and lipoprotein A levels while increasing high-density lipoprotein (HDL) levels—all indicators of improved prognosis and reduced CVD risk. Importantly, no significant adverse events were observed in either trial.[32]

Inclisiran was subsequently approved by the FDA in December 2021 (**Table 2**).[29] The subcutaneous (SUBQ) injection, intended for use in combination with a statin or a statin plus add-on therapy, is initially administered as a single 284 mg injection and then re-dosed at 3 months and every 6 months thereafter.[29,32] No dosage adjustments are required for kidney or liver impairment. Monitoring parameters include a lipid profile at baseline and a fasting lipid profile 4 to 12 weeks after initiation and every 3 to 12 months thereafter.[28,29] There are no significant drug–drug interactions, and adverse reactions are largely categorized as injection site in nature (erythema, pain, rash at injection site; 8% of patients), although arthralgia (5%) and bronchitis (4%) have also been reported.[29]

Like PCSK9 inhibitors, the approval of inclisiran represents an important advancement in lipid management, filling a therapeutic niche for high-risk patients who are unable to achieve desired LDL levels with conventional oral treatments. Inclisiran's convenient, infrequent dosing scheme and lack of appreciable side effects have important implications for patient adherence and outcomes[32]; especially given the high discontinuation rates of statins.[33] Improved adherence might be realized if injections could be administered by a member of the health care team, including nurses.

HEART FAILURE

HF is anticipated to affect approximately 8 million Americans by the year 2030.[34] HF is defined as a structural disorder within the heart that impairs the function of ventricular filling or ejection of blood. HF classification is primarily dependent on LVEF, expressed as a percentage of the amount of oxygenated blood that is pumped out of the heart with each contraction.[34,35] The American College of Cardiology Foundation/AHA/Heart Failure Society of America guidelines define HF with reduced ejection fraction (HFrEF) as LVEF of ≤40% and HF with preserved ejection fraction (HFpEF) as LVEF of greater than 50%.[34] More recently, HF with LVEF of 41% to 49% is classified as HF with mildly reduced EF (HFmrEF).[34] An important predictor of prognosis, LVEF guides pharmacologic management for improving survival. Landmark clinical trials in HF have primarily been conducted in patients with HFrEF producing guideline-directed medical therapy (GDMT). However, more recent studies have provided evidence for specific pharmacologic treatments in patients with HFpEF.

Table 2
Small interfering ribonucleic acid for treatment of familial hypercholesterolemia

Drug	Route	FDA-Labeled Indications	How Supplied	Time to Peak	Half-Life Elimination	Clinical Pearls
Inclisiran (Leqvio)	SUBQ	Heterozygous familial hypercholesterolemia Secondary prevention of CVD events	284 mg/1.5 mL prefilled syringe*	~4 h	~9 h	Avoid areas of active skin disease or injury No dose adjustments for those with kidney/liver impairment Avoid in pregnancy No significant drug-drug interactions Monitor fasting lipid profile 4–12 weeks after initiation, and every 3–12 months thereafter

* Recommended starting dose.

Source: Leqvio (inclisiran) [prescribing information]. East Hanover, NJ: Novartis Pharmaceuticals Corporation; December 2021.

Conventional Approach to Treatment of Heart Failure with Reduced Ejection Fraction

GDMT for patients with HFrEF aims to attenuate the body's evolved compensatory responses that result from inadequate cardiac output. Neurohumoral mechanisms such as increased activation in the sympathetic nervous system and renin angiotensin aldosterone system (RAAS) and alterations in other vasomodulating peptide hormones all work to increase cardiac output. These responses prevent acute CV complications and temporarily balance the circulatory system to maintain homeostasis. However, overtime, these compensatory mechanisms lead to cardiac remodeling and ultimately disease progression.[36,37]

Each pharmacologic pillar of GDMT possesses benefits to increase survival and prevent HF exacerbations that lead to hospitalization and death. Evidence-based therapies that provide clinical benefits in HFrEF include RAAS inhibitors with or without a neprilysin inhibitor, beta-blockers, mineralocorticoid receptor antagonists (MRA), and more recently, sodium-glucose cotransporter-2 (SGLT2) inhibitors. The initiation of quadruple therapy reduces CV death or HF hospitalization by up to 62% and adds an estimated 1.4 to 6.3 additional years of life.[36]

RAAS inhibitors, such as angiotensin-converting enzyme inhibitors (ACEI) and angiotensin II receptor blockers (ARBs), prevent RAAS-mediated vasoconstriction resulting in increased pressure on the heart to eject blood from the ventricle as well as the release of aldosterone which induces cardiac fibrosis and remodeling.[37] The angiotensin receptor-neprilysin inhibitor (ARNI) valsartan/sacubitril (Entresto) has both RAAS inhibitor properties and helps increase free vasodilatory peptides by preventing the breakdown of neprilysin which naturally inactivates them.[37] In PARADIGM-HF, the use of valsartan/sacubitril as compared with enalapril, an ACEI, resulted in a 20% reduction of CV death, HF exacerbation leading to hospitalization, and sudden cardiac death.[38] Based on these results, current treatment guidelines recommend that prescribers initiate ARNIs (or switch patients from an ACE or ARB to an ARNI) in patients with symptomatic HFrEF.[37]

Guidelines support the use of only three beta-blockers (ie, metoprolol succinate, bisoprolol, and carvedilol) to reduce morbidity and mortality in patients with HFrEF.[39] Selective beta-blockers, metoprolol succinate, and bisoprolol, target beta-1 adrenergic receptors located on the heart, which is provoked by the sympathetic nervous system in response to decreased cardiac output. Preventing further loss of heart contractility in HFrEF is essential to suppress ventricular remodeling and essentially slow down disease progression. Carvedilol exhibits beta-1, beta-2, and alpha-1 blocking activity, resulting in vasodilation and lowered blood pressure.[39]

MRAs such as spironolactone and eplerenone reduce morbidity and mortality in patients with HFrEF.[37] Aldosterone is a naturally occurring hormone that is upregulated during the activation of the RAAS system in response to decreased cardiac output. Upregulated aldosterone is responsible for the formation of cardiac fibrosis and remodeling, leading to structural dysfunction and complications, such as atrial fibrillation.[37] MRA therapy is believed to prevent and reverse the structural damage caused by HFrEF and the cardiovascular sequelae that follow.[40]

A Repurposed Treatment Option for Heart Failure with Reduced Ejection Fraction and Heart Failure with Preserved Ejection Fraction

SGLT2 inhibitors, dapagliflozin (Farxiga) and empagliflozin (Jardiance), are the latest addition to GDMT for HFrEF. Initially developed as glucose-lowering agents for the treatment of type 2 diabetes, multiple studies revealed a cardiovascular benefit,

Table 3
Sodium glucose co-transport 2 inhibitors for treatment of heart failure

Drug	Route	FDA-Labeled Indications	How Supplied	Time to Peak	Half-Life Elimination	Clinical Pearls
Empagliflozin (Jardiance)	PO	Reduce risk of CV death and HF-related hospitalization in adults with HF	10 mg* 25 mg	1.5 h	~12.4 h	Administer in morning with or without food
						Contraindicated in dialysis
						Avoid in pregnancy
Dapagliflozin (Farxiga)	PO	Reduce risk of CV death and HF-related hospitalization in adults with HFrEF	5 mg 10 mg*	2 h	~12.9 h	Monitor for genital mycotic infections and urinary tract infections
						Assess volume depletion before and during therapy

* Recommended starting dose.
Source(s): Jardiance (empagliflozin) [prescribing information]. Ridgefield, CT: Boehringer Ingelheim Pharmaceuticals Inc; August 2021. Farxiga (dapagliflozin) [prescribing information]. Wilmington, DE: AstraZeneca Pharmaceuticals LP; July 2022.

including reduced HF hospitalizations, in patients with type 2 diabetes and established CVD or at high risk for CVD.[41,42]

As a result, two large phase III trials, DAPA-HF and EMPEROR-Reduced, were undertaken to assess the efficacy of dapagliflozin and empagliflozin, respectively, on outcomes for patients with an LVEF ≤40% and NYHA class II–IV HF on GDMT. At a median follow-up of 16 to 18 months, both studies showed a 25% reduction in the composite of CV death or HF exacerbations leading to hospitalization when compared with placebo.[43,44] A meta-analysis of both studies showed that SGLT2 inhibitor therapy significantly reduced all-cause mortality when compared with placebo.[45] These results led to the FDA-approval of expanded indications for both dapagliflozin (May 2020) and empagliflozin (August 2021) to reduce the risk of CV death and HF-related hospitalization in adults with HFrEF (**Table 3**).[46,47] In 2022, the FDA amended empagliflozin's approval to include adults with HFpEF and HFmrEF.[47,48] This change was based on the results of the phase III EMPEROR-Preserved trial, which enrolled patients with an LVEF greater than 40% and NYHA class II–IV HF on GDMT. Over a median follow-up of ~26 months, empagliflozin showed a 29% reduction in risk of HF hospitalization, though no benefit was observed in all-cause mortality.[48] The new indication for empagliflozin represents a positive step forward for patients with HFpEF, which has few treatment options.

The mechanisms by which SGLT2 inhibitors aid in HF are yet to be fully understood. A combination of metabolic (ie, natriuresis and increased insulin sensitivity), hemodynamic (ie, osmotic diuresis and plasma/interstitial volume reduction), and organ-specific effects (ie, reduction in LV mass) are thought to contribute to the positive effects observed in trials.[49]

SGLT2 inhibitors are orally administered and prescribed at a starting dose of 10 mg once daily for patients with HF (with or without diabetes type 2).[46,47] Neither dapagliflozin nor empagliflozin has been studied in patients with an estimated glomerular filtration rate (eGFR) <25 mL/min/1.73 m^2 and eGFR <20 mL/min/1.73 m^2, respectively. Thus, caution is recommended when initiating or continuing therapy in patients with chronic kidney disease and contraindicated in those receiving dialysis.[46,47,50] No dosage adjustments are required for liver impairment. However, blood glucose, kidney function, and volume status should be monitored. Serious side effects include acute kidney injury, recurrent urinary tract infections (8%–9%), and genitourinary fungal infections (2%–6%), which could warrant discontinuation of therapy.[46,47] SGLT2 inhibitors such as canagliflozin and ertugliflozin have not yet been FDA-approved, thus should not be prescribed for HF.[34]

SUMMARY

The development of new pharmacologic agents is essential to reduce the significant morbidity and mortality associated with CVD. As the landscape of treatment continues to evolve, it is critical that nurses understand the basic pharmacology, potential adverse effects, and special considerations associated with new pharmacologic agents to provide appropriate patient education, ensure safe monitoring of patients, and ultimately improve patient outcomes.

CLINICS CARE POINTS

- Nurses should educate patients who are prescribed mavacamten to report side effects such as dizziness, syncope, or worsening heart failure symptoms that may be associated with this medication.

- One strategy to increase adherence for lipid lowering medications such as inclisiran that are dosed infrequently is to have nurses or other clinicians administer the subcutaneous injection during a clinical encounter.
- Patients with chronic heart failure who are taking SGLT2 inhibitors (such as dapagliflozin or empagliflozin) should be monitored for signs/symptoms of over-diuresis, worsening kidney function, and urinary tract or genitourinary fungal infections.
- The FDA has recently expanded indications for valsartan/sacubitril, spironolactone, and dapagliflozin to include individuals with heart failure with preserved ejection fraction (EF) greater than 40%.

DISCLOSURE

The authors have no relevant disclosures.

REFERENCES

1. Tsao CW, Aday AW, Almarzooq ZI, et al. Heart disease and stroke statistics – 2023 update: a report from the American heart association. Circulation 2023;147:e00.
2. Maron BJ, Gardin JM, Flack JM, et al. Prevalence of hypertrophic cardiomyopathy in a general population of young adults. Echocardiographic analysis of 4111 subjects in the CARDIA Study (Coronary Artery Risk Development in [young] adults. Circulation 1995;92(4):785–9.
3. Semsarian C, Ingles J, Maron MS, et al. New perspectives on the prevalence of hypertrophic cardiomyopathy. J Am Coll Cardiol 2015;65(12):1249–54.
4. Ommen SR, Mital S, Burke MA, et al. 2020 AHA/ACC Guideline for the diagnosis and treatment of patients with hypertrophic cardiomyopathy: a report of the American college of cardiology/American heart association joint committee on clinical practice guidelines. Circulation 2020;142(25):e558–631.
5. Maron BJ, Maron MS, Semsarian C. Genetics of hypertrophic cardiomyopathy after 20 years: clinical perspectives. J Am Coll Cardiol 2012;60(8):705–15.
6. Spudich JA. Three perspectives on the molecular basis of hypercontractility caused by hypertrophic cardiomyopathy mutations. Pfluegers Arch 2019;471(5):701–17.
7. Elliott PM, Anastasakis A, Borger MA, et al. 2014 ESC Guidelines on diagnosis and management of hypertrophic cardiomyopathy: the task force for the diagnosis and management of hypertrophic cardiomyopathy of the European Society of Cardiology (ESC). European Society of Cardiology (ESC) 2014;35(39):2733–79.
8. Maron BJ. Clinical course and management of hypertrophic cardiomyopathy. N Engl J Med 2018;379(7):655–68.
9. Camzyos (mavacamten) [prescribing information]. Brisbane, CA: MyoKardia Inc; 2022.
10. Green EM, Wakimoto H, Anderson RL, et al. A small-molecule inhibitor of sarcomere contractility suppresses hypertrophic cardiomyopathy in mice. Science 2016;351(6273):617–21.
11. Del Rio CL, Ueyama Y, Baker DC, et al. In vivo cardiac effects of mavacamten (MYK-461): evidence for negative inotropy and improved compliance. Circulation 2018;136(suppl 1). Article 20593 (abstr).
12. Heitner SB, Jacoby D, Lester SJ, et al. Mavacamten treatment for obstructive hypertrophic cardiomyopathy: a clinical trial. Ann Intern Med 2019;170(11):741–8.
13. Olivotto I, Oreziak A, Barriales-Villa R, et al. EXPLORER-HCM study investigators. Mavacamten for treatment of symptomatic obstructive hypertrophic

cardiomyopathy (EXPLORER-HCM): a randomised, double-blind, placebo-controlled, phase 3 trial. Lancet 2020;396(10253):759–69.

14. Rader F. Mavacamten for treatment of symptomatic obstructive hypertrophic cardiomyopathy – EXPLORER-HCM. Presented at the American College of Cardiology Annual Scientific Session; April 3, 2022; Washington DC. Available at: https://www.acc.org/latest-in-cardiology/clinical-trials/2020/08/28/16/14/explorer-hcm. Accessed October 15, 2022.

15. Ho CY, Mealiffe ME, Bach RG, et al. Evaluation of mavacamten in symptomatic patients with nonobstructive hypertrophic cardiomyopathy. J Am Coll Cardiol 2020;75(21):2649–60.

16. Desai MY, Owens AT, Geske JB, et al. Dose-blinded myosin inhibition in patients with obstructive HCM referred for septal reduction therapy: Outcomes through 32-weeks. Circulation 2022. https://doi.org/10.1161/CIRCULATIONAHA.122.062534. Online ahead of print.

17. Chuang C, Collibee S, Ashcraft L, et al. Discovery of aficamten (CK-274), a next-generation cardiac myosin inhibitor for the treatment of hypertrophic cardiomyopathy. J Med Chem 2021;64(19):14142–52.

18. Elliott P. Aficamten: A cardiac myosin inhibitor for obstructive hypertrophic cardiomyopathy. EMJ Cardiol 2022;10(Suppl 1):2–5.

19. de Ferranti SD, Rodday AM, Mendelson MM, et al. Prevalence of familial hypercholesterolemia in the 1999 to 2012 United States National Health and Nutrition Examination Surveys (NHANES). Circulation 2016;133:1067–72.

20. Beheshti SO, Madsen CM, Varbo A, et al. Worldwide prevalence of familial hypercholesterolemia: Meta-analyses of 11 million subjects. J Am Coll Cardiol 2020;75:2553–66.

21. McGowan MP, Dehkordi SHH, Moriarty PM, et al. Diagnosis and treatment of heterozygous familial hypercholesterolemia. J Am Heart Assoc 2019;8(24):e013225.

22. Sturm AC, Knowles JW, Gidding SS, et al. Clinical genetic testing for familial hypercholesterolemia: JACC scientific expert panel. J Am Coll Cardiol 2018;72(6):662–80.

23. Williams RR, Hunt SC, Schumacher MC, et al. Diagnosing heterozygous familial hypercholesterolemia using new practice criteria validated by molecular genetics. Am J Cardiol 1993;72(2):171–6.

24. Risk of fatal coronary heart disease in familial hypercholesterolemia. Scientific Steering Committee on behalf of the Simon Broome Register Group. BMJ 1991;303(6807):893–6.

25. Austin MA, Hutter CM, Zimmern RL, et al. Genetic causes of monogenic heterozygous familial hypercholesterolemia: a huge prevalence review. Am J Epidemiol 2004;160:407–20.

26. Gidding SS, Champagne MA, de Ferranti SD, et al. American Heart Association Atherosclerosis, Hypertension, and Obesity in Young Committee of Council on Cardiovascular Disease in Young, Council on Cardiovascular and Stroke Nursing, Council on Functional Genomics and Translational Biology, and Council on Lifestyle and Cardiometabolic Health. The agenda for familial hypercholesterolemia: a scientific statement from the American Heart Association. Circulation 2015;132(22):2167–92.

27. Lui DTW, Lee ACH, Tan KCB. Management of familial hypercholesterolemia: current status and future perspectives. J Endocr Soc 2020;5(1):bvaa122.

28. Grundy SM, Stone NJ, Bailey AL, et al. 2018 AHA/ACC/AACVPR/AAPA/ABC/ACPM/ADA/AGS/APhA/ASPC/NLA/PCNA Guideline on the management of blood cholesterol: executive summary: a report of the American College of Cardiology/

American Heart Association task force on clinical practice guidelines. J Am Coll Cardiol 2019;73(24):3168–209.

29. Leqvio (inclisiran) [prescribing inf. East Hanover, NJ: Novartis Pharmaceuticals Corporation; 2021. ormation].

30. Fitzgerald K, White S, Borodovsky A, et al. A highly durable RNAi therapeutic inhibitor of PCSK9. N Engl J Med 2017;376(1):41–51.

31. Ray KK, Landmesser U, Leiter LA, et al. Inclisiran in patients at high cardiovascular risk with elevated LDL cholesterol. N Engl J Med 2017;376(15):1430–40.

32. Ray KK, Wright RS, Kallend D, et al. Two phase 3 trials of inclisiran in patients with elevated LDL cholesterol. N Engl J Med 2020;382(16):1507–19.

33. Avorn J, Monette J, Lacour A, et al. Persistence of use of lipid-lowering medications - a cross national study. JAMA 1998;279(18):1458–62.

34. Heidenreich PA, Bozkurt B, Aguilar D, et al. 2022 ACC/AHA/HFSA guidelines for management of heart failure. Circulation 2022;145:e894–1032.

35. Bozkurt B, Coats AJS, Tsutsui H, et al. Universal definition and classification of heart failure: a report of the heart failure society of America, heart failure association of the European society of cardiology, Japanese heart failure society and writing committee of the universal definition of heart failure. J Card Fail 2021; 27:387–413.

36. Vaduganathan M, Claggett BL, Jhund PS, et al. Estimating lifetime benefits of comprehensive disease-modifying pharmacological therapies in patients with heart failure with reduced ejection fraction: a comparative analysis of three randomised controlled trials. Lancet 2020;396:121–8.

37. Maddox TM, Januzzi JL Jr, Allen LA, et al. 2021 Update to the 2017 ACC expert consensus decision pathway for optimization of heart failure treatment: answers to 10 pivotal issues about heart failure with reduced ejection fraction. J Am Coll Cardiol 2021;77(6):772–810.

38. McMurray JJ, Packer M, Desai AS, et al. Angiotensin-neprilysin inhibition versus enalapril in heart failure. N Engl J Med 2014;371:993–1004.

39. Cleland JGF, Bunting KV, Flather MD, et al. Beta-blockers for heart failure with reduced, mid-range, and preserved ejection fraction: an individual patient-level analysis of double-blind randomized trials. Eur Heart J 2018;39:26–35.

40. Aldactone (spironolactone) [prescribing information]. New York, NY: Pfizer Inc; 2021.

41. Wiviott SD, Raz I, Bonaca MP, et al. Dapagliflozin and cardiovascular outcomes in type 2 diabetes. N Engl J Med 2019;380:347–57.

42. Zinman B, Wanner C, Lachin JM, et al. Empagliflozin, cardiovascular outcomes, and mortality in type 2 diabetes. N Engl J Med 2015;373:2117–28.

43. McMurray JJV, Solomon SD, Inzucchi SE, et al. Dapagliflozin in patients with heart failure and reduced ejection fraction. N Engl J Med 2019;381:1995–2008.

44. Packer M, Anker SD, Butler J, et al. Cardiovascular and renal outcomes with empagliflozin in heart failure. N Engl J Med 2020;383:1413–24.

45. Zannad F, Ferreira JP, Pocock SJ, et al. SGLT2 inhibitors in patients with heart failure with reduced ejection fraction: a meta-analysis of the EMPEROR-Reduced and DAPA-HF trials. Lancet 2020;396:819–29.

46. Farxiga (dapagliflozin) [prescribing information]. Wilmington, DE: AstraZeneca Pharmaceuticals LP; 2023.

47. Jardiance (empagliflozin) [prescribing information]. Ridgefield, CT: Boehringer Ingelheim Pharmaceuticals Inc; 2021.

48. Anker SD, Butler J, Filippatos G, et al. Empagliflozin in heart failure with a preserved ejection fraction. N Engl J Med 2021;385:1451–61.

49. Packer M, Anker SD, Butler J, et al. Effects of sodium-glucose cotransporter 2 inhibitors for the treatment of patients with heart failure: proposal of a novel mechanism of action. JAMA Cardiol 2017;2(9):1025–9.

50. Vardeny O, Vaduganathan M. Practical guide to prescribing sodium-glucose cotransporter 2 inhibitors for cardiologists. J Am Coll Cardiol HF 2019;7: 169–72.

A Primer on Pacemakers and Defibrillators for Nurses

T. Jennifer Walker, MSN, RN, ANP-BC*,
Anderson Bradbury, MSN, RN, AGNP-C

KEYWORDS

- Pacemaker • Defibrillators • ICD • Cardiac resynchronization therapy • CRT
- Nurses

KEY POINTS

- Because the number of patients with cardiac implantable electronic devices (CIEDs) rises each year, it is essential for nurses to stay updated on the fundamentals of pacing and novel cardiac device therapies.
- Novel devices such as the leadless cardiac pacemaker and the subcutaneous implantable cardioverter defibrillator are designed to overcome challenges related to transvenous leads.
- CIEDs offer the significant benefit of improving quality of life and survival, but complications can arise in approximately 10% of device patients.

INTRODUCTION

Nurses in various clinical settings frequently encounter patients with cardiac implantable electronic devices (CIEDs). "Cardiac implantable electronic device" is a term that includes cardiac devices that treat and manage arrhythmias, such as pacemakers, implantable cardioverter defibrillators (ICDs), and cardiac resynchronization therapy (CRT). It is estimated that over 3 million people in the United States have a pacemaker, and over 0.8 million people have an ICD.[1] The number of people with CIEDs continues to increase because of expanding indications for devices and the aging population. Nurses must have a good fundamental knowledge of pacemakers and ICDs to effectively care for cardiac device patients.

Technological advances in device therapies over the past 60 years have changed the landscape for patients in need of pacing support or sudden death prevention. New modalities aim to improve device size and battery longevity and reduce

Department of Cardiac Electrophysiology, University of North Carolina, 100 Eastowne Drive, Chapel Hill, NC 27514, USA
* Corresponding author.
E-mail address: Jennifer.Walker@unchealth.unc.edu

Nurs Clin N Am 58 (2023) 405–419
https://doi.org/10.1016/j.cnur.2023.05.007
0029-6465/23/© 2023 Elsevier Inc. All rights reserved.

nursing.theclinics.com

complications associated with leads and generators. This essential guide provides nurses with a comprehensive overview of the principles of pacing and ICDs, as well as innovative technologies such as leadless cardiac pacemakers (LCPs) and subcutaneous ICDs (S-ICDs). This guide also includes nursing implications and clinical pearls to help nurses effectively manage patients with CIEDs.

PACEMAKERS

Pacemakers provide heart rate support and are indicated for the treatment of symptomatic bradycardia (heart rate <60 bpm).[2] Although it may be physiologically normal for some people to have a heart rate less than 60 bpm, others may experience symptoms of fatigue, weakness, lightheadedness, shortness of breath, pre-syncope, or syncope related to a slow heart rate. Bradycardia is often caused by disorders of the sinus or atrioventricular (AV) node, such as sinus node dysfunction, advanced second-degree AV block, or third-degree AV block.[2] Sinus or AV nodal disease commonly affects people who are elderly because of degeneration of the electrical conduction system over time. Bradycardia can also be caused by medications such as beta-blockers, calcium channel blockers, digoxin, and antiarrhythmic drugs. Medications with heart rate slowing effects should be withheld for the symptomatic patient. Current guidelines recommend pacemakers as a Class I indication for treatment of symptomatic sinus node dysfunction, advanced second-degree AV block, or third-degree AV block (**Table 1**).[2]

A traditional pacemaker is typically implanted under conscious sedation. The generator is placed in the pre-pectoral region, with one to 3 leads implanted transvenously. The patient may receive a single chamber (lead inserted into one chamber, commonly the right ventricle [RV]), dual chamber (leads inserted into the right atrium and RV), or biventricular (leads inserted to pace the right and left ventricles) device.

Pacing Functions

Pacemakers have 2 main functions, to pace and to sense. Pacing refers to the ability to depolarize the myocardial tissue by delivering an electrical impulse, which leads to contraction (capture) of the atria or ventricle. Sensing refers to the ability of the pacemaker to "sense" the intrinsic activity of the heart, which helps the pacemaker determine whether to pace or inhibit.

Failure of the pacemaker to adequately capture or sense can cause symptoms such as lightheadedness, shortness of breath, pre-syncope, or syncope. Nurses should interpret the 12-lead electrocardiogram (ECG) or telemetry strips to confirm normal pacemaker function and promptly identify pacemaker malfunction.

Pacing Modes and Code

The programmed mode determines how the pacemaker responds to a sensed intracardiac signal. The standardized coding system consists of five letter positions to denote pacemaker function (**Table 2**).[3] The first letter position refers to the chamber paced, and the second position refers to the chamber sensed (A = atrium, V = ventricle, D = dual, or O = none). The third letter position indicates whether the pacemaker will trigger (T) or inhibit (I) a pacing stimulus in response to a sensed event. The letter D (dual) refers to inhibition and trigger, which can only be used in dual chamber pacing. For example, if the third position is programmed to dual (D), the atria are inhibited when there is sensed atrial activity, but the pacemaker will trigger a ventricular stimulus. This mode of pacing helps maintain AV synchrony. The fourth letter position refers to rate-adaptive or rate-responsive pacing. Through physiologic and

Table 1
Indications for device-based therapy

Pacemaker[2]	ICD[7]	CRT[2]
• Symptomatic third-degree or advanced second-degree AV block • Asymptomatic third-degree or advanced second-degree AV block with pauses $\geq$ 3.0 s • Symptomatic bradycardia because of SN dysfunction • Symptomatic chronotropic incompetence • Required drug therapy that results in bradycardia	• Sustained ventricular arrhythmias • Primary prevention of SCD in patients with left ventricular dysfunction (LV ejection fraction $\leq$ 30 to 35%) despite GDMT • Survivors of cardiac arrest • Inherited or infiltrative cardiomyopathies (eg, hypertrophic cardiomyopathy, cardiac sarcoidosis • Cardiac channelopathies (eg, Long-QT syndrome, Brugada)	• Left ventricular ejection fraction $\leq$ 35% in sinus rhythm, New York Heart Association class II symptoms or higher (slight to severe limitation of physical activity), and left bundle branch block with QRS duration $\geq$ 150 ms on GDMT for heart failure

Abbreviations: AV, atrioventricular; GDMT, guideline-directed medical therapy; SN, sinus node; SCD, sudden cardiac death.
This is a summary of common indications. For all indications, refer to the appropriate guidelines.
Data from Refs.[2,7]

Table 2
Pacemaker coding system[3]

Position	I	II	III	IV	V
Category	Chamber Paced	Chamber Sensed	Response to Sensing	Rate Modulation	Multisite Pacing
	O= None	*O*= None	*O*= None	*O*= None	*O*= None
	A = Atrium	*A* = Atrium	*T* = Triggered	*R* = Rate Modulation	*A* = Atrium
	V= Ventricle	*V*= Ventricle	*I*= Inhibited		*V*= Ventricle
	D = Dual (A + V)	*D* = Dual (A + V)	*D* = Dual (T + I)		*D* = Dual (A + V)

Data from Mulpuru and colleagues.

activity sensors, the pacemaker can adapt the heart rate to support the patient during increased cardiopulmonary and metabolic effort. This is helpful for patients who have chronotropic incompetence, which is the inability to increase the heart rate adequately during activity. The absence of the letter R means rate-responsiveness is not turned on. Finally, the fifth letter position is used to indicate whether multisite pacing is present (ie, more than one pacing site in the atria or ventricle, or pacing in the atria or ventricles).[3]

Temporary Cardiac Pacing

Temporary cardiac pacing can be achieved with transcutaneous, transvenous, or epicardial pacing (typically used post-cardiac surgery). These modalities provide heart rate support in the setting of acute hemodynamic instability until there is resolution of reversible causes or as a therapeutic bridge to permanent pacing.

Patients with acute bradycardia should be evaluated for reversible causes, including myocardial infarction, cardiac surgery, Lyme disease, hypothermia, electrolyte abnormalities, drugs or toxins, or medications (eg, beta-blocker, digoxin, non-dihydropyridine calcium channel blockers, antiarrhythmics, methyldopa, risperidone).[4] Withdrawal of offending medications or treatment of reversible causes may improve the patient's heart rate and clinical condition and potentially avoid the need for a pacemaker.

Nurses should promptly recognize signs of acute decompensation in the patient with bradycardia, such as hypotension, bradycardia, altered mental status, syncope, chest discomfort, and poor perfusion. Medical management for acute bradycardia with symptoms or hemodynamic compromise includes atropine, isoproterenol, dopamine, or dobutamine to increase heart rate.[4] If medical therapy fails to improve the patient's condition, transcutaneous pacing can be quickly initiated by nurses until temporary transvenous pacing can be implemented.[4]

Nursing Considerations for Temporary Pacing

Nurses caring for a patient with transcutaneous pacing should maintain patient comfort with sedation or analgesia if possible, ensure proper pad placement in the anterior–posterior position, and monitor pacing settings.[5] In addition, the nurse should interpret telemetry for adequate pacemaker capture and assess the patient for signs of improved cardiac output, such as improved vital signs and mentation.[5]

Temporary transvenous and epicardial pacing leads are connected to an external pacemaker. The venous site dressing should be kept clean and dry, and the external pacemaker should be placed in a safe location to prevent accidental setting changes or disconnection of leads. Pacing rate, output, sensitivity, and capture thresholds are programmed and checked as part of the nursing assessment.[6]

IMPLANTABLE CARDIOVERTER DEFIBRILLATORS

Sudden cardiac death (SCD) is caused by ventricular tachycardia or ventricular fibrillation and accounts for approximately 50% of cardiac deaths.[7] Risk factors for SCD include advanced age, coronary artery disease, cardiomyopathy, genetic disorders, or channelopathies (eg, Brugada syndrome, long QT syndrome).[7] Although survival after SCD has increased in the past decade, the overall survival rate remains low. Only 10.8% to 11.4% of people survive an out-of-hospital cardiac arrest.[8]

ICDs improve survival from SCD by providing early defibrillation to terminate ventricular arrhythmias. ICDs can also provide pacing support for patients with bradycardia. Current guidelines recommend ICDs in patients with sustained ventricular arrhythmias, left ventricular (LV) dysfunction (LV ejection fraction $\leq$ 30 to 35%), or survivors of cardiac arrest for the prevention of SCD (see **Table 1**).[7]

Schrage and colleagues investigated the association between primary prevention ICD use in patients with heart failure and reduced ejection fraction and reaffirmed that ICD recipients compared with non-ICD recipients had reduced 1 year and 5 year all-cause mortality.[9] Despite the compelling survival benefits of ICDs, only 10% of the 16,702 eligible patients in the study had an ICD.[9] Low rates of ICD utilization are multifactorial and are attributed to gender disparities, low patient and provider knowledge, and gaps in transitions of care.[10] Nurses can help bridge this gap by providing patient education regarding heart failure and SCD, and facilitating close follow-up after hospital discharge.

Additional Implantable Cardioverter Defibrillator Functions

In addition to providing early arrhythmia therapies to prevent SCD, ICDs offer heart failure diagnostics to identify patients at risk for worsening heart failure. Pulmonary congestion is estimated by measuring of thoracic impedance. Thoracic impedance is derived from a constant electrical signal passing through the tissue between the lead and the device generator. Because intrathoracic fluid and pulmonary congestion increase, the electrical signal travels through the tissue more easily. Thus, a low thoracic impedance indicates an increase in pulmonary congestion.[11] Measurement of thoracic impedance can provide early warning of possible worsening heart failure when used with other parameters, such as decreased patient activity level or rapid heart rates.[12]

CARDIAC RESYNCHRONIZATION THERAPY

Heart failure causes negative structural and electrical changes within the heart, also referred to as negative cardiac remodeling. These changes can manifest as a decline in systolic or diastolic function, chamber dilation, fibrosis, or electrical abnormalities such as first-degree AV block or bundle branch block (QRS duration > 120 ms).[2] Bundle branch blocks cause delayed ventricular activation, or "ventricular dyssynchrony," and increase the risk for worsened heart failure and SCD.[2]

Cardiac resynchronization therapy aims to "resynchronize" the heart by simultaneously pacing the right and left ventricles. This is accomplished by implanting one lead into the RV and one lead into a posterolateral branch of the coronary sinus to pace the LV.

Cardiac resynchronization therapy can be used with pacemakers (CRT-P) or defibrillators (CRT-D). Studies have correlated a percentage of biventricular pacing greater than 91% of the time with the most benefit in terms of reduced heart failure hospitalization and mortality.[13]

Patients with New York Heart Association class II symptoms or higher (slight to severe limitation of physical activity), LV ejection fraction $\leq$ 35%, sinus rhythm, and left bundle branch block with QRS duration $\geq$ 150 ms gain the most benefit from CRT (see **Table 1**).[2] In conjunction with guideline-directed medical therapies, CRT has been shown to improve heart failure symptoms and functional capacity, as well as reduce heart failure hospitalizations and mortality.[14]

NOVEL DEVICES: LEADLESS CARDIAC PACEMAKERS AND SUBCUTANEOUS IMPLANTABLE CARDIOVERTER DEFIBRILLATORS

Despite advances in technology, there are considerable limitations with pulse generators and endocardial leads. Pulse generators can cause pocket complications such as infection, hematoma, pain, and erosion, whereas transvenous leads pose a risk for cardiac perforation, deep venous thrombosis, tricuspid valve insufficiency, and endocarditis.[15] Patients with lead fractures or lead insulation breaks may require a lead extraction procedure, which carries a significant mortality risk. To overcome lead-related and pocket-related complications, the leadless cardiac pacemaker and the S-ICD were developed.

Leadless Cardiac Pacemaker

A leadless, self-contained cardiac pacemaker was first conceptualized over 50 years ago.[16] Tremendous advances in technology led to the Food and Drug Administration approval of the Micra leadless transcatheter pacing system in 2016 (Medtronic, Minneapolis, MN, **Fig. 1**) followed by the approval of the AVEIR leadless pacemaker in 2022 (Abbott, Chicago, IL).[17]

The battery longevity of the LCP is estimated to be 15 years, compared with 12.5 years for the traditional pacemaker.[16] The LCP is implanted in the RV to provide single-chamber pacing. Of note, only 15% to 30% of pacemaker patients are candidates for RV-only pacing, including patients with chronic atrial fibrillation and AV block, or sinus node dysfunction and infrequent pauses (**Table 3**).[16] The majority of patients with bradyarrhythmias benefit from a traditional pacemaker that offers dual chamber pacing (pacing of the atria and ventricles) to maintain AV synchrony. Furthermore, right-ventricular pacing alone can be detrimental to patients with heart failure because of ventricular dyssynchrony.[16]

The LCP implant procedure is minimally invasive and differs from the traditional pacemaker implant. The LCP is delivered through a catheter-based approach via the femoral vein. The device is actively fixed to the RV and then released from the delivery catheter.[16] The absence of a pulse generator means the patient will not have a dressing on the chest. Instead, nurses should monitor the patient's groin

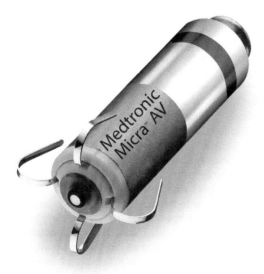

Fig. 1. MICRA transcatheter pacing system (Images used with permission from Medtronic, plc © 2022.)

Table 3 Candidates for leadless cardiac pacemakers and subcutaneous ICD	
Consider Leadless Cardiac Pacemaker in Ref.[16]:	Consider Subcutaneous ICD in Ref.[7]:
• Permanent atrial fibrillation • After AV node ablation • May be reasonable in sedentary patients, significant comorbidities, or vascular issues • Carotid sinus hypersensitivity • Maintenance of AV synchrony (dual chamber pacing) is not necessary	• Difficult vascular access (eg, hemodialysis, complex cardiac anatomy) • High risk for infection • Long QT syndrome • Hypertrophic cardiomyopathy • Patients with prosthetic heart valves • Women because of possible cosmetic advantages • Does not require pacing support

Abbreviation: AV, atrioventricular.
  Data from Refs. [7,16].

for complications such as hematoma, bleeding, pseudoaneurysm, or arteriovenous fistula.

In a comprehensive review comparing LCPs to traditional pacemakers, LCPs are associated with a lower overall rate of complications. However, LCPs have a higher rate of device dislodgement (2.3% vs 0%), cardiac perforation, and pericardial effusion than the traditional pacemaker (1.5% vs 0.1%).[16] These increased risks are potentially related to the design of the screw-in active fixation mechanism of the LCP. This method requires the implanting provider to achieve the right balance in securing the device while preventing cardiac perforation.[16]

Subcutaneous Implantable Cardioverter Defibrillator

To overcome lead-related challenges, the EMBLEM MRI S-ICD (Boston Scientific, 2012, **Fig. 2**) was developed. The S-ICD system is completely subcutaneous, which obviates the risk of lead-related complications such as venous occlusion, thromboembolism, or endocarditis.[18] The main limitation of the S-ICD is that it cannot provide anti-bradycardia pacing or anti-tachycardia pacing (ATP; quick, painless bursts of pacing to attempt termination of ventricular tachycardia) compared with a traditional ICD. In essence, it functions like a "shock box" to terminate ventricular arrhythmias that cause sudden death.

The 2017 American Heart Association/American College of Cardiology/Heart Rhythm Society Guideline for Management of Patients with Ventricular Arrhythmias and the Prevention of Sudden Cardiac Death recommends the S-ICD device in patients at risk for sudden death with difficult vascular access or susceptible to infection (Class I indication).[7] The S-ICD is also reasonable for patients with long QT syndrome, hypertrophic cardiomyopathy, patients with prosthetic heart valves, or women because of possible cosmetic advantages (**Table 3**).[7]

The S-ICD generator is implanted subcutaneously in the left lower chest between the fourth and sixth intercostal spaces at the mid-axillary line to anterior axillary line. The device is connected to a sensor that is placed subcutaneously and vertically along the sternum. The S-ICD generator is twice as large with a shorter anticipated battery life compared with the traditional transvenous ICD (5.6 vs 7 years).[19] The larger size of the generator requires a longer, deeper incision, which typically causes more pain for the patient. Assessing for pain and providing prophylactic pain medications can help minimize postoperative discomfort for the patient.[18]

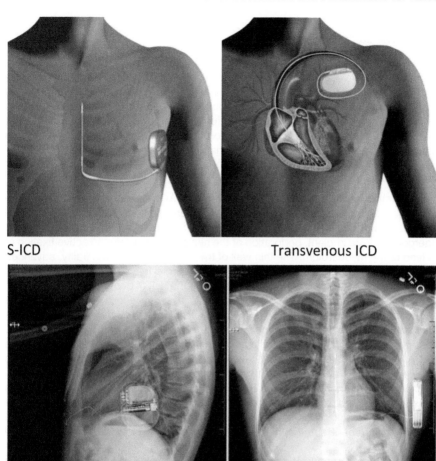

S-ICD   Transvenous ICD

S-ICD Chest Xray (lateral view)   S-ICD Chest Xray (PA view)

Fig. 2. EMBLEM MRI S-ICD. (Image provided courtesy of Boston Scientific. ©2023 Boston Scientific Corporation or its affiliates. All rights reserved.)

Table 4
Device-related complications[20,24,25,27]

Acute Complications	Nonacute Complications
Lead dislodgement/malposition	Pocket/device infection
Pneumothorax	Pocket pain
Hemopericardium/Tamponade	Retained, nondissolved suture
Pocket hematoma	Endocarditis
	Subclavian DVT (arm swelling)
	Lead fracture or failure
	Device erosion
	Diaphragm stimulation
	Device manipulation/Twiddler's syndrome
	Hypertrophic scar/keloid formation
	Tricuspid valve dysfunction

Abbreviation: DVT, deep vein thrombosis.
Data from Refs.[20,24,25,27]

DEVICE-RELATED COMPLICATIONS

CIEDs offer the significant benefit of improving quality of life and survival, but complications can arise in approximately 10% of device patients.[20] Complications are categorized as acute complications, which occur within the first 30 days of implant, or as chronic complications (**Table 4**). Key components of the nursing assessment after a device implant include monitoring the site for bleeding or hematoma and assessing the affected extremity for adequate perfusion. Nurses should be aware of any acute changes in vital signs or assessment that may indicate a complication.

Acute Complications

Cardiac tamponade is a rare but potentially fatal complication encountered in the periprocedural setting. Cardiac tamponade occurs when significant bleeding into the pericardial sac puts pressure on the heart and prevents adequate cardiac output. In patients undergoing device implant, perforation of the heart may occur during active fixation of the lead to the myocardium. The thin wall of the RV apex, along with frailty, advanced age, BMI <20, female sex, heart failure, prior myocardial infarction, hemodialysis, and chronic obstructive pulmonary disease, increases the risk of perforation.[21,22]

Prompt recognition of cardiac tamponade is essential for patient survival. The symptoms can be subtle initially, but the patient may quickly deteriorate into cardiogenic shock. The patient may appear anxious or pale, with symptoms of dyspnea, chest pain, and hiccups.[22] The hallmark signs of cardiac tamponade (Beck's triad) are hypotension, distended jugular veins, and diminished or muffled heart sounds on auscultation.[23]

Nursing management consists of hemodynamic support with volume resuscitation or vasopressors and oxygen therapy.[23] Echocardiography is the gold standard for the diagnosis of cardiac tamponade. Nurses should anticipate and prepare for pericardiocentesis or emergent surgical management to drain the blood from the pericardial sac.[24]

A more common complication encountered in the acute post-implant setting is lead malposition or dislodgement. Lead dislodgement is suspected when there is loss of capture or improper sensing on a 12-lead ECG or telemetry. A chest radiograph is performed post-implant to assess and document proper lead placement, and treatment involves a repeat procedure to reposition the lead.

Pneumothorax occurs in approximately 1% of patients and results from subclavian venous puncture because of the proximity of the apex of the lung.[3] Patients may report shortness of breath with signs of tachypnea or tachycardia, or they may be asymptomatic. A chest radiograph is obtained post-implant to rule out pneumothorax. Small pneumothoraxes may be observed for resolution, but large pneumothoraxes may require a chest tube for treatment.

Intermediate and Long-Term Complications

Device pocket hematoma can occur in the acute and subacute postoperative phases of healing and occurs in 1% to 9% of device implants.[25–27] Patients present with pain and swelling around the device. On examination, the area may be warm, fluctuant, erythematous, or ecchymotic. Risk factors for hematoma include increased age, heart failure, kidney failure, coronary artery disease, and coagulopathies.[25] Patients taking blood thinners such as antiplatelet therapy, direct-acting oral anticoagulants (DOAC), or vitamin K antagonists (eg, warfarin) are at increased risk for hematoma.[25] Although hematomas do not affect mortality, they are associated with an increased length of stay and an increased likelihood of infection.[26,27]

One-third of patients with a CRT device may complain of diaphragmatic stimulation secondary to the LV lead inappropriately capturing the phrenic nerve.[28] These patients describe a jumping or bouncing sensation in the left upper abdomen that may be positional. Reprogramming the device can typically resolve the diaphragmatic stimulation.

Because device longevity of CIEDs reaches several years, various complications may arise over time. These complications include lead malfunction and dislodgment, infection, and generator erosion.[20] Leads are the most common component to fail because of repetitive stress by the cardiac cycle and chest muscle movement.[3]

Device infection is a feared complication because it increases cardiovascular mortality.[20] The risk for infection is higher with temporary pacemakers and generator changes compared with a new device implant. Additional risk factors for device infection include diabetes, steroid use, heart failure, renal failure, and pocket hematoma.[3] Although some infections are superficial and limited to the pocket, deeper infections involving the leads or valves can lead to bacteremia or endocarditis. Treatment of an infected device is complex and may include long-term IV antibiotics and extraction of the device system.

Nine percent of patients who require a high burden of RV pacing may develop pacemaker-induced cardiomyopathy.[29] Pacemaker-induced cardiomyopathy is defined as a greater than 10% reduction in LV ejection fraction after device implant in a patient who RV paces at least 20% of the time.[29] Patients often present with signs and symptoms of decompensated heart failure, such as dyspnea on exertion, lower extremity edema, elevated jugular venous pressure, pulmonary crackles on auscultation, and pulmonary edema on a chest radiograph.[29] The cornerstones of treatment of pacemaker-induced cardiomyopathy include guideline-directed medical therapies for heart failure and the upgrade of the current device to CRT.

REMOTE MONITORING OF CARDIAC IMPLANTABLE ELECTRONIC DEVICES

Along with regular in-office visits, most device patients have the option to be monitored remotely.[12] Remote monitoring (RM) refers to automatic data transmission that is triggered by device alerts, and remote interrogation (RI) is the routine and scheduled transmission of device data.[12] Remote monitoring obtains data regarding normal device, battery, and lead function, as well as ICD therapies (shocks), device-related malfunctions, or negative trends in arrhythmia burden or heart failure diagnostics.[30] The ability to remotely acquire data from CIEDs has improved patient care. Studies have associated RM with a shorter mean time to first diagnosis of clinical events (eg, battery depletion, lead malfunction), and an earlier time to diagnosis of new arrhythmia events.[12]

While RM previously included trans-telephonic monitoring through handheld phone adaptors, this method is being phased out. Currently, RM is facilitated through a home monitor (transmitter) that is placed next to a patient's bed and is connected to the device company through a telephone line, WIFI, or cell phone service.[12] The bedside monitor automatically connects to the CIED wirelessly to transmit data, often at night while the patient is asleep.[12] Information from RM is sent to the providers' office for interpretation.

PATIENT EDUCATION

Nurses play a vital role in providing patients with the information needed to live well with a cardiac device. Education should be focused on the indication for device implant, basic device function, and RM. Although specific details may vary between different institutions, discharge education should include these essential components.

- Basic incision care (keeping the area clean and dry)

- Signs and symptoms to report (eg, pain, redness, swelling, warmth, drainage, or hematoma at the site)
- Arm and activity restrictions
- Driving restrictions
- ICD patients should have a plan for what to do in case of ICD shocks (whom to notify, when to seek emergency care)
- Contact information for the device clinic and electrophysiology clinic
- Device ID card from the manufacturer
- Follow-up wound check and clinic appointments

SPECIAL CONSIDERATIONS

Many patients with CIEDs eventually require magnetic resonance imaging (MRI) evaluation for the diagnosis of other medical conditions. CIEDs are categorized as MRI-safe or MRI-conditional, and nonsafe or nonconditional systems. These designations are determined by the device manufacturers and pertain to the generator and the leads. Previously, any nonconditional system would preclude a patient from undergoing an MRI because of concerns for device displacement, lead malfunction/thermal lead injury, and lethal arrhythmias.[31] However, recent studies have shown that the risk of damage to the system or harm to the patient undergoing an MRI with nonconditional systems is minimal and is often outweighed by the benefit an MRI evaluation would offer the patient.[31] Given the low risk of complications for the patient and device, MRIs can be safely done in device patients with careful planning and collaboration between cardiology and the specialist requesting the MRI.

FUTURE DIRECTIONS

The exciting development of the LCP and the S-ICD is only a sample of what science and technology could bring to arrhythmia management. Emerging therapies focus on improving cardiac efficiency and reducing hardware. Because of the negative effects of chronic right ventricular pacing, multisite pacing and alternative pacing sites are being explored.[12] Pacing from the His bundle is currently one strategy that mimics physiologic conduction, but lead stability can be challenging in this location.[12] One promising therapy is the gene-based or cell-based biological pacemaker, which would eliminate the need for batteries.[12] Creative concepts such as adding a substernal pacing lead to an S-ICD or combining the LCP with an S-ICD to offer supportive pacing are being studied.[19]

A fully dissolvable temporary pacemaker is currently being tested in animal clinical trials.[32] The flexible, leadless pacemaker weighs less than 0.5 g and is placed on the external surface of the heart to offer temporary pacing support.[32] The device is battery-free and powered by a remote power source similar to the wireless charging of a smartphone. This dissolvable pacemaker offers temporary pacing support as a bridge to permanent pacemaker implantation or after cardiac surgery. The device dissolves 5 to 7 weeks after implanting without the need for surgical removal.[32]

SUMMARY

In summary, CIEDs are an increasingly common therapy for a multitude of cardiac pathologies, including sinus node dysfunction, heart block, ventricular arrhythmias, SCD prevention, and systolic heart failure. Although the concepts of pacing have been around for more than half a century, innovative devices like the LCP and the S-ICD have shifted the paradigm. Nurses encounter patients with CIEDs in all aspects of the health care setting. Because exciting CIED therapies are on the horizon, nurses must stay up-to-date to optimize outcomes for CIED patients.

CLINICS CARE POINTS

- Permanent and temporary pacemakers are indicated for the treatment of symptomatic bradycardia. Reversible causes of bradycardia (eg, myocardial infarction, Lyme disease, medications) should be ruled out before implanting a permanent pacemaker.

- Leadless cardiac pacemakers are delivered via femoral venous access and implanted in the RV to provide single-chamber pacing (no chest incision). Monitor the groin site for bleeding, hematoma, or infection because of femoral venous access. Although the complication rates are low with LCPs, they are associated with a higher rate of cardiac perforation compared with traditional pacemakers.

- ICDs prevent SCD by providing early defibrillation to treat ventricular arrhythmias. ICDs also provide pacing support and valuable heart failure diagnostics that recognize worsening heart failure.

- Patients may experience more localized pain after an S-ICD implant because of the larger device size and longer incision. Providing prophylactic pain medications can help minimize postoperative discomfort for the patient.[18]

- Patients with cardiac resynchronization therapy may report diaphragmatic stimulation or "hiccups" because of the proximity of the left ventricular lead to the diaphragm. This is not dangerous and can typically be eliminated with device reprogramming.

- Cardiac tamponade is a rare but potentially fatal complication after a device implant. Nurses should recognize the hallmark signs of cardiac tamponade: Hypotension, distended jugular veins, and diminished or muffled heart sounds on auscultation.[23]

- Given the low risk of complications for the patient and device, MRIs can be safely done in device patients with careful planning and collaboration between cardiology and the specialist requesting the MRI.

- Remote monitoring and interrogation can provide detailed information about device function, arrhythmias, and presenting rhythm. A useful benefit of remote interrogation is that in patients with atrial fibrillation—the rhythm can be assessed remotely, which often eliminates the need to obtain an ECG.

DISCLOSURES

Ms J. Walker reports research salary support from the Bristol Myers Squibb Foundation, United States.

REFERENCES

1. Benjamin MM, Sorkness CA. Practical and ethical considerations in the management of pacemaker and implantable cardiac defibrillator devices in terminally ill patients. SAVE Proc 2017;30(2):157–60.
2. Tracy CM, Epstein AE, Darbar D, et al. 2012 ACCF/AHA/HRS Focused update of the 2008 guidelines for device-based therapy of cardiac rhythm abnormalities. JACC (J Am Coll Cardiol) 2012;60(14):1297–313.
3. Mulpuru SK, Madhavan M, McLeod CJ, et al. Cardiac pacemakers: function, troubleshooting, and management. J Am Coll Cardiol 2017;69(2):189–210.
4. Kusumoto FM, Schoenfeld MH, Barrett C, et al. 2018 ACC/AHA/HRS Guideline on the evaluation and management of patients with bradycardia and cardiac

conduction delay: Executive summary: A report of the American College of Cardiology/American Heart Association Task Force on Clinical Practice 'slines, and the Heart Rhythm Society. Circulation 2019;140(8). https://doi.org/10.1161/CIR.0000000000000627.

5. Adams A, Adams C. Transcutaneous pacing: An emergency nurse's guide. J Emerg Nurs 2021;47(2):326–30.
6. Mooney M. Managing patients with transvenous & transcutaneous pacemakers in nursing. In: Study.com. Published October 18, 2020. Available at: https://study.com/academy/lesson/managing-patients-with-transvenous-transcutaneous-pacemakers-in-nursing.html. Accessed November 17, 2022.
7. Al-Khatib SM, Stevenson WG, Ackerman MJ, et al. 2017 AHA/ACC/HRS Guideline for management of patients with ventricular arrhythmias and the prevention of sudden cardiac death. Circulation 2018;138(13):e272–391.
8. Sawyer KN, Camp-Rogers TR, Kotini-Shah P, et al. Sudden cardiac arrest survivorship: A scientific statement from the American Heart Association. Circulation 2020;141(12):e654–85.
9. Schrage B, Uijl A, Benson L, et al. Association between use of primary-prevention implantable cardioverter-defibrillators and mortality in patients with heart failure: A prospective propensity score–matched analysis from the Swedish heart failure registry. Circulation 2019;140(19):1530–9.
10. Goldstein SA, Li S, Lu D, et al. Implantable cardioverter defibrillator utilization and mortality among patients ≥65 years of age with a low ejection fraction after coronary revascularization. Am J Cardiol 2021;138:26–32.
11. Theuns DAMJ, Radhoe SP, Brugts JJ. Remote monitoring of heart failure in patients with implantable cardioverter-defibrillators: Current status and future needs. Sensors 2021;21(11):3763.
12. Madhavan M, Mulpuru SK, McLeod CJ, et al. Advances and future directions in cardiac pacemakers. J Am Coll Cardiol 2017;69(2):211–35.
13. Esteves A, Parreira L, Mesquita D, et al. Optimal percentage of biventricular pacing to obtain CRT response: How high is high enough. EP Europace 2021;23(Supplement_3). euab116.460.
14. Gold MR, Rickard J, Daubert JC, et al. Redefining the classifications of response to cardiac resynchronization therapy. JACC (J Am Coll Cardiol): Clinical Electrophysiology 2021;7(7):871–80.
15. van der Zee S, Doshi S. Permanent leadless cardiac pacing. American College of Cardiology. Published March 23, 2016. Available at: https://www.acc.org/latest-in-cardiology/articles/2016/03/23/08/09/http%3a%2f%2fwww.acc.org%2flatest-in-cardiology%2farticles%2f2016%2f03%2f23%2f08%2f09%2fpermanent-leadless-cardiac-pacing. Accessed November 17, 2022.
16. Tjong FVY, Reddy VY. Permanent leadless cardiac pacemaker therapy: A comprehensive review. Circulation 2017;135(15):1458–70.
17. Ibrahim R, Khoury A, El-Chami MF. Leadless pacing: Where we currently stand and what the future holds. Curr Cardiol Rep 2022;24(10):1233–40.
18. Vedachalam S, Cook S, Koppert T, et al. Approaches to minimizing periprocedural complications during subcutaneous implantable cardioverter-defibrillator placement. J Innov Card Rhythm Manag 2020;11(5):4100–5.
19. van Dijk VF, Boersma LV. The subcutaneous implantable cardioverter defibrillator in 2019 and beyond. Trends Cardiovasc Med 2020;30(6):378–84.
20. Palmisano P, Guerra F, Dell'Era G, et al. Impact on all-cause and cardiovascular mortality of cardiac implantable electronic device complications. JACC (J Am Coll Cardiol): Clinical Electrophysiology 2020;6(4):382–92.

21. Akbarzadeh MA, Mollazadeh R, Sefidbakht S, et al. Identification and management of right ventricular perforation using pacemaker and cardioverter-defibrillator leads: A case series and mini review. Journal of Arrhythmia 2017; 33(1):1–5.
22. Piccini JP, Cunnane R, Steffel J, et al. Development and validation of a risk score for predicting pericardial effusion in patients undergoing leadless pacemaker implantation: experience with the Micra transcatheter pacemaker. EP Europace 2022;24(7):1119–26.
23. Stashko E, Meer JM, Danitsch D. Cardiac tamponade (Nursing). In: StatPearls. StatPearls Publishing; 2022. http://www.ncbi.nlm.nih.gov/books/NBK568727/. Accessed November 17, 2022.
24. Khalid M, Murtaza G, Ayub MT, et al. Right ventricle perforation post pacemaker insertion complicated with cardiac tamponade. Cureus 2018;10(3). https://doi.org/10.7759/cureus.2266.
25. Notaristefano F, Angeli F, Verdecchia P, et al. Device-pocket hematoma after cardiac implantable electronic devices. Circ: Arrhythmia and Electrophysiology 2020;13(4). https://doi.org/10.1161/CIRCEP.120.008372.
26. Sridhar ARM, Yarlagadda V, Kanmanthareddy A, et al. Incidence, predictors and outcomes of hematoma after ICD implantation: An analysis of a nationwide database of 85,276 patients. Indian Pacing Electrophysiol J 2016;16(5):159–64.
27. Tarakji KG, Korantzopoulos P, Philippon F, et al. Infectious consequences of hematoma from cardiac implantable electronic device procedures and the role of the antibiotic envelope: A WRAP-IT trial analysis. Heart Rhythm 2021;18(12): 2080–6.
28. Shah R, Qualls Z. Diaphragmatic stimulation caused by cardiac resynchronization treatment. CMAJ (Can Med Assoc J) 2016;188(10):E239.
29. Koo A, Stein A, Walsh R. Pacing-induced cardiomyopathy. CPC-EM 2017;1(4): 362–4.
30. Zeitler EP, Piccini JP. Remote monitoring of cardiac implantable electronic devices (CIED). Trends Cardiovasc Med 2016;26(6):568–77.
31. Gupta SK, Ya'qoub L, Wimmer AP, et al. Safety and clinical impact of MRI in patients with non–MRI-conditional cardiac devices. Radiology: Cardiothoracic Imaging 2020;2(5):e200086.
32. Choi YS, Yin RT, Pfenniger A, et al. Fully implantable and bioresorbable cardiac pacemakers without leads or batteries. Nat Biotechnol 2021;39(10):1228–38.

Mechanical Circulatory Support Therapy in the Cardiac Intensive Care Unit

Sarah E. Schroeder, PhD, ACNP-BC, MSN RN, AACC

KEYWORDS

- Mechanical circulatory support • Left ventricular assist device
- Cardiac intensive care unit • LVAD management

KEY POINTS

- Heart failure continues to be highly prevalent and comes with a high cost, despite ongoing guideline recommendations for management.
- Mechanical circulatory support (both temporary and durable devices) continues to have a presence in the management of the critically ill cardiac or respiratory patient.
- Gold standard practice for blood pressure monitoring in a durable left ventricular assist device (dLVAD) is by obtaining an opening pressure by Doppler.
- Survival for dLVAD recipients has increased significantly irrespective of their cardiac transplantation candidacy due to ongoing advancements of the devices themselves.
- Cardiac nurses are crucial in reinforcing bedside education to the MCS patient to prepare for a successful discharge.

INTRODUCTION

Heart failure (HF) is highly prevalent,[1–3] uses significant health care resources, and has a detrimental survival rate of less than 25% if symptoms persistent despite treatment with guideline-directed medical therapy (GDMT).[4] Advanced HF accounts for 5% to 10% of the current 6.5 million individuals in the United States living with HF, and by 2030, HF will account for 3% of the total population.[1,5] Advanced HF is defined as refractory HF symptoms despite GDMT, with progressive decline in activity tolerance, persistent volume overload resulting in adverse events and hospitalizations, and less than 2 years life expectancy.[6,7] Cardiac transplantation remains the gold standard treatment for advanced HF; however, not all individuals meet criteria or are too sick to reach cardiac transplantation. One treatment option for qualifying individuals with advanced HF, regardless of transplant eligibility, is the use of mechanical circulatory

Mechanical Circulatory Support Nurse Practitioner and Program Manager, Bryan Heart, 1600 South 48th Street, Suite 600, Lincoln, NE 68506, USA
E-mail address: sarah.schroeder@bryanheart.com

Nurs Clin N Am 58 (2023) 421–437
https://doi.org/10.1016/j.cnur.2023.05.008
nursing.theclinics.com
0029-6465/23/© 2023 Elsevier Inc. All rights reserved.

support (MCS) therapy, which is a compilation of fully implantable or temporary mechanical devices aimed at managing cardiogenic shock oftentimes found in advanced HF. This type of shock may be associated with acute myocardial infarction (MI), right-sided HF, or advanced HF despite GDMT.

Fully implantable devices are also called durable left ventricular assist devices (dLVAD). Temporary devices may include right-sided support (with a temporary right ventricular assist device [tRVAD]) or left-sided support (with a temporary LVAD [tLVAD]). Individuals undergoing a durable LVAD surgery or placement of a tLVAD/tRVAD need close monitoring and stabilization in the intensive care unit (ICU). Nurses trained in cardiac surgery recovery and ICU care management are crucial to the success of any patient with cardiogenic shock who requires MCS.

The purpose of this article is to provide guidance for nurses who care for MCS patients in the ICU. Key areas discussed are the history of durable LVADs; indications for short- and long-term support MCS options, total artificial heart devices, and cardiac transplantation; and nursing care of patients with MCS including implications for nursing assessment, shared decision-making, and supportive education for patients, family, and caregivers.

INDICATIONS FOR MECHANICAL CIRCULATORY SUPPORT

As an evolving treatment for advanced HF, MCS devices have changed overtime becoming smaller and more durable to decrease adverse events associated with MCS therapy. Durable LVADs were initially developed as a bridge to transplant (BTT), not intended to be permanent. After additional research, indications for durable LVADs expanded to include destination therapy (DT) for individuals who do not qualify for cardiac transplantation, yet still experience advanced HF symptoms. Recent terminology has changed from BTT and DT to short-term versus long-term strategies, respectively.

Temporary ventricular assist device strategies are indicated for acutely ill individuals with cardiogenic shock that need an immediate intervention to decrease mortality. **Table 1** differentiates between the durable LVAD devices and tLVAD/tRVAD devices currently used for cardiogenic shock.

NEXT-GENERATION LEFT-SIDED MECHANICAL CIRCULATORY SUPPORT

In 2001, the first-generation pulsatile fully implantable durable LVAD was designed as BTT which improved overall survival to 52% as compared with 25% for those on medications alone.[8] Significant adverse events (including infection, bleeding, and stroke) were predominant,[8] leading to changes in pump dynamics. Subsequently, second-generation axial-flow durable LVADs were developed as smaller and more durable devices, with the overall goal of improving clinical characteristics and outcomes for individuals meeting candidacy for short-term therapy (BTT) or for individuals ineligible for cardiac transplantation with advanced HF meeting criteria for long-term therapy (DT) (**Fig. 1**).

The most recent generation of durable LVADs include a centrifugal device that has the best hemocompatibility of all available pumps, resulting in fewer adverse events (stroke, pump malfunction, and bleeding) and improved 1-year survival nearing 85%.[9] **Table 2** describes the pivotal MCS studies.

Up until June 2021, patients with advanced HF were treated with one of three pumps: the Heartmate II or the HeartWare HVAD system (both axial-flow pumps), or the HeartMate 3 (a durable LVAD functions with a fully levitated magnet to propel blood out of the pump). In June 2021, the HeartWare HVAD system was removed

Table 1
Differentiation between durable and temporary mechanical circulatory support devices[21]

MCS Device	Indication	Cannulation Strategies	Risks of Device
Durable			
HeartMate II	LVAD	Left ventricular apex (inflow cannula) Ascending aorta (outflow graft)	Thrombus Pump malfunction Stroke Bleeding
HeartWare (HVAD)	LVAD	Left ventricular apex (inflow cannula) Ascending Aorta (outflow graft)	Thrombus Pump malfunction Stroke Bleeding
HeartMate 3	LVAD	Left ventricular apex (inflow cannula) Ascending aorta (outflow graft)	Thrombus (low) Pump malfunction (low) Stroke Bleeding
Temporary			
Tandem Heart/ Lifesparc	tRVAD tLVAD BiVAD	Right neck with Protek Duo catheter to RIJ-pull from RA, bypass RV and push in to PA system Femoral artery Femoral artery femoral vein RIJ	Bleeding Device dislodgement Thrombus Shunt development Tamponade
Centrimag	tRVAD tLVAD BiVAD	RIJ; may be placed surgically Femoral artery, axillary artery Femoral artery and vein; axillary artery and vein	Device migration Kinked tubing Pump thrombus Suction events
Impella	tRVAD tLVAD BiVAD	Femoral vein; axillary vein Femoral artery; axillary artery Femoral artery or axillary artery; femoral vein or axillary vein	Hemolysis Device migration leading to malposition Injury to aortic valve Arrhythmias

Abbreviations: PA, pulmonary artery; RA, right atrium; RIJ, right internal jugular.

from the market due to the increased risk of neurologic events (strokes) and mortality.[10] The HeartMate II is no longer being implanted due to the superiority of the HeartMate 3. With the development of this third-generation device, adverse events have decreased. **Table 3** describes each durable LVAD currently in use.

RIGHT-SIDED MECHANICAL CIRCULATORY SUPPORT DEVICES

Acute right-sided HF may result from ischemia related to an acute MI (primarily right ventricular infarct) or postsurgical complications, acute hypoxia from significant pulmonary embolism, inflammation from arrhythmias, myocarditis, or infection (eg, sepsis/critical illness).[11] Right-sided HF is manifested by hypoperfusion, decreased consciousness, diaphoresis, tachycardia, and cool extremities.[11] A Swan-Ganz catheter is beneficial in management of right-sided HF for monitoring and guiding medical treatment. When using a Swan-Ganz catheter, right HF is seen with elevated central venous pressure greater than 12 mm Hg, central venous pressure/pulmonary capillary wedge pressure ratio greater than 0.8, and a pulmonary artery pulsatility index less

First Generation Devices	Second Generation Devices	Third Generation Devices

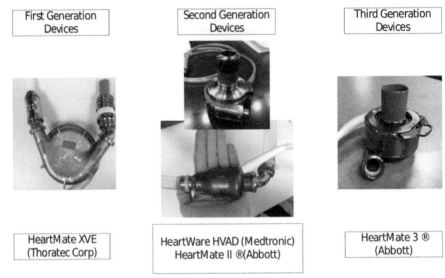

HeartMate XVE (Thoratec Corp)	HeartWare HVAD (Medtronic) HeartMate II ®(Abbott)	HeartMate 3 ® (Abbott)

Fig. 1. First-, second-, and third-generation left ventricular assist devices (*Created by* SE Schroeder, 2022).

than 1 (calculated by systolic pulmonary artery pressure—diastolic pulmonary artery pressure/central venous pressure).[12]

Medical management for acute right-sided HF should focus on decreasing volume overload (with diuretics or continuous renal replacement therapy if failing diuretics) and the use of vasoactive agents to help with contractility and maintenance of perfusion (**Table 4**). If vasoactive agents are unsuccessful in maintaining perfusion tRVADs are indicated. The goal with tRVAD use is to pull blood from the inferior vena cava or right atrium, bypass the right ventricle to allow for rest, and propel blood in the pulmonary artery system to promote forward blood flow. These devices could be removed as early as 24 hours, but oftentimes tRVADs remain in place in for a minimum of 72 hours after which weaning attempts are implemented to determine if the patient is ready for deactivation and removal.

When considering placement of a tRVAD, the medical team determines if the patient meets indications for device placement, goal blood pressure parameters, device type and cannulation strategies, and anticoagulation strategies. Nursing considerations include positioning of the patient based on the type of the device used (log-rolling, skin assessment for pressure ulcers, and having additional help with repositioning to ensure stability of the lines), monitoring for the effects of hemolysis (dark tea-colored urine, worsening kidney function), and monitoring for abnormal tRVAD numbers that warrant discussions with the providers on the case (alarms, malpositioned devices, or abnormal blood pressure).

TOTAL ARTIFICIAL HEART

There is a small subset of patients who suffer from biventricular failure, whereby a total artificial heart may be considered. However, this is only used as a BTT strategy at a cardiac transplantation center. Early research on the total artificial heart (late 1960s) was largely unsuccessful due to poor cardiac transplantation survival rates. As survival improved in cardiac transplantation over the next decade, total artificial heart therapy

Table 2
Pivotal trials for mechanical circulatory support

Trial	Year	Purpose of the Trial	Devices Used
REMATCH Randomized Evaluation of Mechanical Assistance for the Treatment of Congestive Heart Failure[8]	2001	Compare long-term LVAD implantations to optimal guideline-driven medical therapy in individuals with end-stage heart failure who otherwise do not qualify for cardiac transplantation	Medications vs HeartMate XVE
HM2 vs XVE trial Advanced Heart Failure Treated with Continuous Flow Left Ventricular Assist Device[22]	2009	Reported results of randomized trial and clinical outcomes in those receiving a pulsatile-flow LVAD vs a continuous-flow LVAD	Heartmate II vs Heartmate XVE (2:1 ratio)
HM2 Destination Therapy Trial (HM2 DT) Outcomes in Advanced Heart Failure Patients with Left Ventricular Assist Devices for Destination Therapy[23]	2012	Compare outcomes between the primary patient cohort (BTT) to the later enrolled patient cohort (DT)	HeartMate II
HVAD ADVANCE Trial Use of an Intrapericardial, Continuous-Flow, Centrifugal Pump in Patients Awaiting Heart Transplantation[24]	2012	To assess the effectiveness of the HVAD LVAD system on survival, functional outcomes, quality of life, and adverse events	HVAD as BTT
ENDURANCE Trial Intrapericardial Left Ventricular Assist Device for Advanced Heart Failure[25]	2017	To assess the safety, efficacy, and outcomes following the implantation of a centrifugal-flow pump compared with an axial flow pump	HVAD vs HM2
ENDURANCE2 Trial HVAD: The ENDURANCE Supplemental Trial[26]	2018	Post hoc analysis to prospectively investigate the significance of blood pressure management regarding strokes in those receiving an HVAD LVAD	HVAD vs HM2 LVAD (2:1 ratio)
Momentum 3 Trial A Fully Magnetically Levitated Left Ventricular Assist Device-Final Report[9]	2019	To investigate the efficacy and end points between a centrifugal-flow LVAD and axial-flow LVAD	HM3 vs HM2 (1:1 ratio)

Abbreviations: BTT, bridge to transplant; DT, destination therapy; HM2, Heartmate II; HM3, HeartMate 3; HVAD, HeartWare HVAD system; LVAD, left ventricular assist device; XVE, HeartMate XVE (first generation).

Table 3
Similarities and differences of durable left ventricular assist devices currently used

Device	Type of Flow	Parameters	Concerns
Heartmate II	Axial, continuous	Flow ranges 3–8 LPM Speed 8800–10,000 RPM Pulse index (PI) ranges 3–8 Power ranges 5–8 W	Pump malposition with weight loss Pump thrombus ± stroke risk Bleeding (epistaxis, GI bleeding, head bleeds) Infection at driveline site
HeartWare HVAD System	Centrifugal, continuous	Flow ranges 4–6 LPM Speed ranges 2400–4000 RPM Peak to trough 2–4 L/min/beat Power ranges 3–7 W	Pump malposition with weight loss Pump thrombus ± stroke risk Bleeding (epistaxis, GI bleeding, head bleeds) Infection at driveline site
HeartMate 3	Centrifugal with full magnetically levitation, continuous	Flow ranges 3–8 Speed 4800–6000+ Pulse index (PI) ranges 3–8 Power ranges 3–7 W	Pump malposition with weight loss Pump thrombus ± stroke risk (although lower) Bleeding (lower) Infection at driveline site

Abbreviations: GI, gastrointestinal; LPM, liters per minute; PI, pulsatile index; RPM, revolutions per minute; W, watts

still stuttered due to the significant mortality risk. When total artificial hearts began to be used as a BTT in selected populations, momentum with gained with 79% survival to cardiac transplantation.[13] Despite attempts to discharge patients with total artificial hearts from the hospital, this device is used mostly on an inpatient basis at cardiac transplantation centers. Nurses working with these devices require special training, including dressing change frequency, management of cannulas, anticoagulation strategies, and situations that could arise requiring further guidance from the medical team.

HEART TRANSPLANTATION

Based on the American College of Cardiology (ACC)/American Heart Association (AHA) guidelines,[14] indications for cardiac transplantation in adults are fairly universal in the United States. These include end-stage HF (New York Heart Association functional class III to IV symptoms and ACC/AHA stage D symptoms), refractory cardiogenic shock with use of temporary devices, severe cardiogenic shock requiring dependence on inotrope therapy (eg, Dobutamine or Milrinone), end-stage congenital heart disease, recurrent or refractory ventricular arrhythmias, or recurrent angina without surgical revascularization options.[14] Contraindications to transplantation include worsening end-organ dysfunction (irreversible kidney, liver or pulmonary disease) or relatively recent hematologic or solid organ malignancy within the last 5 to 7 years based on each individual transplant center's guidelines. Obesity with a body mass index greater than 35 and advanced age greater than 70 years of age are also carefully considered in each center.[14]

Table 4
Vasoactive drugs for management of acute heart failure[27,28]

Drug	Mechanism of Action	Dosing	Special Considerations
Dobutamine (IV)	Inotrope Raises blood pressure Increases cardiac output	2–10 mcg/kg/min	May cause tachycardia; less effect of RV and LV offloading Increases myocardial demand
Dopamine (IV)	Inotrope Coronary vasodilation Increases blood pressure *High doses = vasoconstriction	1–20 mcg/kg/min	Increased heart rates Arrhythmias HTN
Epinephrine (IV)	Vasopressor Inotrope Increases blood pressure Adds protection to the right ventricle	0.01–0.2 mcg/kg/min	Hyperglycemia Hypoperfusion at high doses to the periphery and gastric mucosa
Milrinone (IV)	Inotrope Pulmonary vasodilator Decreases HR	0.125–0.750 mcg/kg/min	May cause arrhythmias; may induce hypotension
Nitric oxide (INHL)	Pulmonary vasodilator	0–40 parts per million	Dizziness Bradycardia Blue lips
Nitroglycerin (IV)	Afterload reduction Vasodilator Decreases blood pressure	5–100 mcg/min	Hypotension Syncope Headache Flushing
Nitroprusside (IV)	Afterload reduction Vasodilator Decreases blood pressure	0.3–0.5 mcg/kg/min	Hypotension Cyanide toxicity Nausea Bradycardia
Norepinephrine (IV)	Inotrope Vasoconstriction Increases blood pressure	0.02–1 mcg/kg/min	HTN Arrhythmias Bradycardia Headache
Vasopressin (IV)	Inotrope Vasoconstriction Increases blood pressure	0.01–0.04 units/min	Arrhythmias Mesenteric ischemia Nausea Bronchospasm Bradycardia

Abbreviations: HR, heart rate; HTN, hypertension; INHL, inhaled; IV, intravenous; LV, left ventricle; mcg/kg/min, micrograms per kilogram per minute; mcg/min, micrograms per minute; RV, right ventricle; units/min, units per minute.
Doses over 10mcg/kg/min may be used but are rare due to adverse events.
* represents High Doses= Dopamine dosing > 10 micrograms per kilogram per minute.

The United Network of Organ Sharing (UNOS) is responsible for ongoing management of organ allocations through the United States. Each individual placed on the UNOS transplant wait list is given a "status" ranking describing the severity of illness and the urgency in needing organ allocation.[14] The UNOS allocation guidelines recently changed in October 2018 to reduce weight list mortality, improve organ allocation equity, and improve geographical organ sharing. **Table 5** describes new

Table 5
United Network of Organ Sharing recently revised allocation status criteria[15,16]

Status	Criteria for Listing
1	• Veno-arterial extracorporeal membranous oxygenation (VA-ECMO) • dLVAD with life-threatening ventricular arrhythmias • Non-dischargeable biventricular (BiVAD) mechanical circulatory support
2	• Use of an intra-aortic balloon pump (IABP) • Non-dischargeable dLVAD • Falling or malfunctioning dLVAD • Ventricular arrhythmias without MCS in place • BiVAD, total artificial heart, VAD for single ventricle • Temporary RVAD or LVAD
3	• Dependency on multiple inotropes or single high-dose inotrope with continuous hemodynamic monitoring • VA-ECMO after 7 d or IABP/percutaneous temporary MCS • Dischargeable dLVAD for discretionary 30 d • Single inotrope with continuous hemodynamic monitoring • Non-dischargeable dLVAD on support > 14 d • dLVAD without complications
4	• Dischargeable dLVAD • Retransplant • Intractable angina with known unrevascularizable coronary artery disease • Hypertrophic, restrictive cardiomyopathy • Amyloidosis • Chronic inotrope use without hemodynamic monitoring
5	• Multiorgan waitlist (at least one additional organ waitlist)
6	• All other remaining candidates who are actively listed on a waitlist

Abbreviations: BiVAD, biventricular ventricular assist device; dLVAD, durable left ventricular assist device; IABP, intra-aortic balloon pump; MCS, mechanical circulatory support; RVAD, right ventricular assist device; VA-ECMO, veno-arterial extracorporeal membranous oxygenation.

allocation criteria.[15] Nurses working with cardiac transplant candidates will require special training for management and care of the cardiac transplanted patient.

There has been much discussion on the effects of the revised six-tiered allocation system from UNOS for patients with durable LVADs implanted that are waiting for a suitable donor. The year before the change in the allocation system, there was a significant utilization of durable LVADs. However, following the change in allocation, the usage of durable LVAD dropped significantly. There was a significant increase in usage of temporary devices. Also, following the change in the allocation system, more transplant recipients were already in the hospital as compared with prior years where a majority of individuals were being called into the hospital for transplantation.[15] The effects of the allocation system on durable LVAD therapy have resulted in the perception of de-incentivizing the benefits of durable LVAD whereby individuals with durable LVADs in place have a lower transplant waitlist status as compared with those who receive the benefits of temporary devices.[16]

Another important factor to consider is where donor hearts come from. Traditionally, primary sources of organ donors came from donation after brain death. Brain death is established by a battery of tests, including the inability to breathe on their own when off the ventilator. More recently, organ donors are established through donation after circulatory (or cardiac) death. Once circulatory death has been established, organ retrieval takes place and the donor heart is restarted. The heart is then transported in a machine, maintaining a beat throughout transport.[17] With the additional donor options from circulatory death and organs coming from donors with high-risk behaviors, such as drug use and other mechanisms of death,[18] more hearts are now available for transplantation.

CARE OF PATIENTS WITH MECHANICAL CIRCULATORY SUPPORT

Patients with MCS, whether it is a durable LVAD or a temporary device, require care in the cardiac ICU. Nurses need to know what preparations are needed to ready patients for a durable LVAD surgery as well as patients undergoing an urgent temporary device.

Care of Patients with Durable Left Ventricular Assist Devices

Preoperatively, as time allows, patients undergoing surgery for a durable LVAD require education to understand the implantation of the device and the postoperative care and management. This education may be delivered by an LVAD coordinator or the bedside nursing staff. Special training is required to educate the patients and their care givers. Other preoperative preparations include placement of surgical lines (a Swan-Ganz catheter, a central line, and an arterial line). Laboratory values should be reviewed the morning of surgery to monitor for abnormalities affecting the implantation of the LVAD, including infection or worsening end-organ dysfunction (eg, kidneys or liver). A Foley catheter is often placed preoperatively to monitor urinary output. The nurse should ensure that the patient (or next of kin) has signed the informed consent for surgery.

Following durable LVAD implantation, there are several nursing tasks to perform, and based on staffing in the cardiac ICU, there may be two nurses assigned to care for patients in the immediate postoperative period. Blood pressure management, monitoring for acute bleeding, balancing acid-base levels, and monitoring for the appropriate function of the newly implanted LVAD are among the many responsibilities for the cardiac ICU nurse(s) to monitor. Owing to the flow pattern through a durable LVAD, regardless of the axial or centrifugal flow, oftentimes there are no palpable pulses and certain types of automatic blood pressure cuffs do not accurately measure systolic and diastolic pressures. Therefore, the gold standard for blood pressure monitoring is through the mean arterial pressures (MAP) obtained by Doppler. **Box 1** displays the steps for obtaining an opening pressure by Doppler or MAP.

Postoperatively patients who have undergone durable LVAD placement need a MAP maintained between 60 and 90 mm Hg. Thus, multiple intravenous (IV) medications may be used for blood pressure parameter management as well as maintaining contractility and protection of the right ventricle. These medications may include

---

Box 1
Steps for obtaining mean arterial pressures by Doppler

1. Place a traditional blood pressure cuff on the upper or lower arm

2. Locate a palpable pulse in the wrist (radial or ulnar) or in the antecubital area; Pulse may sound different in an MCS patient compared to a non-MCS patient

3. Pump up the blood pressure cuff 10 mm Hg past the disappearance of the sound

4. Slowly let out the air of the sphygmomanometer, paying close attention to the first sound heard, equaling the Doppler opening pressure (known as the MAP).

epinephrine, vasopressin, dobutamine and/or milrinone, norepinephrine, or dopamine. Postoperatively patients will have dressings to the midsternal incision, covering the durable LVAD exit site (in the abdomen), and over the chest tubes designed to drain any additional bleeding and healing fluids. All dressings should be monitored for signs of infection or bleeding.

Significance of chest tube output is determined based on criteria from the surgeon performing the surgery. Nursing staff in the cardiac ICU will monitor chest tube outputs according to the policies of the nursing floor and postoperative surgical orders. The durable LVAD should be attached to electrical wall power unless the individual is transported off the floor for a specific reason. Patients with durable LVADs may also be on battery power support to promote activity and rehabilitation. Foley catheters are used for monitoring urine output. However, the Foley catheter should be removed in a timely manner to limit risk of infection.

Ventricular arrhythmias are common in patients with durable LVADs due to a variety of situations including interference from the inflow cannula affecting conduction or causing additional stimuli in the myocardium. Keep in mind that at baseline, patients with LVADs are more prone to arrhythmias overall due to their advanced HF. On return from the operating room, patients usually have a 12-lead electrocardiogram (ECG) to ensure that there are no acute changes (ST segment elevation and depression). Unfortunately, due to the electrical internal interference caused from a durable LVAD, the ECG is generally nondiagnostic due to the artifact (fuzziness) noted within the isoelectric line. This does not mean that an ECG should not be done; it just means that there

Table 6
Pump parameter differences based on the clinical scenario

	Flow	Speed	PI	Power	Other
Tamponade	↓	↓ ↑	↓	→	Not enough blood getting in to pump
Right Ventricular Failure	↓	→	↓	→	Not enough forward flow
Suction Events	↓	↓	↓	↑ →	Usually due to arrhythmias or not enough flow getting in to LV
Hypotension	↓	→	↓	→	Low flow in= Low flow out
Hypertension	↓	→	↑	→	High pressure= low pump output
Arrhythmias	↓	→	↓	→	Will be tolerated fairly well; likely will NOT lose consciousness

*Remember that all devices are a little different. This table represents the HeartMate 3 device from clinical practice as this is the only pump currently being implanted in the United States at the moment; LV, left ventricle; PI, Pulse Index.

are differences noted within this patient population that should be considered during interpretation.

Understanding parameters that come from each particular durable LVAD used is important in the management and treatment of patients. **Table 6** describes adverse events that may be seen in patients with durable LVADs, including cardiac tamponade, right ventricular failure, suction events, hypotension, hypertension, arrhythmias, and other pump malfunctions.

Although not well described in the literature, inhaled nitric oxide may be delivered in the immediate postoperative period to increase pulmonary vasodilation and decrease right ventricular afterload. This limits the risk of right ventricular failure. Several factors influence readiness to wean from the ventilator and extubation to alternative oxygen delivery, including hemodynamic stability with minimal inotrope support, stable right ventricular function, and normalized arterial blood gases.[19] To limit bacterial blood stream infections, readiness for removal of surgical lines needs to be assessed daily. Patients recovering from cardiac surgery need to undergo pulmonary toileting and lung volume expansion with the use of nebulized bronchodilators, suctioning, and incentive spirometry to minimize pulmonary dysfunction. A key reminder in effective airway clearance is appropriate pain management to facilitate airway dilation and removal of secretions.[19]

A variety of anticoagulants are used in the ICU to decrease the risk of thrombus in the pump itself. These include vitamin K antagonists (eg, warfarin or Coumadin), IV anticoagulation (eg, heparin), and oral antiplatelet agents (eg, aspirin). All of these medications are essential to maintain functionality of a durable LVAD. Heparin is generally initiated postoperatively within 48 hours and monitored either by the activated partial thromboplastin (aPTT) or anti-factor Xa laboratory values. Heparin prevents further clot formation. While on heparin, oftentimes warfarin is usually started for long-term management of anticoagulation. Because it takes approximately 3 days for the warfarin to reach a therapeutic range, both are given simultaneously. Warfarin dosing varies among patients as it depends on dietary intake, liver function, and other patient factors. An important nursing consideration when caring for patients on warfarin is to monitor the international normalized ratio (INR). The target INR is based on the patient's history of bleeding, intolerance to medications, or drug allergies. Most patients with durable LVADs have a target INR of 2 to 3. This means the blood is 2 to 3 times "thinner" than usual. Aspirin is oftentimes started within 24 hours after a durable LVAD implant. Aspirin decreases platelet aggregation thereby preventing thrombus formation inside the pump, limiting risk of stroke.

Nutrition is another important aspect of care in the post-implant recovery phase. Increasing caloric consumption as well as protein intake assists healing. Adequate nutrition will also help in stabilizing an appropriate bowel regimen and mitigating pain.

Activity postimplantation is important. Sternal precautions should be in place for a minimum of 8 weeks to allow for proper bone healing. Physical activity will increase breathing efforts to assist in pulmonary toileting, decrease risks of pneumonia, and promote improved bowel motility to establish a healthy bowel regimen. Generally, being active sooner rather than later postoperatively helps patients get home faster.

Upon stabilization, patients with a durable LVAD will move out of the ICU to a lower level of care (eg, Progressive Care or Cardiac Care units)to prepare for discharge readiness. Nurses educate patients and care givers about post-discharge care of the LVAD as they work toward obtaining a better quality of life than pre-implantation (see below).

Care of Patients with Temporary Devices

Temporary mechanical devices are useful in situations such as acute MI, persistent or worsening cardiogenic shock, or sequelae that come from pulmonary emboli or sepsis. Based on the patient's needs, a tLVAD or tRVAD may be placed to improve perfusion and overall outcomes post-MI. Regardless of where the device is placed, there are factors that should be considered when caring for a patient with a temporary device in place.

Indications for Temporary Devices: Patients presenting with an acute MI run the risk of death due to lack of blood flow through the coronary arteries. Following reperfusion therapy (eg, a coronary artery stent or fibrinolytic therapy such as tissue plasminogen activator) for an acute MI, the myocardium may be stunned due to the limited flow, resulting in decreased perfusion for up to 30 days. If this is severe, the patient may undergo placement of a temporary LVAD. The type of device and location of access is based on surgeon or the interventional cardiologist's preference (see **Table 1**).

For example, typical locations for access to arteries for left-sided devices include the right or left femoral arteries, and in certain situation, one of the axillary arteries may also be used. The femoral artery access site places limitations to ambulation, whereas the axillary arteries allow the patient the freedom to walk around. As with any arterial access site, the nurse should monitor the patient for bleeding.

Some devices are also placed during a surgical intervention due to the patient needing increased perfusion following post-cardiotomy shock to temporarily enhance recovery. Access for RVADs with any right-sided HF or presentation for pulmonary emboli with cardiac compromise may include the subclavian or internal jugular veins as well as the femoral veins. As with the left-sided devices, nurses should still monitor for bleeding.

MONITORING AND SURGICAL LINES

Any patient that has a temporary mechanical device should also have a central line for delivery of highly potent medications for hypotension such as epinephrine, vasopressin, dobutamine, milrinone, norepinephrine, or dopamine (see **Table 4**, for more information about vasoactive medications). An arterial line is also highly recommended for more precise blood pressure monitoring when vasoactive agents are being administered. A Foley catheter should be in place to monitor for any early signs of hemolysis (noted by tea-colored urine). Hemolysis generally indicates that the device has broken the hemoglobin cells, posing risk for kidney dysfunction. Refer to **Box 2** for a description of various laboratory values that need to be monitored.

Temporary mechanical devices are placed usually for about 72 hours. However, some patients may keep them in for a few weeks despite not necessarily being

---

Box 2
Laboratory values to monitor

- Complete blood count to monitor for infection and anemia
- Lactic dehydrogenase to monitor for risk of thrombotic events or hemolysis
- Complete metabolic profile to monitor for worsening kidney and liver function
- Lactic acid to monitor for adequate end organ perfusion
- Anticoagulation laboratories (Protime/International Normalized Ratio [PT/INR] or aPTT) depending on the anticoagulant used

indicated by the individual temporary device companies. Nurses who care for patients with temporary mechanical devices undergo educational training to care for these complex patients. Furthermore, most patients with temporary devices are also mechanically ventilated and in the ICU.

SHARED DECISION-MAKING

Multidisciplinary care for patients undergoing temporary or durable (more permanent) devices is crucial to ensure that shared decision-making is used. Shared decisions are important between patients, their families and caregivers, and the medical team. Sometimes these decisions (especially those requiring temporary devices during life-threatening situations) are time sensitive, and patients are unable to speak for themselves. Thus, family members or significant others are involved in the decision-making who act in the best interest of their loved one. Those involved in decision-making need to understand the gravity of the medical condition, the significant risk of mortality when undergoing placement of a temporary device, and the potential adverse effects that come with temporary device such as respiratory failure, worsening multisystem organ failure, increased risk of stroke, and/or death. The family members or significant others need to be well-informed to make the best decision for their loved one in this urgent state.

Decision-making regarding a durable LVAD is different in which there is generally more time to consider the pros and cons of receiving a device. Many members of the multidisciplinary team such as providers, a host of therapists, and other consultants work with the patient and family members/caregivers to carefully consider the patient's candidacy for implantation of a durable LVAD. Social workers are often involved as well as members of the palliative care team to ensure the patients and caregivers understand what life will be like after LVAD placement. In fact, most patients undergo a psychosocial evaluation to aid in the cognitive and emotional readiness for those considering implantation of a durable LVAD. The multidisciplinary approach to candidacy for a durable LVAD is designed to systematically approach candidacy, determining which individuals would benefit from this therapy.[20] Each implanting center that implants durable LVADs develops their own approach to multidisciplinary team discussions.

IMPLICATIONS FOR NURSING ASSESSMENT
Preoperative Nursing Care

When preparing a patient for a durable or a temporary device, before going to the operating room, the nurse should ensure that the consent(s) have been signed, laboratory values have been reviewed for baseline abnormalities, the surgical lines and Foley catheter have been placed, and antibiotics are ready for administration. Various personnel may be responsible for bringing the durable LVAD equipment to the operating room preoperatively including perfusion staff, LVAD coordinators, or other biomedical technicians who work in the LVAD program. Situations that may arise that would cancel or postpone device implantation include infection, respiratory failure with or without mechanical ventilation, persistent and significant ventricular arrhythmias, acute stroke, or worsening end-organ dysfunction. If any of these situations are noted before the device implantation, they should be reported immediately to the cardiothoracic surgeon.

When preparing a patient for temporary mechanical device support, nurses need to realize that this is a very serious, life-threatening situation that requires a critical care management and collaboration among many members of the care team to successfully care for these patients. Members of the care team include, but are not limited to, nursing staff, advanced practice providers, cardiologists, and cardiothoracic surgeons. Preoperatively, nurses should monitor for signs of worsening end-organ dysfunction (eg, worsening kidney or liver function). As discussed, scenarios involving temporary device implantation require nurses to assist family and caregivers in understanding what is going on with their loved ones and bringing them together for discussions with the providers. Nurses may consult with the hospital chaplain and other supportive staff as appropriate, especially when the situation is unexpected.

Postoperative Nursing Care

In the immediate postoperative phase following a durable LVAD implantation, the priority for care is hemodynamic stabilization with use of different vasoactive agents. From there, respiratory therapy assists in management of mechanical ventilation. Nurses are responsible for monitoring laboratory values. Chest tube drainage should be monitored to assess bleeding as well as urinary output. The medical team will provide parameters of what is expected (for chest tube output and urinary output). Nurses working in the cardiac ICU also need to understand various scenarios that would cause alterations in the LVAD parameters, which should be reported to the LVAD team members. Precautions need to be taken regarding the sternotomy incision to promote healing. Following the immediate postoperative period, patients begin having drains and tubes removed, including mechanical ventilation. As discussed, activity and nutrition are of upmost importance to help patients progress to discharge. Patients and their caregiver(s) will also need a significant amount of education about how to manage their power sources, secure their driveline exit sites to minimize infection, and to use all of their remaining LVAD equipment for home. Nurses play an important role in reinforcing the education by the LVAD team with the hands-on aspect of LVAD equipment.

Postoperative care for a temporary mechanical device has a slightly different focus due to the critical nature of the patient. Nurses need to monitor for acute bleeding at the cannulation sites, migratory patterns of these cannulas which could indicate inappropriate function of the mechanical device, end-organ dysfunction (worsening kidney or liver dysfunction) or significant hemolysis (tea-colored urine or unexplained anemia). Once the temporary device has been discontinued, the usual care of the patient is resumed.

IMPLICATIONS FOR DISCHARGE EDUCATION

When preparing the patient and family/caregivers for discharge, there is an extensive amount of education that is required for the successfully caring for the durable LVAD at home. As discussed, this education will likely be delivered by the members of the durable LVAD team and reinforced by the nursing staff in the cardiac ICU and step-down units. Education will include driveline dressing management, showering, management of the pocket controller, understanding alarms, exchanging of power sources from batteries to nighttime power sources, recharging the batteries, and other key steps in management of the durable LVAD to ensure success. This educational process varies between each center depending on specific programmatic protocols. The literature reinforces the importance of involvement of family and caregivers (if available) to promote success post-LVAD implantation leading to discharge. Early on, it is important that the patient feels empowered to manage their durable LVAD. Reinforcing independence helps promote improved quality of life following implantation of a durable LVAD. Nursing staff in the cardiac ICU and step-down unit should use the LVAD coordinators in strategizing plans for establishing patient success with education and LVAD management in the home.

SUMMARY

MCS as an advanced therapy has been used for over 20 years for candidates undergoing durable and temporary mechanical devices. Recent literature suggests that patients who have undergone durable LVAD implantation have improved survival of nearly 85% in the first year following placement of a third-generation ventricular assist device,[10] which has dramatically improved from 25 years ago when there was 20% to 25% survival rate with only medications.[4] Cardiac ICU nurses are integral in the care of individuals undergoing a durable LVAD implantation or acutely having a temporary device placed. Understanding the key concepts of management for this unique and complex patient population is important to optimize success of MCS therapy.

CLINICS CARE POINTS

- The key to survival of a patient suffering from a cardiogenic shock or heart failure is early recognition and intervention.
- MCS patients may not have a palpable pulse or blood pressure by automated cuff. In this setting, doppler pulses and blood pressures are gold standard.
- Blood pressure management in durable MCS is key in preventing adverse events such as strokes.
- MCS patients need to be connected to a power source at all times to ensure appropriate function of the device.

DISCLOSURE

Investigator Grant awarded by Abbott, 2023.

REFERENCES

1. Tsao CW, Aday AW, Almarzooq ZI, et al. Heart Disease and Stroke Statistics—2022 Update: A Report From the American Heart Association. Circulation 2022; 145(8). https://doi.org/10.1161/CIR.0000000000001052.
2. Lee JA, Yanagawa B, An KR, et al. Frailty and pre-frailty in cardiac surgery: a systematic review and meta-analysis of 66,448 patients. J Cardiothorac Surg 2021; 16(1):184.
3. Chen-Scarabelli C, Saravolatz L, Hirsh B, et al. Dilemmas in end-stage heart failure. J Geriatr Cardiol JGC 2015;12(1):57–65.
4. Mozaffarian D, Benjamin EJ, Go AS, et al. Heart Disease and Stroke Statistics—2016 Update: A Report From the American Heart Association. Circulation 2016; 133(4).
5. Bytyçi I, Bajraktari G. Mortality in heart failure patients. Anadolu Kardiyol Derg Anatol J Cardiol 2015;15(1):63–8.
6. AbouEzzeddine OF, Redfield MM. Who Has Advanced Heart Failure? Definition and Epidemiology: who has advanced heart failure? Congest Heart Fail 2011; 17(4):160–8.
7. Trachtenberg B, Cowger J, Jennings DL, et al. HFSA Expert Consensus Statement on the Medical Management of Patients on Durable Mechanical Circulatory

Support. J Card Fail 2023. https://doi.org/10.1016/j.cardfail.2023.01.009. S10719 16423000398.

8. Rose EA, Gelijns AC, Moskowitz AJ, et al. Long-Term Use of a Left Ventricular Assist Device for End-Stage Heart Failure. N Engl J Med 2001;345(20):1435–43.

9. Mehra MR, Uriel N, Naka Y, et al. AA Clinical Update on Vasoactive Medicat Ventricular Assist Device — Final Report. N Engl J Med 2019;380(17):1618–27.

10. Medtronic. Medtronic To Stop Distribution and Sale of HVAD (TM) System.; 2021. Available at: https://news.medtronic.com/2021-06-03-Medtronic-to-Stop-Distribution-and-Sale-of-HVAD-TM-System. Accessed February 22, 2023.

11. Konstam MA, Kiernan MS, Bernstein D, et al. Evaluation and Management of Right-Sided Heart Failure: A Scientific Statement From the American Heart Association. Circulation 2018;137(20). https://doi.org/10.1161/CIR.0000000000000560.

12. Fahad Salam M. Current and Emerging Strategies for RV Shock Management in The Setting of RV Infarct. 2022. ACC: Expert Analysis. Available at: https://www.acc.org/Latest-in-Cardiology/Articles/2021/11/01/12/41/Current-and-Emerging-Strategies-for-RV-Shock-Management. Accessed February 24, 2023.

13. Cook JA, Shah KB, Quader MA, et al. The total artificial heart. J Thorac Dis 2015;7(12):2172–80.

14. Alraies MC, Eckman P. Adult heart transplant: indications and outcomes. J Thorac Dis 2014;6(8):1120–8.

15. Liu J, Yang BQ, Itoh A, et al. Impact of New UNOS Allocation Criteria on Heart Transplant Practices and Outcomes. Transplant Direct 2020;7(1):e642.

16. Li SS, Funamoto M, Wolfe S, et al. Effects of the New Heart Allocation System on Choice of Mechanical Circulatory Support as a Bridge to Transplant. J Heart Lung Transplant 2022;41(4):S15.

17. Rajab TK, Singh SK. Donation After Cardiac Death Heart Transplantation in America Is Clinically Necessary and Ethically Justified. Circ Heart Fail 2018;11(3):e004884.

18. Copeland H, Knezevic I, Baran DA, et al. Donor heart selection: Evidence-based guidelines for providers. J Heart Lung Transplant 2023;42(1):7–29.

19. Schroeder SE, Schettle SD. A guide to mechanical circulatory support: a primer for ventricular assist device (VAD) clinicians. Chapter: postoperative management of the VAD patient. Switzerland: Springer, Cham; 2022.

20. Rhoades B, Hamm H, Stewart S. A guide to mechanical circulatory support: a primer for ventricular assist device (VAD) clinicians. Chapter: patient optimization prior to MCS. Switzerland: Springer, Cham; 2022.

21. Saffarzadeh A, Bonde P. Options for temporary mechanical circulatory support. J Thorac Dis 2015;7(12):2102–11.

22. Slaughter MS, Rogers JG, Milano CA, et al. Advanced heart failure treated with continuous-flow left ventricular assist device. N Engl J Med 2009;361(23):2241–51.

23. Park SJ, Milano CA, Tatooles AJ, et al. Outcomes in Advanced Heart Failure Patients With Left Ventricular Assist Devices for Destination Therapy. Circ Heart Fail 2012;5(2):241–8.

24. Aaronson KD, Slaughter MS, Miller LW, et al. Use of an intrapericardial, continuous-flow, centrifugal pump in patients awaiting heart transplantation. Circulation 2012;125(25):3191–200.

25. Rogers JG, Pagani FD, Tatooles AJ, et al. Intrapericardial Left Ventricular Assist Device for Advanced Heart Failure. N Engl J Med 2017;376(5):451–60.

26. Milano CA, Rogers JG, Tatooles AJ, et al. HVAD: The ENDURANCE Supplemental Trial. JACC Heart Fail 2018;6(9):792–802.

27. Shankar A, Gurumurthy G, Sridharan L, et al. A Clinical Update on Vasoactive Medication in the Management of Cardiogenic Shock. Clin Med Insights Cardiol 2022;16. 117954682210750.
28. Farmakis D, Agostoni P, Baholli L, et al. A pragmatic approach to the use of inotropes for the management of acute and advanced heart failure: An expert panel consensus. Int J Cardiol 2019;297:83–90.

Special Populations

Cardiovascular Disease in Women: An Update for Nurses

John R. Blakeman, PhD, RN, PCCN-K[a],*, Ann L. Eckhardt, PhD, RN[b]

KEYWORDS

• Women • Cardiovascular disease • Nursing • Signs and symptoms • Heart disease

KEY POINTS

• Women have different risk factors for cardiovascular disease (CVD) than men and diagnostic tests have varying efficacy because of physiologic differences in women.
• Women are more likely to experience ischemia related to microvascular dysfunction with no obstructed coronary arteries.
• Chest pain is the most common symptom of acute coronary syndrome regardless of sex or gender, but women may not report chest pain because the experience is characterized as discomfort, heaviness, or pressure.
• Some women may see an obstetrician-gynecologist (OB-GYN) provider for primary care, so it is important that OB-GYN providers provide primary prevention and monitoring for CVD.

INTRODUCTION AND BACKGROUND

Cardiovascular disease (CVD) is the leading cause of death for women.[1] Even so, women have historically been under-represented in CVD clinical trials and research.[2,3] In clinical practice, women have often been undertreated and experienced worse outcomes than men with CVD.[2,3] Moreover, women's experiences of CVD are often labeled as "atypical," whereas men's experiences are more often called "typical,"[4] which leads to delay in diagnostic testing and treatment.

Since the turn of the twenty-first century, increased focus has been placed on CVD in women. It is critical that nurses and other health care providers understand the experiences of women diagnosed with CVD. Women have different cardiovascular risk factors, and the accuracy of diagnostic tests differs based on sex. Registered nurses must recognize the unique needs of women with CVD and the symptom profile in women to provide high-quality care and patient education. The goal of this paper is

[a] Mennonite College of Nursing, Illinois State University, Campus Box 5810, Normal, IL 61790, USA; [b] Department of Graduate Nursing, College of Nursing and Health Innovation, University of Texas at Arlington, Pickard Hall 516, 411 S. Nedderman Dr, Arlington, TX 76019, USA
* Corresponding author.
E-mail address: jrblak1@ilstu.edu

Nurs Clin N Am 58 (2023) 439–459
https://doi.org/10.1016/j.cnur.2023.05.009
nursing.theclinics.com

to review the latest information about CVD in women, including risk factors, symptoms, diagnostic testing, and educational priorities.

We use the term women broadly throughout this article, incorporating aspects of sex and gender. We note, however, that sex and gender are different variables,[5] and can independently affect CVD.[6–8] We also acknowledge that additional special considerations exist for transgender women, gender nonconforming and nonbinary individuals who may be chromosomally female, intersex individuals, and many others.[9] In this paper, we have specifically focused on the experience of cisgender, chromosomally female individuals—that is, women who were born female and identify as women. However, we encourage readers to seek out resources supporting the experiences of all individuals, regardless of identity category.

COMMON CARDIOVASCULAR PROBLEMS IN WOMEN

At the root of most CVD is atherosclerosis, an inflammatory process involving the accumulation of lipids and white blood cells in the walls of the arteries. Because atherosclerosis progresses, plaques form, ultimately leading to a narrowing of the blood vessel lumen; plaque rupture or erosion may lead to acute thrombosis, which causes cardiovascular events like acute coronary syndrome (ACS) (unstable angina, non-ST-elevation myocardial infarction, and ST-elevation myocardial infarction), stroke, and acute ischemic limb.[10] Thus, preventing atherosclerosis is a priority for prevention. Although it is beyond the scope of this paper to detail the complex pathophysiology and epidemiology of every CVD experienced by women, below we have highlighted particularly salient issues pertinent to women for leading cardiovascular conditions, including coronary artery disease (CAD), stroke, and heart failure.

Coronary Artery Disease

At the most basic level, CAD occurs when atherosclerotic plaques progress and one or more coronary arteries become narrowed, reducing blood flow to the myocardium. If one of these atherosclerotic plaques ruptures or erodes, ACS may occur.[10] However, it is increasingly recognized that microvascular dysfunction is common in women, present in as many as 2 in 3 women who undergo clinically indicated coronary angiography.[11] Instead of major coronary arteries (eg, left anterior descending, left circumflex) being stenosed, small, more distal arterioles may become narrowed or obstructed, causing ischemia with no obstructive coronary arteries, or INOCA.[11] Women may present with common symptoms of CAD, undergo coronary angiography, and be told that their coronary vessels are "normal," even though they have unrecognized microvascular dysfunction.[11] Unfortunately, even though the larger coronary arteries in these women are not involved, they are still more likely to die from a cardiovascular problem within 10 years and have up to 10 times higher odds of hospital admission with heart failure with preserved ejection fraction (HFpEF).[11–13] Additionally, women are often more likely to develop long term, chronic angina because of this microvascular dysfunction, and this form of angina may be more challenging to treat.[11] Thus, nurses' attention to the possibility of microvascular disease in women is essential.

Two additional related conditions affecting women more often than men include Takotsubo syndrome and spontaneous coronary artery dissection (SCAD).[14,15] Takotsubo syndrome is also called Takotsubo cardiomyopathy, apical ballooning syndrome, broken heart syndrome, and stress cardiomyopathy. Although emotional triggers (eg, death of a loved one, loss of job) have often been linked to Takotsubo syndrome, as many as one-third of patients cannot identify such a stressor.[15] Thus, nurses must recognize that Takotsubo syndrome is possible, even without an identifiable stressor. **Table 1** highlights information about these 2 diagnoses. Given that these conditions have only recently received significant research attention, clinical evidence about diagnoses continues to emerge.

Stroke

Stroke is slightly more common in women (lifetime risk 25.1%) than in men (lifetime risk 24.7%), and it is the fifth most common cause of death for women in the United States.[16,17] However, Black women in the United States have higher mortality from stroke and the highest overall prevalence of stroke (4.9%), compared with White, non-Hispanic women (2.5%), Hispanic women (1.7%), and Asian women (1.0%).[1] Some reasons why Black women are at higher risk of stroke include a higher prevalence of risk factors, including chronic inflammation from psychosocial and environmental stressors, hypertension, smoking, diabetes, obesity, and sickle cell disease.[1,18]

Heart Failure

Although men and women can experience heart failure with reduced ejection fraction (HFrEF, ejection fraction $\leq$ 40%), heart failure with mildly reduced ejection fraction (ejection fraction 41%–49%), and HFpEF (ejection fraction $\geq$50%), women are almost three times more likely than men to be diagnosed with HFpEF.[19] Comorbidities such as long-standing hypertension, obesity, diabetes, chronic kidney disease, atrial fibrillation, and amyloidosis contribute to the development of HFpEF.[19] Other risk factors for heart failure may affect women more severely than men, including depression, anxiety, and psychosocial stress.[20]

In addition to HFpEF, peripartum cardiomyopathy (a cause of HFrEF) is also a consideration for pregnant women, occurring in 0.01% to 0.1% of pregnancies brought to delivery.[19] Peripartum cardiomyopathy tends to happen in the third trimester or early postpartum period, more often affecting Black women and those older than 30 years of age, along with women who experience hypertensive disorders of pregnancy and exhibit common cardiovascular risk factors.[19] Although the incidence is low, it is still a consideration for nurses and other health care providers, especially those working in peripartum settings.

RISK FACTORS FOR CARDIOVASCULAR DISEASE IN WOMEN

Several factors increase the risk of CVD, irrespective of sex and gender. Nurses are ideally positioned to educate women about these various risk factors and to implement evidence-based strategies to help women reduce their CVD risk. **Box 1** highlights these important risk factors. Many of these risk factors have been documented and emphasized for decades. Still, they remain essential, given that the prevalence and incidence of many of these risk factors in the United States population have continued to grow or remain at higher-than-desirable levels.[1,3] For example, nearly 43% of women in the United States have hypertension, one of the most important risk factors for CVD development and progression, and hypertension remains uncontrolled in approximately two-thirds of these people.[1] Of note, hypertension is markedly more prevalent in Black women (57.6%) than in Asian women (42.1%), Hispanic women (40.8%), and White, and non-Hispanic women (40.5%) in the United States.[1] Nurses play an essential role in accurately measuring blood pressure, and many blood pressure measurements are taken improperly.[21] **Table 2** highlights key recommendations for measuring blood pressure precisely and the consequences of imprecise measurement. Additionally, Hispanic and Black women in the United States have a higher

Table 1
Key features of spontaneous coronary artery dissection and Takotsubo syndrome

	Spontaneous Coronary Artery Dissection	Takotsubo Syndrome
Overall problem	• Dissection of the coronary artery, followed by the development of a hematoma in the wall of the coronary artery or blockage of blood flow because of a disruption in the arterial wall	• Acute but transient development of left-ventricular dysfunction (reduced left ventricular ejection fraction), generally followed by improvement in ejection fraction
Prevalence in women vs men	• At least 3 in 4 patients with SCAD are women • Often affects younger women (age 40–50) • Exact prevalence metrics are difficult to establish, given under-recognition/underdiagnosis	• Affects women about five times more than men • Exact prevalence metrics are difficult to establish given under-recognition/underdiagnosis
Common precipitating events[a]	• Connective tissue disorders (eg, Marfan syndrome, Ehlers-Danlos syndrome) • Emotional stressors • Fibromuscular dysplasia • Hormonal therapies (eg, birth control, hormone replacement therapy) • Perimenopause • Physical stressors • Pregnancy	• Emotional stressors (eg, loss of job, death of a loved one) • Physical stressors (eg, acute illness)
Theories about etiology[b]	• Hemorrhage from within the wall of the vessel • Hormones, pregnancy, unknown arteriopathies, inflammation, and genetics may all play a role • Tear of the intimal layer of the artery	• A surge of catecholamines may explain part of the pathophysiology
Signs and Symptoms	• Chest pain/discomfort • Diaphoresis • Elevated cardiac troponin • Nausea and/or vomiting • Shortness of breath • ST-segment and t-wave abnormalities	• Chest pain/discomfort • ECG with ST-segment and t-wave abnormalities • Elevated cardiac troponin • Left-ventricular wall motion abnormality on echocardiography (usually apical, basal, or focal) • Shortness of breath • Symptoms consistent with acute heart failure
Notes for nurses	• Both may mimic CAD/ACS, leading to misdiagnosis • Clinicians must keep diagnoses in mind when patients present with consistent symptoms, especially when other precipitating events are present and/or when other common diagnoses are ruled out	

Abbreviations: ACS, acute coronary syndrome; CAD, coronary artery disease; ECG, electrocardiogram; SCAD, spontaneous coronary artery dissection.
[a] Both spontaneous coronary artery dissection and Takotsubo syndrome may occur in individuals without any obvious precipitating events.
[b] The true etiology/pathophysiologic basis for these diagnoses is not fully understood at this time.
Data from Refs.[14,15]

Box 1
Selected important risk factors for cardiovascular disease development and progression

- Advancing age
- Chronic kidney disease
- Diabetes mellitus
- Diet high in saturated fats and trans fats
- Elevated LDL-C levels (general goal is LDL-C < 70 mg/dL in individuals with existing atherosclerotic disease, < 100 mg/dL in high-risk individuals, and < 130 mg/dL in other populations)
- First-degree relative (eg, biologic parent, biologic sibling) with history of premature atherosclerotic cardiovascular disease (age < 55 for males and < 65 for females)
- Hypertension
- Metabolic syndrome (elevated glucose, hypertension, large waist circumference, low levels of HDL, and elevated triglycerides)
- Overweight (BMI 25.0–29.9 kg/m^2) and obesity (BMI $\geq$ 30 kg/m^2)
- Sedentary lifestyle
- Sleep disorders (eg, obstructive sleep apnea) and getting less than 7 or > 10 hours of sleep per night
- South Asian ancestry (higher cardiovascular risk than other ethnicities)
- Tobacco use, including smoking, vaping, and using smokeless products
- Triglyceride level > 175 mg/dL on 3 or more occasions

Abbreviations: BMI, body mass index; LDL-C, low-density lipoprotein cholesterol; HDL, high-density lipoprotein cholesterol.

Data from Refs.[1,32,59]

Table 2
Clinics care points: recommendations for accurate blood pressure measurement

Recommendation	Consequences of Not Following the Recommendation
Use the correct size blood pressure cuff	A cuff too small for the arm may add 2–10 mm Hg
Apply the blood pressure cuff to a bare arm, not over clothing	Taking blood pressure over clothing may add 5–50 mm Hg
Ensure the arm is supported and placed at heart level	An unsupported arm may add 10 mm Hg
Ensure the legs are not crossed and the feet are flat on the floor	Crossing legs may add 2–8 mm Hg
Do not talk during the measurement	A patient talking or actively listening to someone talk can add 10 mm Hg
Ensure the patient empties their bladder prior to measurement	A full bladder may add 10 mm Hg
The patient's back should be supported, as should their feet	Unsupported back/feet may add 6.5 mm Hg

Data from Ref.[57]

prevalence of overweight and obesity (78%) than the national average of 68%.[3] Diabetes mellitus is experienced by about 14% of Hispanic women and 13% of Black women, compared with the national average of 9%.[3]

Although these universal risk factors are always important and harm CVD health, women's CVD risk increases substantially during the postmenopausal period.[22] Menopause does not cause CVD, but hormones such as estrogen are present in higher quantities before menopause and may play a protective role before menopause.[23] Other changes that occur with the onset of menopause, such as weight gain, a higher incidence of depression, sleep disturbances, and higher LDL and apolipoprotein B levels, also increase CVD risk.[23] Premature menopause—that is, menopause that occurs before age 40—in particular increases a woman's long-term risk of CVD.[23]

Aside from the accelerated risk around the onset of menopause, women are also at an increased risk for CVD given several sex-related and gender-related factors, as shown in **Box 2**. In the United States, women have a nearly 13% chance of developing breast cancer in their lifetime, compared with 0.13% for men.[24] Treating breast cancer with chemotherapeutic agents and/or radiation may increase the lifetime risk of CVD, including CAD, heart failure, and arrhythmias.[25] The use of hormonal contraceptives, especially by women with other CVD risk factors, may also increase the risk of thrombosis, but the specific hormonal formulation of these products appears to affect the degree of overall CVD risk.[26] Women are also at increased risk of other autoimmune problems that increase CVD risk, including conditions like rheumatoid arthritis and systemic lupus erythematosus.[26] Systemic scleroderma, which may lead to inflammation and scarring across the cardiovascular system, is almost five times more common in women than men.[27]

Pregnancy-related complications also increase CVD risk. Gestational hypertension, preeclampsia, and eclampsia increase cardiovascular risk in women, especially in the presence of additional risk factors.[28] Women with preeclampsia during their first

---

Box 2
Selected sex-related and gender-related cardiovascular risk factors for women

- Pregnancy-related hypertension (gestational hypertension, preeclampsia, and eclampsia)
- Preterm delivery or delivery of a child with a low birth weight
- Polycystic ovarian syndrome (related to higher incidence of metabolic syndrome and diabetes mellitus)
- Menopause prior to age 40
- Certain hormonal contraceptives, especially when used by patients with additional cardiovascular risk factors
- Inflammation from autoimmune disorders, including systemic lupus erythematosus and rheumatoid arthritis. Sclerosis is caused by the autoimmune condition scleroderma.
- Breast cancer treatment with chemotherapeutic agents, especially doxorubicin and epirubicin. Additional agents with cardiovascular risk potential include cisplatin, 5-fluorouracil, tamoxifen, letrozole, anastrozole, and paclitaxel.
- Breast cancer treatment with radiation, especially when the heart is in the path of radiation.
- Adverse life events, especially physical, sexual, and emotional abuse
- Smoking or drug use as a method of weight loss or weight maintenance

Data from Refs.[7,23,25,26,28]

pregnancy are almost two times more likely to experience CVD than those who do not. Other pregnancy-related problems, such as gestational diabetes mellitus and preterm delivery, also increase CVD risk.[22]

In addition to biologically driven, sex-specific factors increasing cardiovascular risk, various gender-driven factors affect CVD, and the gender construct stands as an independent risk factor for CVD. For example, O'Neil and colleagues[7] pointed out that physical activity, which is protective and promotes health, has traditionally been encouraged for young boys, whereas young girls have historically been directed to participate in less physically demanding activities. To lose weight and maintain their body image, young women are more likely to smoke cigarettes; also, stress created by harassment and discrimination affects women's cardiovascular health (CVH) more significantly than men.[7] Moreover, depression and other emotional stress, which may originate from issues related to gender, often influence women's CVH more significantly than men.[25]

PREVENTION OF CARDIOVASCULAR DISEASE IN WOMEN

Prevention of CVD falls into different categories: primordial prevention, primary prevention, secondary prevention, and tertiary prevention. Each of these levels of prevention focuses on different time frames and has different goals, as outlined in **Fig. 1**. **Table 3** highlights examples of prevention at every level. Of note, authors define and classify levels of prevention in slightly different ways, but the overall message remains intact, regardless of specific definitions.

Primordial Prevention

Primordial prevention is perhaps the truest form of prevention in that it involves interventions that prevent the development of *risk factors* for CVD, ultimately preventing CVD.[29] Primordial prevention involves individual-level and population-level interventions that improve overall health and living conditions and reduce the incidence of CVD risk factors. The idea is that by eliminating risk factors for CVD in the population, especially through middle age, CVD can be largely eliminated.[30] Improving parents' health today and eliminating CVD risk factors in this group may reduce the risk of CVD in the next generation.[31]

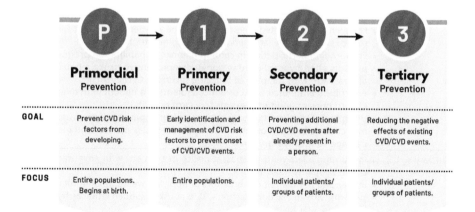

	Primordial Prevention	**Primary** Prevention	**Secondary** Prevention	**Tertiary** Prevention
GOAL	Prevent CVD risk factors from developing.	Early identification and management of CVD risk factors to prevent onset of CVD/CVD events.	Preventing additional CVD/CVD events after already present in a person.	Reducing the negative effects of existing CVD/CVD events.
FOCUS	Entire populations. Begins at birth.	Entire populations.	Individual patients/ groups of patients.	Individual patients/ groups of patients.

Fig. 1. This figure illustrates the 4 levels of prevention.

Table 3
Selected examples of cardiovascular disease prevention at each level

Level of Prevention	Examples
Primordial[a]	• Advocating with policymakers and food companies to reduce the amount of sodium included in the nation's food supply • Advocating for policies that lead to the elimination of secondhand smoke in public places and the elimination of tobacco use altogether • Developing exercise and healthy eating programs in schools • Enhancing maternal health to support fetal health • Expanding access to healthy food and clean water • Facilitating access to high-quality health care at all stages of life, across all geographical areas (rural, suburban, and urban) • Improving social determinants of cardiovascular health (education, health care access, socioeconomic status, environment, social support) • Maintaining a healthy weight, normal glucose, blood pressure, and cholesterol levels from birth • Promoting equity, diversity, and inclusion initiatives that in turn reduce discrimination, bias, and psychobiological stress • Providing access to health education and wellness programs by meeting individuals where they live and work (churches, workplaces, barber shops/hair salons, community facilities) • Supporting the mental health of the population through interventions to reduce stigma, improve access to mental health care, and reduce stress
Primary[a,b]	• Encouraging participation in weight management programs to lose weight (if overweight or obese) • Facilitating the cessation of smoking and tobacco use at the individual level (education, behavioral interventions, medications) • Measuring blood pressure, glucose, and cholesterol to identify those with hypertension, prediabetes/diabetes, and dyslipidemia • Treating dyslipidemia with lifestyle change (reduced intake of trans fats and saturated fats, exercise) and pharmacotherapy (statins and PCSK9 inhibitors in qualifying patients) • Treating hypertension with lifestyle changes (weight loss, increased physical activity, reduced sodium intake, following the DASH eating plan) and medication, as indicated • Using risk assessment tools to quantitatively assess an individual's risk of future CVD and to make decisions on strategies to mitigate that risk
Secondary	• Encouraging adherence to prescribed lifestyle interventions and risk factor control after a CVD event/diagnosis • Following goal-directed medical therapy for a patient with heart failure to reduce subsequent exacerbations and hospitalization • Encouraging participation in cardiopulmonary rehabilitation programs for patients after myocardial infarction or comprehensive stroke rehabilitation after stroke (with the goal of reducing recurrent CVD events) • Prescribing antiplatelet and/or anticoagulants in a patient with diagnosed CVD to prevent additional events (eg, stroke, ACS) • Using high-sensitivity troponin assays to identify patients with myocardial infarction or injury in order to intervene in a timely manner and reduce damage to the myocardium
Tertiary	• Implanting a left-ventricular assist device in a patient with advanced cardiomyopathy/heart failure • Implanting permanent defibrillators or applying wearable defibrillators to patients with an ejection fraction < 35% at risk of sudden lethal arrhythmias like ventricular tachycardia

(continued on next page)

Table 3 (continued)	
Level of Prevention	Examples
	• Encouraging participation in cardiopulmonary rehabilitation programs for patients with CVD or comprehensive stroke rehabilitation after stroke (with the goal of preventing further morbidity and mortality and improving quality of life) • Performing stent placement or coronary artery bypass surgery in appropriate patients with CAD to improve blood flow to the myocardium

Abbreviations: ACS, acute coronary syndrome; CAD, coronary artery disease; CVD, cardiovascular disease; DASH, dietary approaches to stop hypertension; PCSK9, proprotein convertase subtilisin/kexin type 9.

[a] Primordial and primary prevention interventions may also be beneficial as a means of secondary and tertiary prevention, because these primordial and primary prevention strategies target cardiovascular health promotion and risk factor reduction overall, which is beneficial for the cardiovascular system regardless of prevention level.

[b] Hypertension and hyperlipidemia can be viewed as cardiovascular diseases as well as risk factors for other cardiovascular diseases/events, such as coronary artery disease and acute coronary syndrome; thus, interventions for hypertension and hyperlipidemia could be included in primary and/or secondary prevention.

Data from Refs.[3,18,19,26,28,29,32]

Primary Prevention

Although primordial prevention focuses on preventing risk factors from ever developing, primary prevention focuses on the early identification and management of causal risk factors for CVD before a CVD event.[32] The use of risk assessment tools, such as the American Heart Association/American College of Cardiology Atherosclerotic Cardiovascular Disease (ASCVD) risk estimator, has been encouraged to assess an individual's 10 year and lifetime risk of CVD.[33] To achieve primordial and primary prevention, attention can be turned from cardiovascular disease to CVH and the strategies that promote optimal cardiovascular wellness and reduce the development of atherosclerosis and CVD.[34] The 8 critical components of CVH have come to be known by the American Heart Association as Life's Essential 8, outlined in **Box 3**.

Secondary and Tertiary Prevention

Though primordial and primary prevention occur before CVD onset, secondary and tertiary prevention are employed once an individual has experienced a CVD event or has been diagnosed with CVD. Secondary prevention focuses on reducing the chance of another CVD event in an individual with known CVD. In contrast, tertiary prevention strategies aim to reduce the long-term complications and worsening of existing CVD, hopefully reducing mortality and improving quality of life.[35]

Prevention strategies are important across all populations of women. However, given their increased risk of CVD, attention to prevention is especially important for women with pregnancy-related complications, such as hypertensive disorders, premature delivery, and low birth weight babies.[28] A systematic review and meta-analysis of data from over 1 million women also suggests that breastfeeding may reduce women's long-term risk of CVD.[36] Additionally, work is needed to engage women of all backgrounds in secondary and tertiary prevention. For example, women are less likely than men to participate in cardiopulmonary rehabilitation after being diagnosed with acute cardiovascular conditions, even though they can derive

---

Box 3
The American Heart Association's Life's Essential 8: Strategies for ideal cardiovascular health

- Do not use nicotine (including cigarettes and vaping products)
- Maintain a healthy weight (BMI < 25 kg/m^2 for ages 20 years and above; below the 85th percentile for ages 2–19 years)
- Engage in physical activity ($\geq$150 min/wk of moderate or greater intensity exercise for ages 20 years and above; $\geq$ 420 min/wk of moderate or greater intensity exercise for ages 6–19 years)
- Consume a heart-healthy diet (following DASH-style and/or Mediterranean diet patterns)
- Reduce non-HDL cholesterol (<130 mg/dL for ages 20 years and above; < 100 mg/dL for ages 9–19 years)
- Maintain a normal blood pressure (SBP < 120 mm Hg and DBP < 80 mm Hg for ages 13 years and above; blood pressure less than the 90th percentile for ages < 13 years)
- Maintain normal fasting plasma glucose levels and/or HbA1c (serum glucose < 100 mg/dL and HbA1c < 5.7% for ages 12 years and above)
- Achieve an average of 7 to < 9 hours of sleep per night (too little and too much sleep confer cardiovascular risk)

Abbreviations: BMI, body mass index; DBP, diastolic blood pressure; SBP, systolic blood pressure.

Data from Ref.[34]

---

benefits.[37] Psychosocial and referral issues likely contribute to the lack of participation by women, and nurses are positioned to find ways to facilitate access to these programs.[37]

WOMEN'S CARDIOVASCULAR DISEASE SYMPTOM PRESENTATION

Symptoms play an important role in the CVD experience, alerting patients and health professionals to the presence of CVD, including time-sensitive problems like stroke and ACS. Moreover, symptom recognition and care seeking play an important role in secondary and tertiary prevention, given that when patients accurately recognize and attribute the symptoms they are experiencing to a cardiovascular condition, they seek care more rapidly.[38,39] Further, accurate assessment and triage of symptoms by nurses and other health care providers reduces delays in intervening for CVD.[10]

Although early stroke identification is important, the symptoms of stroke in men and women are largely the same (**Box 4**). Given the prevalence of ACS and the lack of awareness of ACS symptoms in women, this section focuses specifically on symptoms of ACS in women. Cushman and colleagues[40] found that women's knowledge of common ACS symptoms declined significantly from 2009 to 2019, especially related to shortness of breath, tightness of the chest, pain that spreads to the shoulders/neck/arms, and fatigue. Knowledge of chest pain as an ACS symptom also declined for some groups, including Black, Hispanic, and Asian women and those ages 25 to 44 years.[40] Regardless of racial or ethnic group, only 51.5% of women recognized chest pain as a symptom of ACS, whereas 27.9% recognized shortness of breath, 6.6% recognized fatigue, and 5.7% recognized tightness of the chest.[40] Additionally, patients sometimes delay seeking care for symptoms when their expectations about symptoms do not match their actual symptom experience.[41,42] For example, a woman may expect ACS symptoms to be overwhelming, excruciating,

---

Box 4
Common stroke symptoms: BE-FAST[a]

- The following symptoms occur in a large majority of ischemic strokes. The sudden onset of the below symptoms is particularly concerning.

- B = Balance (trouble with balance, coordination, standing)

- E = Eyes (blurred vision; double vision; loss of vision in one or both eyes, especially when there is no pain)

- F = Facial Drooping (droop on one side of the face or numbness)

- A = Arm Weakness (weak or numb arm; when raised, one arm drops or drifts)

- S = Speech Difficulty/Trouble (unable to form words or speak coherently; slurred speech; cannot repeat a simple sentence)

- T = Time to call emergency services/seek care (early intervention for stroke is critical)

[a]This box represents common stroke symptoms. Symptom experiences may vary, and exceptions to the symptoms included in this box are possible.

Data from Ref.[60]

---

or debilitating in nature when, in fact, these symptoms range in their overall severity and may be only moderate or mild in severity and intensity and develop gradually. Women also report concerns about bothering others, having too many competing life responsibilities, embarrassment, and the belief that symptoms are not serious as reasons for delaying care for symptoms consistent with ACS.[38,43]

Women experience prodromal and acute symptoms of ACS, highlighted in **Table 4**. Women seek care for prodromal symptoms of ACS, affording clinicians an early opportunity to intervene, but these symptoms are not always recognized as cardiac in nature.[44,45] When women tell health professionals about symptoms consistent with possible CAD or ACS, they have reported sometimes feeling that their symptoms were trivialized, not fully assessed, or were quickly attributed to other health conditions, such as weight or other comorbidities.[44,46]

Women and men differ in the overall frequency with which they experience *some* ACS symptoms, and women tend to experience a larger number of ACS symptoms. However, women and men experience ACS symptoms that are more similar than different, and even when the frequency of a particular symptom differs between men and women, the overall magnitude of this difference is small.[4,47,48] A recent meta-analysis showed that men experience chest pain slightly more than women (79% vs 74%); however, chest pain is still the most common acute ACS symptom, regardless of sex or gender.[47] Recent evidence suggests that men and women sometimes incorrectly associate several ACS symptoms with different genders.[43] In a study comparing the ACS symptoms associated with men and women in a nationwide sample, almost 80% of participants selected a chest symptom (eg, discomfort, pain, pressure) as the most common ACS symptom for men, whereas less than 50% selected a chest symptom as the most common for women.[43] Further, women (46.9%) in this study were significantly more likely than men (17.3%) to endorse that men and women have either "fairly different" or "very different" ACS symptoms.[43]

Beyond patients' knowledge and attribution of symptoms, the assessment of symptoms by nurses and other health care professionals is crucial. When asking patients about common CAD and ACS symptoms like chest pain, it is wise for nurses to ask patients if they are experiencing symptoms using a variety of descriptors, given the

Table 4
Common prodromal and acute symptoms of acute coronary syndrome experienced by women

Category of Symptom	Characteristics	Common Symptoms in the Category
Prodromal ACS Symptoms	• Occur in the days, weeks, and months prior to ACS • May fluctuate in severity and frequency leading up to ACS • Serves as a warning of an impending ACS event • Rarely experience one prodromal symptom in isolation (generally experience a combination of symptoms)	• Unusual or overwhelming fatigue • Changes in sleep/trouble sleeping • Anxiety • Frequent indigestion • Racing heart or palpitations • Change in thinking/remembering or cognition • Discomfort in the chest • Tingling in the arms/hands
Acute ACS Symptoms	• Occur at time of ACS event • Range in severity and degree of distress they cause • Though patients often expect that acute symptoms like chest pain will be excruciating or debilitating, may be only mildly to moderately intense and minimally debilitating • Rarely experience one acute symptom in isolation (generally a combination of symptoms)	• Chest symptoms (eg, pressure, tightness, discomfort, heaviness) • Shortness of breath • Diaphoresis • Nausea/vomiting • Arm, shoulder, and/or upper back pain • Dizziness/lightheadedness • Fatigue (unusual or new onset) • Neck and/or jaw pain • Palpitations • Indigestion

Abbreviation: ACS, acute coronary syndrome.
Data from Refs.[47,48,58]

recognition that "chest pain" as a CAD and ACS symptom is an umbrella term for many sensations,[49] as shown in **Box 5**. It has been demonstrated that women sometimes deny having chest *pain* because they are experiencing a different sensation, such as chest heaviness or discomfort, potentially leading to a missed opportunity to identify CAD or impending ACS.[50] In addition to using a variety of descriptors to assess symptoms, it is essential to note that fatigue is an important possible CAD symptom,[51] as endorsed by over 70% of women before ACS.[52] Indeed, fatigue is a common symptom of many different problems, so it may be challenging to determine whether fatigue is cardiac-related. However, nurses should be aware that fatigue (especially unusual or overwhelming) is a common symptom of heart disease and ACS.

DIAGNOSTIC TESTING FOR LOW-RISK CHEST PAIN IN WOMEN

Women with low-risk chest pain require diagnostic testing but typically do not require hospitalization or urgent cardiac testing. Low-risk chest pain is defined as symptoms suggestive of ACS but with a <1% risk of a major adverse cardiac event (MACE) within 30 days. To determine the likelihood of MACE, a detailed history and physical exam are needed, along with basic diagnostic testing—12-lead electrocardiogram (ECG) and troponin.[49]

Basic Diagnostic Testing

Unless a noncardiac cause is immediately apparent, all women experiencing chest symptoms should get a 12-lead ECG immediately. A normal 12-lead ECG does not rule out ACS but is an important diagnostic tool. If symptoms persist, serial ECGs may be indicated. If the history and physical exam suggest a noncardiac cause that can be diagnosed through a chest radiograph (eg, pneumonia), then it is appropriate

---

Box 5
Tips for recognizing diverse descriptions and experiences of "chest pain" related to coronary artery disease and acute coronary syndrome[a]

- The term chest pain may not truly capture the sensation experienced by individuals with CAD or ACS, given that the sensation is not always considered by patients to be "painful" or a type of "pain."
- Chest pain related to CAD/ACS is often described using a variety of narrative terms:
  - Pressure, squeezing, gripping, heaviness, tightness, dullness, aching, discomfort
- Chest pain related to CAD/ACS is more often:
  - Centrally located or located on the left side of the chest
- Obtaining a complete history of chest symptoms is important, considering:
  - Location, character/quality, quantity/severity, timing, setting/situation, aggravating or relieving factors, associated factors or symptoms, and the patient's perception of the symptoms
- Shoulder, arm, neck, back, upper abdominal, and jaw pain/pressure/tightness/discomfort, and shortness of breath are potentially chest pain equivalents. As such, these symptoms may occur with CAD/ACS, even absent a chest symptom.

Abbreviations: ACS, acute coronary syndrome; CAD, coronary artery disease. [a]This box represents common chest pain characteristics. Symptom experiences may vary, and exceptions to the characteristics included in this box are possible.

Data from Ref.[49]

to obtain a chest radiograph and rule out other diagnoses. In addition to a 12-lead ECG and possibly a chest radiograph, troponin should be measured. High sensitivity cardiac troponin is the preferred biomarker; however, a basic troponin is also of diagnostic value if the facility does not have high-sensitivity lab troponin testing. Troponin is specific to myocardial injury, and the addition of CK-MB is not of diagnostic value.[49] Women may experience smaller elevations in troponin compared with men, necessitating different criteria for the upper reference limit of this test.[53] Additionally, elevated troponin may not be detected for 2 to 4 hours after initial symptom onset and may take as long as 8 to 12 hours,[54] so women who seek medical attention quickly may initially have a normal troponin. For ongoing symptoms or in women presenting shortly after symptom onset, serial troponin measurements may be indicated.[53,54] A follow-up evaluation with the further diagnostic testing presented below is often warranted.

Further Diagnostic Testing

When considering diagnostic testing for women, anatomical differences may impact the sensitivity of the testing. Women are at higher risk for microvascular changes in distal vessels as opposed to large obstructive plaques in major coronary arteries, making exercise stress tests less sensitive in women.[13] However, recent consensus statements support the use of exercise stress tests as a cost-effective strategy for low-risk women who have a normal resting ECG.[13,49] In women at higher risk, a stress echocardiogram improves diagnostic accuracy (eg, dobutamine stress echocardiography). Compared with an exercise stress test, the stress echocardiogram has better sensitivity and specificity for detecting obstructive CAD.[13]

Both exercise stress tests and stress echocardiograms are functional tests of CAD. Although the sensitivity of these modalities is adequate for most low-risk women, they are not as sensitive as tests that detect anatomical CAD (eg, cardiac computed tomography angiography [CTA]). The cardiac CTA is a noninvasive test with high diagnostic accuracy. Women with a positive CTA are more likely to have a clinically significant event than those with a positive exercise stress test. Cardiac CTA allows evaluation of plaque characteristics, including identification of coronary artery calcium (CAC) lesions. Cardiac CTA allows clinicians to provide treatment recommendations based on plaque characteristics and patient risk factors.[13] This personalized approach to treatment better meets the needs of individual patients. CAC testing can also be a standalone test, often called a heart scan. This specialized CT scan is used in low-risk and intermediate-risk individuals to detect plaques and may be recommended as a screening test if certain risk factors are present. A CAC score of 0 means that it is unlikely that the woman has obstructive plaques.

Many other valuable diagnostic tests, including PET scans and nuclear myocardial perfusion stress tests, are available; however, low-risk individuals rarely need costly workups. For low-risk women who can exercise, beginning with an exercise stress test is acceptable. If further evaluation is needed, additional testing can be ordered as appropriate. If symptoms persist, it is reasonable to assess coronary microvascular dysfunction, which may be the cause of ischemia symptoms.[13] Recent guidelines consider the anatomical differences in women and men as recommendations are made for diagnostic testing. **Table 5** outlines the differences in some common outpatient diagnostic tests.

PATIENT AND FAMILY EDUCATION

Patient and family education is a cornerstone of nursing practice. Education about CVD prevention and CVH promotion should be provided to patients and their family

Table 5
Common imaging tests for the evaluation of chest symptoms

Test	Notes	Indications	Nursing Considerations
12-Lead electrocardiogram	• First line for all patients with chest symptoms • Records the electrical signals in the heart to detect ischemia • Not a routine screening test in adults who do not have suspected ischemic symptoms	• All patients with symptoms suggestive of heart disease, including chest symptoms, dizziness, rapid pulse, and shortness of breath, among others	• Make sure the patient remains still during the reading • Shave chest, arm, or leg hair as appropriate
Chest X ray (CXR)	• Used to rule out other causes of chest symptoms	• Patients with complaints that may be related to the heart or lungs	• Assess for potential pregnancy
Exercise stress test	• First-line option for low-risk patients with chest symptoms • Lower diagnostic accuracy in women	• Patients with complaints of chest pain who are physically able to exercise	• The patient must be able to exercise • Assess for musculoskeletal, pulmonary, or other conditions that may prevent the patient from exercising at a high enough intensity to reach target heart rate
Stress echocardiogram	• Often used in patients when imaging is a recommended adjunct (eg, intermediate-risk women) • Better accuracy than an exercise stress test • Exercise or pharmacologic measures can be used to increase HR	• Intermediate-risk women with complaints of chest symptoms • Low-risk women who are unable to complete an exercise stress test, for whom testing is deemed necessary	• Patient-dependent factors may limit usefulness (eg, morbid obesity) • Adequate pre-procedure education is necessary because the medication used to speed the heart may make the patient uncomfortable or experience a panic attack

Table 5
(continued)

Test	Notes	Indications	Nursing Considerations
Coronary Calcium or Heart Scan	• A specialized CT scan is used in low-risk to intermediate-risk people • Detects and measures calcium-containing plaques in coronary arteries • Women with more plaque are at higher risk for MACE	• Screening for heart disease risk • May be recommended if a woman has certain risk factors	• Education about what to expect during the scan (eg, potential use of medication to slow the heart; placement of electrodes on the chest) • Depending on the score, patient education on modifiable risk factors
Computed Tomography Angiography (CTA)	• High diagnostic accuracy because it allows visualization of coronary arteries	• Not recommended as a first-line screening test in low-risk women because of higher cost • Used to assess intermediate risk patients or patients whose stress test was inconclusive	• Check for an iodine allergy • Educate the patient on what to expect during the test (eg, insertion of an IV; injection of dye; feeling when dye is injected)
Nuclear myocardial perfusion testing/Nuclear stress test	• High diagnostic accuracy • Shows cardiac perfusion and areas of decreased perfusion • Exercise or pharmacologic measures can be used to increase HR	• Not a first-line screening in low-risk patients because of cost	• Review medications because some may need to be stopped prior to the procedure (eg, beta blockers) • Educate the patient on what to expect and any preprocedural preparations (eg, avoid caffeine; IV insertion; injection of dye)
Cardiac PET scan	• Best approach to diagnose cardiac microvascular dysfunction • Shows myocardial and coronary blood flow	• May be used in women with continued chest pain after obstruction is ruled out	• Patient education about what to expect and preprocedural preparation are necessary (eg, NPO x4-6 h)

Abbreviations: CT, computed tomography; MACE, major adverse cardiovascular event; NPO, nothing by mouth; PET, positron emission tomography.
Data from Refs.[13,49]

members (and/or support persons).[55] Engaging family members and caregivers may increase the likelihood that positive behavior change will occur and create a synergistic effect in which a patient's close friends and family develop healthier habits themselves.[55] Additionally, it is recognized that many women receive primary care from their obstetrician-gynecologist (OB-GYN) or women's health nurse practitioner and thus may not have routine contact with any other provider.[26] As such, nurses and providers in OB-GYN practices must recognize the opportunity that they have to address cardiovascular risk and health with their patients.[26]

One evidence-based strategy for patient and family education is the development of SMART (specific, measurable, action-oriented, realistic, and timely) goals. Working collaboratively with patients, nurses and other health care providers can develop goals that are achievable and measure the short-term success of the patient. An example of an exercise SMART goal is: Starting Monday, 9/26 for 1 month, I want to walk at least 30 minutes, 3 times each week. The SMART goal provides a specific, measurable time frame, and the goal itself is action-oriented. Too often, education is centered around teaching patients what they should do without providing any goals or actions. Action-oriented goals can be discussed at a follow-up appointment to determine whether the goal needs to be revised. The Preventive Cardiovascular Nurses Association has a Heart Healthy Toolbox complete with information on SMART goals and many other patient education materials.[56]

SUMMARY

Indeed, much progress has been made in understanding women's experiences with CVD. However, more work is needed to improve CVD outcomes in women. Continued emphasis on CVD prevention, especially through primordial and primary prevention, will be critical, as will better understanding the underlying pathophysiology and causes of problems like SCAD and Takotsubo syndrome. Eliminating knowledge deficits will continue to be a focus for nurses and patients alike. It is imperative that women recognize CVD symptoms and recognize that CVD is the leading cause of death for women. Prompt, evidence-based workup of patients with symptoms consistent with CAD and ACS remains essential.

Nurses are charged with taking the best available evidence and applying it to their real-world practice. Nurses are well positioned to listen carefully to women, regardless of background—hearing their stories, concerns, and experiences and seeking to have open, transparent conversations that engage women in their own care. By improving knowledge deficits through active engagement and by implementing behavior change strategies, nurses can help improve the CVH of all women.

CLINICS CARE POINTS

- In addition to universal risk factors for cardiovascular disease, such as high blood pressure and smoking, women may experience additional sex- and gender-specific risk factors, including pregnancy-related and hormone-based risk factors. See **Box 2** for details.

- Following blood pressure measurement guidelines will better ensure accurate blood pressure readings. Inaccurate blood pressure measurement could lead to a missed diagnosis of hypertension or a diagnosis of hypertension in a patient who is not actually hypertensive. See **Table 2** for details.

- "Life's Essential 8" from the American Heart Association provide opportunities to optimize cardiovascular health in women. These strategies include avoiding nicotine, maintaining a healthy weight, engaging in physical activity, consuming a heart-healthy diet, reducing non-

HDL cholesterol, maintaining a normal blood pressure, maintaining a normal fasting plasma glucose level, and achieving an average of 7 to < 9 hours of sleep per night. See **Box 3** for details.

- Women experience many of the same acute coronary syndrome symptoms as men, and a chest symptom, such as chest pressure or chest tightness, remains the most common for women and men. However, women may experience a larger number of symptoms than men. See **Table 4** and **Box 5** for details.

- Especially when the likelihood of acute coronary syndrome is low, nurses must be aware that spontaneous coronary artery dissection and Takotsubo syndrome are mimics that are more common in women than in men. See **Table 1** for details.

- Nurses should recognize that a normal left ventricular ejection fraction does not rule out heart failure. In fact, many patients have heart failure with preserved (normal) ejection fraction, also labeled HFpEF. Women are more likely than men to be diagnosed with this type of heart failure.

DISCLOSURE

The authors have no conflicts of interest to disclose.

REFERENCES

1. Tsao CW, Aday AW, Almarzooq ZI, et al. Heart disease and stroke statistics-2022 update: A report from the American Heart Association. Circulation 2022;145(8): e153–639.
2. McSweeney JC, Rosenfeld AG, Abel WM, et al. Preventing and experiencing ischemic heart disease as a woman: State of the science: A scientific statement from the American heart association. Circulation 2016;133(13):1302–31.
3. Wenger NK, Lloyd-Jones DM, Elkind MSV, et al. Call to action for cardiovascular disease in women: Epidemiology, awareness, access, and delivery of equitable health care: A presidential advisory from the American Heart Association. Circulation 2022;145(23):e1059–71.
4. DeVon HA, Mirzaei S, Zegre-Hemsey J. Typical and atypical symptoms of acute coronary syndrome: Time to retire the terms? J Am Heart Assoc 2020;9(7): e015539.
5. Blakeman JR. Words matter: Sex and gender as unique variables in research. ANS Adv Nurs Sci 2020;43(3):214–27.
6. Norris CM, Johnson NL, Hardwicke-Brown E, et al. The contribution of gender to apparent sex differences in health status among patients with coronary artery disease. J Womens Health (Larchmt) 2017;26(1):50–7.
7. O'Neil A, Scovelle AJ, Milner AJ, et al. Gender/sex as a social determinant of cardiovascular risk. Circulation 2018;137(8):854–64.
8. Pelletier R, Khan NA, Cox J, et al. Sex versus gender-related characteristics: Which predicts outcome after acute coronary syndrome in the young? J Am Coll Cardiol 2016;67(2):127–35.
9. Streed CG, Beach LB, Caceres BA, et al. Assessing and addressing cardiovascular health in people who are transgender and gender diverse: A scientific statement from the American Heart Association. Circulation 2021;144(6):e136–48.
10. Bhatt DL, Lopes RD, Harrington RA. Diagnosis and treatment of acute coronary syndromes: A review. JAMA 2022;327(7):662–75.
11. Bairey Merz CN, Pepine CJ, Walsh MN, et al. Ischemia and no obstructive coronary artery disease (INOCA). Circulation 2017;135(11):1075–92.

12. Kenkre TS, Malhotra P, Johnson BD, et al. Ten-year mortality in the WISE study (Women's Ischemia Syndrome Evaluation). Circ Cardiovasc Qual Outcomes 2017;10(12):e003863.

13. Rodriguez PF, Kaso ER, Bourque JM, et al. Cardiovascular imaging for ischemic heart disease in women: Time for a paradigm shift. JACC Cardiovasc Imaging 2022;15(8):1488–501.

14. Hayes SN, Kim ESH, Saw J, et al. Spontaneous coronary artery dissection: Current state of the science. Circulation 2018;137(19):e523–57.

15. Singh T, Khan H, Gamble DT, et al. Takotsubo syndrome: Pathophysiology, emerging concepts and clinical implications. Circulation 2022;145(13):1002–19.

16. National Center for Health Statistics. Underlying cause of death 1999-2020: Deaths occurring through 2020. 2022. Available at https://wonder.cdc.gov/controller/datarequest/D76. Accessed July 2, 2022.

17. Rexrode KM, Madsen TE, Yu AYX, et al. The impact of sex and gender on stroke. Circ Res 2022;130(4):512–28.

18. Powell-Wiley TM, Baumer Y, Baah FO, et al. Social determinants of cardiovascular disease. Circ Res 2022;130(5):782–99.

19. Heidenreich PA, Bozkurt B, Aguilar D, et al. 2022 AHA/ACC/HFSA guideline for the management of heart failure: A report of the American College of Cardiology/American Heart Association Joint Committee on Clinical Practice Guidelines. Circulation 2022;145:e895–1032.

20. Medina-Inojosa JR, Vinnakota S, Garcia M, et al. Role of stress and psychosocial determinants on women's cardiovascular risk and disease development. J Womens Health (Larchmt) 2019;28(4):483–9.

21. Elias MF, Goodell AL. Human errors in automated office blood pressure measurements. Hypertension 2021;77(1):6–15.

22. O'Kelly AC, Michos ED, Shufelt CL, et al. Pregnancy and reproductive risk factors for cardiovascular disease in women. Circ Res 2022;130(4):652–72.

23. El Khoudary SR, Aggarwal B, Beckie TM, et al. Menopause transition and cardiovascular disease risk: Implications for timing of early prevention. Circulation 2020;142(25):e506–32.

24. Howlander N, Noone AM, Krapcho M, et al. SEER cancer statistics review, 1975-2017. National Cancer Institute; 2020. Available at. https://seer.cancer.gov/archive/csr/1975_2017/. Accessed June 30, 2022.

25. Mehta LS, Watson KE, Barac A, et al. Cardiovascular disease and breast cancer: Where these entities intersect. Circulation 2018;137(8):e30–66.

26. Brown HL, Warner JJ, Gianos E, et al. Promoting risk identification and reduction of cardiovascular disease in women through collaboration with obstetricians and gynecologists. Circulation 2018;137(24):e843–52.

27. Odonwodo, A., Badri, T., & Hariz, A. (2021). Scleroderma. StatPearls. Available at: https://www.ncbi.nlm.nih.gov/books/NBK537335/.

28. Stuart JJ, Tanz LJ, Rimm EB, et al. Cardiovascular risk factors mediate the long-term maternal risk associated with hypertensive disorders of pregnancy. J Am Coll Cardiol 2022;79(19):1901–13.

29. Gilman MW. Primordial prevention of cardiovascular disease. Circulation 2015;131(7):599–601.

30. Lloyd-Jones D, Albert MA, Elkind M. The American Heart Association's focus on primordial prevention. Circulation 2021;144(15):e233–5.

31. Falkner B, Lurbe E. Primordial prevention of high blood pressure in childhood. Hypertension 2020;75(5):1142–50.

32. Arnett DK, Blumenthal RS, Albert MA, et al. 2019 ACC/AHA guideline on the primary prevention of cardiovascular disease. Circulation 2019;140(11):e596–646.
33. Lloyd-Jones D, Braun LT, Ndumele CE. Use of risk assessment tools to guide decision making in the primary prevention of atherosclerotic cardiovascular disease. Circulation 2019;139:e1162–77.
34. Lloyd-Jones DM, Allen NB, Anderson CAM, et al. Life's essential 8: Updating and enhancing the American Heart Association's construct of cardiovascular health: A presidential advisory from the American Heart Association. Circulation 2022; 146(5). https://doi.org/10.1161/CIR.0000000000001078.
35. World Heart Federation. Prevention. 2022. Available at: https://world-heart-federation.org/what-we-do/prevention. Accessed June 27, 2022.
36. Tschiderer L, Seekircher L, Kunutsor SK, et al. Breastfeeding is associated with a reduced maternal cardiovascular risk: Systematic review and meta-analysis involving data from 8 studies and 1,192,700 parous women. J Am Heart Assoc 2022;11(2):e022746.
37. Khadanga S, Gaalema DE, Savage P, et al. Underutilization of cardiac rehabilitation in women: Barriers and solutions. J Cardiopulm Rehabil Prev 2021;41(4): 207–13.
38. Arrebola-Moreno M, Petrova D, Garcia-Retamero R, et al. Psychological and cognitive factors related to prehospital delay in acute coronary syndrome: A systematic review. Int J Nurs Stud 2020;108:103613.
39. Riegel B, Moser DK, Buck HG, et al. Self-care for the prevention and management of cardiovascular disease and stroke. J Am Heart Assoc 2017;6(9): e006997.
40. Cushman M, Shay CM, Howard VJ, et al. Ten-year differences in women's awareness related to coronary heart disease: Results of the 2019 American Heart Association national survey. Circulation 2021;143(7):e239–48.
41. Smith R, Frazer K, Hyde A, et al. Heart disease never entered my head: Women's understanding of coronary heart disease risk factors. J Clin Nurs 2018;27(21–22): 3953–67.
42. Mirzaei S, Steffen A, Vuckovic K, et al. The association between symptom onset characteristics and prehospital delay in women and men with acute coronary syndrome. Eur J Cardiovasc Nurs 2020;19(2):142–54.
43. Blakeman JR, Eckhardt AL, Kim M. The Lay Public's Knowledge of the Most Common Acute Coronary Syndrome Symptoms Experienced by Women and Men. J Cardiovasc Nurs 2023;38(3):288–98. https://doi.org/10.1097/JCN.0000000000000931.
44. Blakeman JR, Woith WM, Astroth KS, et al. Women's prodromal myocardial infarction symptom perception, attribution, and care seeking: A qualitative multiple case study. Dimens Crit Care Nurs 2022;29(19–20):3882–95.
45. Pate A, Leeman-Castillo BA, Krantz MJ. Treatment-seeking delay among Hispanic and non-Hispanic women with acute myocardial infarction. Health Equity 2019; 3(1):287–96.
46. Arslanian-Engoren C, Scott LD. Women's perceptions of biases and barriers in their myocardial infarction triage experience. Heart Lung 2016;45(3):166–72.
47. van Oosterhout REM, de Boer AR, Maas AHEM, et al. Sex differences in symptom presentation in acute coronary syndromes: a systematic review and meta-analysis. J Am Heart Assoc 2020;9(9):e014733.
48. DeVon HA, Rosenfeld A, Steffen AD, et al. Sensitivity, specificity, and sex differences in symptoms reported on the 13-item acute coronary syndrome checklist. J Am Heart Assoc 2014;3(2):e000586.

49. Gulati M, Levy PD, Mukherjee D, et al. 2021 AHA/ACC/ASE/CHEST/SAEM/SCCT/ SCMR guideline for the evaluation and diagnosis of chest pain. Circulation 2021; 144(22):e368–454.

50. Blakeman JR, Woith WM, Astroth KS, et al. A qualitative exploration of prodromal myocardial infarction fatigue experienced by women. J Clin Nurs 2020; 29(19–20):3882–95.

51. Eckhardt AL, DeVon HA, Piano MR, et al. Fatigue in the presence of coronary heart disease. Nurs Res 2014;63(2):83–93.

52. Blakeman JR, Stapleton SJ. An integrative review of fatigue experienced by women before and during myocardial infarction. J Clin Nurs 2018;27(5–6):906–16.

53. Thygesen K, Alpert JS, Jaffe AS. Fourth universal definition of myocardial infarction (2018). Circulation 2018;138(20):e618–51.

54. Wassie M, Lee M-S, Sun BC, et al. Single vs. serial measurements of cardiac troponin level in the evaluation of patients in the emergency department with suspected acute myocardial infarction. JAMA Netw Open 2021;4(2):e2037930.

55. Goldfarb MJ, Bechtel C, Capers IVQ, et al. Engaging families in adult cardiovascular care: A scientific statement from the American Heart Association. J Am Heart Assoc 2022;11:e025859.

56. Preventive Cardiovascular Nurses Association. (n.d.). Heart Healthy Toolbox. Available at: https://pcna.net/clinical-resources/patient-handouts/heart-healthy-toolbox/.

57. American Medical Association. 7 simple tips to get an accurate blood pressure reading. 2016. Available at: https://targetbp.org/wp-content/uploads/2017/02/ Measuring-blood-pressure-new.pdf. Accessed June 29, 2022.

58. Khan NA, Daskalopoulou SS, Karp I, et al. Sex differences in prodromal symptoms in acute coronary syndrome in patients aged 55 years or younger. Heart 2017;103(11):863–9.

59. Grundy SM, Stone NJ, Bailey AL, et al. 2019 AHA/ACC/AACVPR/AAPA/ABC/ ACPM/ADA/AGS/APhA/ASPC/NLA/PCNA guideline on the management of blood cholesterol. Circulation 2018;73(24):3168–209.

60. Aroor S, Singh R, Goldstein LB. BE-FAST (balance, eyes, face, arm, speech, time): Reducing the proportion of strokes missed using the FAST mnemonic. Stroke 2017;48(2):479–81.

Caring for Sexual and Gender Minority Adults with Cardiovascular Disease

Danny Doan, MPH, Yashika Sharma, MSN, RN,
David López Veneros, MA, RN, Billy A. Caceres, PhD, RN, FAHA*

KEYWORDS

- Sexual and gender minority • Cardiovascular disease • Nursing • Health promotion

KEY POINTS

- Sexual and gender minority (SGM) adults face significant psychosocial stressors across the individual, interpersonal, and structural levels which contribute to disparities in cardiovascular health.
- As the largest health care profession, nurses possess expertise in health promotion and behavior change and therefore can make valuable contributions to improving the cardiovascular health of SGM individuals.
- Nurses must advocate for expanded research, education, and clinical training in SGM health to reduce health disparities in SGM individuals.

INTRODUCTION

Cardiovascular disease (CVD) remains the leading cause of death among adults.[1] CVD accounts for 18 million deaths worldwide every year, which represents approximately 32% of all deaths globally.[2] It is estimated that more than 70% of CVD risk is attributed to modifiable risk factors (eg, tobacco use, obesity).[3] Although racial, ethnic, and sex disparities in CVD have been documented,[4,5] evidence of cardiovascular health disparities due to sexual orientation and gender identity (SOGI) is nascent.[6,7] Sexual and gender minority (SGM; eg, lesbian, gay, bisexual, transgender) individuals are underrepresented within cardiovascular research.[6] Growing evidence suggests that SGM individuals are at higher risk of CVD than the general population.[6,7] However, existing research has focused on CVD risk with very limited investigation of the experiences of SGM adults living with CVD.[6,8]

Several factors have been identified that may contribute to CVD risk among SGM adults. The minority stress model, the predominant explanation for the health

Center for Sexual and Gender Minority Health Research, Columbia University School of Nursing, 560 West 168th Street, New York, NY 10032, USA
* Corresponding author.
E-mail address: bac2134@cumc.columbia.edu

Nurs Clin N Am 58 (2023) 461–473
https://doi.org/10.1016/j.cnur.2023.05.010
0029-6465/23/© 2023 Elsevier Inc. All rights reserved.

nursing.theclinics.com

disparities that have been documented among SGM individuals,[9–11] proposes that SGM individuals experience persistent exposure to minority stressors (ie, unique psychosocial stressors attributed to one's sexual and/or gender minority identity), which contributes to negative health outcomes. Minority stressors are considered additive to general life stressors (eg, financial strain, work stress). The minority stress model has been widely used to examine mental health,[12,13] substance use,[14,15] and human immunodeficiency virus/acquired Immunodeficiency syndrome (HIV/AIDS)[16,17] disparities among SGM individuals. However, with few exceptions,[18–20] there is limited research on the impact of minority stressors on CVD risk in SGM individuals.

In 2020, a scientific statement from the American Heart Association presented an adaptation of the minority stress model that extended it to cardiovascular health.[6] This minority stress model of cardiovascular health posits that SGM adults experience stressors across multiple levels, including at the individual (eg, expectations of rejection), interpersonal (eg, experiences of discrimination), and structural (eg, discriminatory laws) levels. It is hypothesized that greater exposure to these multilevel minority stressors increases CVD risk among SGM individuals through psychosocial (eg, depression, anxiety), behavioral (eg, tobacco use, physical activity), and physiologic (eg, inflammation, hypothalamic–pituitary–adrenal axis) pathways.[6] **Table 1** provides a glossary of terms relevant to SGM health.

Nurses are uniquely suited to address the cardiovascular health disparities that have been observed among SGM adults. Nurses play an important role in the prevention and management of chronic diseases among marginalized populations.[21,22] Reducing health disparities is an important priority for cardiovascular nurses.[23] Because of their expertise in health promotion and behavior change, nurses can make valuable contributions to improving cardiovascular care for SGM patients.[21] Therefore, the purpose of this article was to summarize existing evidence on CVD risk and CVD among SGM adults and present recommendations for providing nursing care to SGM adults with CVD.

DISCUSSION
Tobacco Use

The disproportionately high rates of tobacco use among sexual minority (eg, lesbian, gay, bisexual, and other nonheterosexual) populations have been hypothesized to be a coping response to minority stressors.[24,25] A meta-analysis of 30 studies revealed that the higher prevalence of current cigarette smoking among sexual minority adults relative to heterosexual adults has remained stable since 1987.[26] Compared with both heterosexual men (21.0%) and women (16.6%), bisexual women had the highest prevalence of current cigarette smoking (37.7%).[26] These trends in nicotine exposure are consistent throughout the lifecourse as recent data suggest that gay/lesbian youth (grades 6–12) report higher current e-cigarette and hookah use than their heterosexual peers.[27]

Existing research on tobacco use disparities among gender minority (ie, individuals whose gender identity is not aligned with their sex assigned at birth such as transgender and gender nonbinary) adults is mixed.[7] Analyses of data from the Behavioral Risk Factor Surveillance System (BRFSS) found that all groups of gender minority adults reported higher odds of smokeless tobacco use compared with cisgender (ie, non-transgender) women.[28] Similarly, a recent review of 55 studies revealed a significantly higher prevalence of tobacco use among transgender adults compared with cisgender adults.[29] In addition, qualitative research suggests that tobacco use is a common coping response to exposure to psychosocial stressors among gender minority adults.[30]

Table 1
Glossary of terms for sexual and gender minority health

Bisexual	People who experience sexual, romantic, physical, or spiritual attraction to people of their own gender and toward another gender (the term "bisexual" is sometimes shortened to "bi").
Cisgender	A term used to describe people whose gender identity is congruent with what is traditionally expected from their sex assigned at birth.
Gay	A term used to describe boys/men who are attracted to boys/men but often used and embraced by people with other gender identities to describe their same-gender attractions and relationships. Often referred to as homosexual, although this term is no longer used by the majority of people with same-gender attractions.
Gender identity	A person's inner sense of being a girl/woman, a boy/man, a combination of girl/woman and boy/man, or something else, or having no gender at all. Everyone has a gender identity.
Gender minority	A broad diversity of people who experience an incongruence between their gender identity and what is traditionally expected from their sex assigned at birth, such as transgender and gender nonbinary people.
Gender nonbinary	A term used by some people who identify as a combination of girl/woman and boy/man, as something else, or as having no gender. Often used interchangeably with gender nonconforming.
Lesbian	Used to describe girls/women who are attracted to girls/women; applies for cisgender and transgender girls/women. Often referred to as homosexual, although this term is no longer used by the majority of women with same-gender attractions.
Queer	Used as an umbrella term to represent individuals who identify outside traditional categories for sexual orientation or gender identity. Historically, a derogatory term used against sexual minorities but has been embraced and reclaimed by many as a term of empowerment.
Sex	Biological sex characteristics (chromosomes, gonads, sex hormones, or genitals): male, female, and intersex. Synonymous with sex assigned at birth.
Sex assigned at birth	Usually based on phenotypic presentation (ie, genitals) of an infant and categorized as female or male; distinct from gender identity.
Sexual minority	A broad diversity of people who have a sexual orientation that is anything other than heterosexual/straight and typically includes gay, bisexual, lesbian, queer, or something else.
Sexual orientation	A person's physical, emotional, and romantic attachments in relation to gender. Conceptually separate from gender identity and gender expression. Everyone has a sexual orientation.
Straight/heterosexual	Boys/men or girls/women who are attracted to people of the other binary gender than themselves can refer to cisgender and transgender individuals. Often referred to as heterosexual.
Transgender man	Someone who identifies as male but was assigned female at birth. Also referred to as female to male.
Transgender woman	Someone who identifies as female but was assigned male at birth. Also referred to as male to female.

Diet

Research examining diet among sexual minority adults is largely conflicting.[31] Analyses of data from the National Health and Nutrition Examination Survey (NHANES) found no significant differences in dietary fat intake between sexual minority and their heterosexual adults.[32,33] A review of 13 articles found inconsistent findings when comparing food intake (eg, frequency and quantity of food group consumption) between sexual minority and heterosexual women.[34]

There is growing evidence that gender minority adults are at greater risk of poor diet quality compared with cisgender adults due to a higher prevalence of food insecurity and poverty.[31] Indeed, an online cross-sectional study found that transgender women were less likely than cisgender women to meet recommended daily intake of fruits and vegetables.[35] Further, analyses of longitudinal data have found that gender nonconforming male participants have less favorable diet scores compared with gender-conforming participants of the same sex; however, no differences in diet quality were observed among female-identifying participants.[36]

Physical Activity

Research on physical activity among sexual minority adults suggests that lesbian and bisexual women engage in more hours of physical activity than heterosexual women.[37–41] However, there are contradictory findings regarding differences in physical activity among men. Some studies have found that gay and bisexual men engage in more physical activity than heterosexual men.[40] In contrast, others suggest that sexual minority men are less likely to be physically active than heterosexual men.[37]

The literature on physical activity among gender minority people is limited. The few studies that have examined physical activity in gender minority adults have found that both transgender men and women were less likely to exercise or engage in leisure time physical activities in the past 30 days.[39,42,43] This trend has been observed across the lifecourse with older transgender adults ($\geq$50 years) reporting lower rates of physical activity compared with their cisgender counterparts.[44]

Sleep Health

A review of 31 studies found that 69% of included studies reported that SGM adults had shorter sleep duration compared with heterosexual adults.[45] Further, several studies have found that the odds of reporting poor sleep quality, such as difficulty falling asleep, waking up not feeling well rested, and using medications to sleep, were higher among gay men.[46–48] In contrast, other studies suggest that gay and bisexual men do not have higher odds of short sleep duration (sleeping <7 hours per night) compared with heterosexual men.[49] Moreover, multiple studies have found that lesbian and bisexual women are more likely to report short sleep duration,[39,49] more trouble staying asleep, and greater use of medications to sleep compared with heterosexual women.[47–49]

Several studies have found gender minority adults report higher odds of short sleep duration relative to their cisgender counterparts, which is attributed to minority stress.[39,45] Analyses of data from the National College Health Assessment II found that transgender college students had a higher prevalence of daytime sleepiness, insomnia symptoms, and other sleep disorders compared with cisgender college students.[50] Although evidence is limited, recent studies have found that greater exposure to minority stressors is associated with short sleep duration and greater sleep disturbances in gender minority adults.[51,52]

Obesity

There is consistent evidence that sexual minority women have higher odds of meeting criteria for overweight and obesity compared with heterosexual women.[6,8,53] Recent analyses of objective data from the NHANES found that bisexual men had approximately 1.6 times higher odds of meeting criteria for obesity compared with heterosexual men.[33] However, most of research on obesity disparities between gay and heterosexual men suggests that there are few differences.[6] Research on weight disparities among gender minority adults has largely focused on the influence of gender-affirming hormone therapy (GAHT; eg, estrogen, testosterone) and findings are largely contradictory.[7] A systematic review of 13 studies found that testosterone therapy was associated with significant increases in body mass index among transgender men,[54] but it is unclear if these increases are attributed to greater adipose tissue or lean muscle mass.[54–56]

Hypertension

Although evidence of hypertension disparities among sexual minority adults is conflicting, several studies have found that sexual minority adults have higher odds of hypertension compared with heterosexual adults.[8,20,32,33,57,58] Recent studies have found that sexual minority women have higher systolic and diastolic blood pressure than heterosexual women.[59,60] Findings for gay and bisexual men are mixed. A recent meta-analysis of 20 studies found that although there were no significant differences in blood pressure between gay and heterosexual men, bisexual men were twice as likely as heterosexual men to meet criteria for elevated blood pressure.[61] The few studies that have focused on the effects of GAHT on blood pressure among gender minority adults have revealed mixed findings.[6,62,63]

Diabetes

Multiple studies have found that lesbian and bisexual women are at higher risk of diabetes than heterosexual women.[6,32,64] Findings from gay and bisexual men are conflicting, but most research is null.[6,8] One notable exception is an analysis of NHANES data that found that bisexual men were three times as likely as heterosexual men to meet objective criteria for diagnosis of diabetes in the form of elevated glycosylated hemoglobin.[33]

Studies that have examined the effects of GAHT on glycemic status among gender minority adults report mixed findings.[7] For instance, a systematic review of 13 studies found that only two studies reported increased insulin resistance associated with testosterone therapy among transgender men.[65] Among transgender women, findings were mixed with five of eight studies indicating that transgender women on estrogen experience greater insulin resistance; however, the remaining three studies found that estrogen therapy was not associated with increased insulin resistance among transgender women.[65]

Hyperlipidemia

Research on disparities in hyperlipidemia among sexual minority adults is limited. Findings from a systematic review of 31 studies identified only 9 studies that investigated differences in blood lipids.[8] Out of these nine studies, the majority found no significant differences in hyperlipidemia between sexual minority and heterosexual adults.[8] Management of high cholesterol is of great concern among gender minority individuals due to the potential influence of GAHT on lipids.[66] A meta-analysis of 29 studies found that transgender men had lower high-density lipoprotein cholesterol and higher low-density lipoprotein cholesterol levels at 12 months and ≥24 months following initiation of testosterone therapy.[67] This highlights the importance of providing targeted education about lipid control to gender minority adults on GAHT.

Cardiovascular Disease Diagnoses

Existing evidence of disparities in CVD diagnoses among SGM adults is conflicting and largely based on self-reported data.[6] However, recent studies that have used administrative and electronic record data have found significant disparities in CVD diagnoses and CVD mortality among SGM adults.[68,69] Analyses of mortality data from Canada found that sexual minority adults were 53% more likely to die from CVD compared with heterosexual adults.[68] Further, analyses of electronic health record data from the United States that included over 4900 transgender adults found that transgender women had higher risk of ischemic stroke than cisgender women.[69]

Clinical Relevance

Nurses play an important role in the treatment and management of their patients' health and are uniquely positioned to promote the cardiovascular health of SGM adults.[70] However, a review of 24 studies revealed major gaps in nurses' knowledge of the health needs of SGM adults and many nurses expressed negative attitudes toward this population.[71] This suggests that there is a need for efforts to address explicit bias toward SGM people among nurses. **Fig. 1** summarizes the nursing clinical recommendations for caring for SGM adults with CVD.

Overall, little is known about the experiences of SGM people living with CVD. However, given existing evidence, a focus on tertiary prevention is important to promote optimal function and well-being among SGM adults with CVD. SGM individuals with CVD may require nursing care due to functional limitations that require assistance in completing activities of daily living and managing their CVD. In addition, prior work has shown that SGM adults are more likely to delay care due to fear of discrimination from clinicians and concerns related to health care costs.[72] It is well-documented that SGM people are less likely to rely on informal caregiving from family as they age and more likely to need care from formal caregivers (eg, nurses, home health aides).[73]

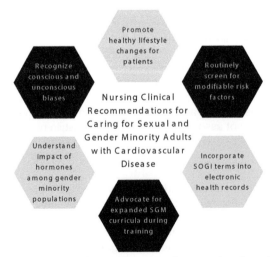

Fig. 1. Nursing clinical recommendations for caring for sexual and gender minority adults with cardiovascular disease.

Because of these reasons, it is not surprising that SGM adults report that advanced care planning is a priority as they age.[73] Given nursing's holistic approach to care, it is important for nurses to assess the availability of informal caregivers as well as other types of support, advanced care planning preferences, financial concerns, and potential fears in accessing health care services among SGM adults with CVD.

Further, there is limited guidance in the research literature regarding best practices for caring for SGM adults with CVD. It is important for nurses and other clinicians to address modifiable risk factors (eg, nicotine exposure, sleep health) to promote optimal cardiovascular health among SGM people. Nurses should be educated on the health disparities that have been documented among SGM individuals. For example, knowing that sexual minority women are more likely to smoke than heterosexual women, nurses should screen for nicotine exposure during clinical encounters with sexual minority women. Efforts to sustain a healthy lifestyle, such as smoking cessation and promoting sleep hygiene, can result in meaningful changes to the cardiovascular health of SGM patients.[6] Nurses should use validated assessment instruments to screen SGM patients for mental health problems (eg, stress, depression)[74] and other risk behaviors (eg, tobacco use,[75] heavy drinking[76]) that have been associated with poor cardiovascular outcomes among adults.[8]

The Fenway Health Institute, a health care organization in the United States focused on optimizing the health and well-being of SGM adults and those affected by HIV, argues that the collection of sexual orientation and gender identity (SOGI) data can help eliminate health disparities among SGM people.[77] As the largest health care profession, nurses can play an important role in advocating for initiatives to incorporate assessment of SOGI data during clinical visits and leading these efforts. SOGI data can help identify hidden disparities among SGM people and may provide direction for tailoring clinical interventions and nursing care. Given the higher prevalence of CVD and CVD mortality found among SGM adults across studies that used administrative and health record data,[68,69] widespread collection of SOGI data has the potential to increase our understanding of CVD in this population. The National Academies of Sciences, Engineering, and Medicine recently released a report describing strategies for accurately and sensitively assessing SOGI in clinical settings.[78] They recommended collecting data on SOGI during routine clinical encounters and using standardized language across national health surveys, such as the NHANES and the BRFSS. Further, they asserted that the use of standardized questions to assess sexual attraction and behavior could improve SOGI data quality and the potential public health impact of research on the health of SGM persons.

Training and curricula are the foundation of the clinical skills, knowledge, and attitudes that are essential to providing high-quality equitable care to patients. Prior work has found that nursing curricula lack sufficient content on SGM health, which can result in insensitive clinical encounters when caring for SGM patients.[73,79,80] This combined with nurses' overall negative attitudes against SGM patients that have been found in prior studies,[81] make these patients particularly vulnerable to receiving inferior care. As recommended by the American Nurses Association, nurses should be trained to not make assumptions regarding a patient's SOGI or their family circumstances, especially regarding surrogate decision-making, visiting privileges, and access to sensitive health information.[82] Therefore, it is important for nurses to be trained in recognizing conscious and unconscious biases to avoid asking SGM patients potentially insensitive questions that may be viewed as intrusive. One strategy to build trust and a more inclusive clinical environment is for nurses to routinely ask patients what their pronouns are and to share one's own pronouns with patients. As SGM health has become a bigger public health concern, there has been a proliferation of resources to help nurses and other clinicians enhance their knowledge of SGM health.[83]

Nurses should specifically be aware of unique issues that may impact the cardiovascular health of gender minority individuals. This is relevant when working with patients currently on GAHT. Although research on the impact of GAHT on CVD risk is mixed, there is consistent evidence that GAHT is associated with improved mental health and well-being among gender minority persons.[84] For instance, multiple studies have found that GAHT is associated with significant reductions in symptoms of anxiety, depression, and suicidality as well as improvements in quality of life and self-esteem in both transgender adolescents and adults.[84–86] Therefore, nurses should collaborate with their gender minority patients and other members of the interdisciplinary team (eg, endocrinologists) to create individualized plans of care that maximize the positive effects of GAHT on mental health and well-being while targeting modifiable risk factors, such as nicotine exposure, to reduce their risk of CVD.

SUMMARY

SGM adults experience unique social and structural disadvantages that influence psychosocial, behavioral, and physiologic risk factors for CVD. Although there has been considerable progress in identifying key drivers of cardiovascular health disparities among SGM individuals, more research is needed to examine the associations between minority stressors and CVD risk factors to inform interventions for this high-risk population. It is evident that nurses need more education to provide high-quality culturally tailored cardiovascular care to SGM adults. Specialized training with standardized health curricula in SGM health would be beneficial for nurses providing care for this population.

CLINICS CARE POINTS

- Nurses should perform the routine screening of modifiable risk factors, psychosocial factors, and health risk behaviors via validated measures among sexual and gender minority adults.
- Nurses should advocate for the collection of sexual orientation and gender identity data and the use of standardized questions to assess sexual attraction and behavior within electronic health records at their institutions.
- Nurses should be trained on recognizing conscious and unconscious biases and refrain from assuming the sexual orientation or gender identity of their patients.

DISCLOSURE

Dr B.A. Caceres was supported by a Mentored Research Scientist Development Award from the National Heart, Lung, and Blood Institute, United States (K01HL146965). Ms Y. Sharma was supported by a predoctoral fellowship from the American Heart Association, United States (Grant number 899585).

REFERENCES

1. Tsao CW, Aday AW, Almarzooq ZI, et al. Heart disease and stroke statistics-2022 update: a report from the American heart association. Circulation 2022;145(8): E153–639.

2. Noncommunicable diseases. Available at: https://www.who.int/news-room/fact-sheets/detail/noncommunicable-diseases. Published September 16, 2022. Accessed November 29, 2022.

3. Yusuf S, Joseph P, Rangarajan S, et al. Modifiable risk factors, cardiovascular disease, and mortality in 155 722 individuals from 21 high-income, middle-income, and low-income countries (PURE): a prospective cohort study. Lancet 2020;395(10226):795–808.

4. Churchwell K, Elkind MSV, Benjamin RM, et al. Call to action: structural racism as a fundamental driver of health disparities: a presidential advisory from the american heart association. Circulation 2020;142(24):E454–68.

5. Havranek EP, Mujahid MS, Barr DA, et al. Social determinants of risk and outcomes for cardiovascular disease. Circulation 2015;132(9):873–98.

6. Caceres BA, Streed CG, Corliss HL, et al. Assessing and addressing cardiovascular health in LGBTQ adults: a scientific statement from the american heart association. Circulation 2020;142(19):e321–32.

7. Streed CG Jr, Beach LB, Caceres BA, et al. Assessing and addressing cardiovascular health in people who are transgender and gender diverse: a scientific statement from the american heart association. Circulation 2021;144(6):E136–48.

8. Caceres BA, Brody A, Luscombe RE, et al. A systematic review of cardiovascular disease in sexual minorities. Am J Public Health 2017;107(4):e13–21.

9. Brooks VR. Minority stress and lesbian women. Lexington, MA: Lexingt Books; 1981.

10. Meyer IH. Prejudice, social stress, and mental health in lesbian, gay, and bisexual populations: conceptual issues and research evidence. Psychol Bull 2003; 129(5):674–97.

11. Testa RJ, Habarth J, Peta J, et al. Development of the gender minority stress and resilience measure. Psychol Sex Orientat Gend Divers 2015;2(1):65–77.

12. Pachankis JE. Uncovering clinical principles and techniques to address minority stress, mental health, and related health risks among gay and bisexual men. Clin Psychol Sci Pract 2014;21(4):313–30.

13. English D, Rendina HJ, Parsons JT. The effects of intersecting stigma: a longitudinal examination of minority stress, mental health, and substance use among black, Latino, and multiracial gay and bisexual men. Psychol Violence 2018; 8(6):669.

14. Caceres BA, Hughes TL, Veldhuis CB, et al. Past-year discrimination and cigarette smoking among sexual minority women: investigating racial/ethnic and sexual identity differences. J Behav Med 2021;44(5):726–39.

15. Goldbach JT, Tanner-Smith EE, Bagwell M, et al. Minority stress and substance use in sexual minority adolescents: a meta-analysis. Prev Sci 2014;15(3):350–63.

16. Flentje A, Heck NC, Brennan JM, et al. The relationship between minority stress and biological outcomes: a systematic review. J Behav Med 2019;43(5):673–94.

17. Rendina HJ, Gamarel KE, Pachankis JE, et al. Extending the minority stress model to incorporate HIV-positive gay and bisexual men's experiences: a longitudinal examination of mental health and sexual risk behavior. Ann Behav Med 2017;51(2):147–58.

18. Poteat TC, Divsalar S, Streed CG, et al. Cardiovascular disease in a population-based sample of transgender and cisgender adults. Am J Prev Med 2021;61(6): 804–11.

19. Mereish EH, Goldstein CM. Minority stress and cardiovascular disease risk among sexual minorities: mediating effects of sense of mastery. Int J Behav Med 2020;27(6):726–36.

20. Caceres BA, Markovic N, Edmondson D, et al. Sexual identity, adverse life experiences, and cardiovascular health in women. J Cardiovasc Nurs 2019;34(5):380.

21. Lanuza DM, Davidson PM, Dunbar SB, et al. Preparing nurses for leadership roles in cardiovascular disease prevention. Eur J Cardiovasc Nurs 2011; 10(Suppl 2). https://doi.org/10.1016/S1474-5151(11)00116-2.

22. State of the world's nursing 2020: investing in education, jobs and leadership. Available at: https://www.who.int/publications/i/item/9789240003279. Published April 6, 2020. Accessed November 29, 2022.

23. Piano MR, Artinian NT, Devon HA, et al. Cardiovascular nursing science priorities: a statement from the american heart association council on cardiovascular and stroke nursing. J Cardiovasc Nurs 2018;33(4):E11–20.

24. Parent MC, Arriaga A, Gobble T, et al. Stress and substance use among sexual and gender minority individuals across the lifespan. Neurobiol Stress 2019;10: 100146.

25. Abrahão ABB, Kortas GT, Blaas IK, et al. The impact of discrimination on substance use disorders among sexual minorities. Int Rev Psychiatry 2022; 34(3–4):423–31.

26. Li J, Berg CJ, Weber AA, et al. Tobacco use at the intersection of sex and sexual identity in the U.S., 2007-2020: a meta-analysis. Am J Prev Med 2021;60(3):415–24.

27. Azagba S, Shan L. Disparities in the frequency of tobacco products use by sexual identity status. Addict Behav 2021;122:107032.

28. Azagba S, Latham K, Shan L. Cigarette, smokeless tobacco, and alcohol use among transgender adults in the united states. Int J Drug Policy 2019;73:163–9.

29. Ruppert R, Kattari SK, Sussman S. Review: Prevalence of addictions among transgender and gender diverse subgroups. Int J Environ Res Public Heal 2021;18:8843.

30. Hinds JT, Chow S, Loukas A, et al. Exploring transgender and gender diverse young adult tobacco use. J Homosex 2021;69(13):2188–208.

31. Caceres BA, Bynon M, Doan D, et al. Diet, food insecurity, and CVD risk in sexual and gender minority adults. Curr Atheroscler Rep 2022;24(1):41–50.

32. Caceres BA, Brody AA, Halkitis PN, et al. Cardiovascular disease risk in sexual minority women (18-59 years old): findings from the national health and nutrition examination survey (2001-2012). Women's Heal Issues 2018;28(4):333–41.

33. Caceres BA, Brody AA, Halkitis PN, et al. Sexual orientation differences in modifiable risk factors for cardiovascular disease and cardiovascular disease diagnoses in men. LGBT Heal 2018;5(5):284.

34. Foley JD, Morris J, Shepard C, et al. Evaluating food intake outcomes among sexual minority women: a systematic review. LGBT Health 2022;9(7):447–62. Available at: https://home.liebertpub.com/lgbt.

35. Smalley KB, Warren JC, Barefoot KN. Differences in health risk behaviors across understudied LGBT subgroups. Heal Psychol 2016;35(2):103–14.

36. VanKim NA, Corliss HL, Jun HJ, et al. Gender expression and sexual orientation differences in diet quality and eating habits from adolescence to young adulthood. J Acad Nutr Diet 2019;119(12):2028–40.

37. Abichahine H, Veenstra G. Inter-categorical intersectionality and leisure-based physical activity in Canada. Health Promot Int 2017;32(4):691–701.

38. Boehmer U, Miao X, Linkletter C, et al. Adult health behaviors over the life course by sexual orientation. Am J Public Health 2012;102(2):292–300.

39. Cunningham TJ, Xu F, Town M. Prevalence of five health-related behaviors for chronic disease prevention among sexual and gender minority adults — 25 U.S. states and Guam, 2016. Morb Mortal Wkly Rep 2018;67(32):888.

40. Fricke J, Gordon N, Downing J. Sexual orientation disparities in physical activity. Med Care 2019;57(2):138–44.

41. Vankim NA, Austin SB, Jun HJ, et al. Physical activity and sedentary behaviors among lesbian, bisexual, and heterosexual women: findings from the nurses' health study II. LGBT Health 2017;26(10):1077–85. Available at: https://home.liebertpub.com/jwh.

42. Downing JM, Przedworski JM. Health of transgender adults in the U.S., 2014–2016. Am J Prev Med 2018;55(3):336–44.

43. Holder J, Morris J, Spreckley M. Barriers and facilitators for participation in physical activity in the transgender population: a systematic review. Phys Act Heal 2022;6(1):136–50.

44. Fredriksen-Goldsen KI, Cook-Daniels L, Kim HJ, et al. physical and mental health of transgender older adults: an at-risk and underserved population. Gerontol 2014;54(3):488–500.

45. Butler ES, McGlinchey E, Juster RP. Sexual and gender minority sleep: a narrative review and suggestions for future research. J Sleep Res 2020;29(1):e12928.

46. Almazan EP. The association between sexual orientation and sleep problems: are there racial and ethnic differences? Clocks Sleep 2019;1:220–5.

47. Duncan DT, Kanchi R, Tantay L, et al. Disparities in sleep problems by sexual orientation among new york city adults: an analysis of the new york city health and nutrition examination survey, 2013–2014. J Urban Heal 2018;95(6):781–6.

48. Galinsky AM, Ward BW, Joestl SS, et al. Sleep duration, sleep quality, and sexual orientation: findings from the 2013-2015 national health interview survey. Sleep Heal 2018;4(1):56–62.

49. Caceres BA, Hickey KT, Heitkemper EM, et al. An intersectional approach to examine sleep duration in sexual minority adults in the United States: findings from the behavioral risk factor surveillance system. Sleep Heal 2019;5(6):621–9.

50. Hershner S, Jansen E, Gavidia R, et al. Associations between transgender identity, sleep, mental health and suicidality among a north american cohort of college students. Nat Sci Sleep 2021;13:383.

51. Caceres BA, Jackman KB, Belloir J, et al. Examining the associations of gender minority stressors with sleep health in gender minority individuals. Sleep Heal 2022;8(2):153–60.

52. Kolp H, Wilder S, Andersen C, et al. Gender minority stress, sleep disturbance, and sexual victimization in transgender and gender nonconforming adults. J Clin Psychol 2020;76(4):688–98.

53. Eliason MJ, Ingraham N, Fogel SC, et al. A systematic review of the literature on weight in sexual minority women. Women's Heal Issues 2015;25(2):162–75.

54. Velho I, Fighera TM, Ziegelmann PK, et al. Effects of testosterone therapy on BMI, blood pressure, and laboratory profile of transgender men: a systematic review. Andrology 2017;5(5):881–8.

55. Suppakitjanusant P, Ji Y, Stevenson MO, et al. Effects of gender affirming hormone therapy on body mass index in transgender individuals: a longitudinal cohort study. J Clin Transl Endocrinol 2020;21. https://doi.org/10.1016/J.JCTE.2020.100230.

56. Nokoff NJ, Scarbro SL, Moreau KL, et al. Body composition and markers of cardiometabolic health in transgender youth compared with cisgender youth. J Clin Endocrinol Metab 2020;105(3). https://doi.org/10.1210/CLINEM/DGZ029.

57. Choi SK, Kittle K, Meyer IH. Health disparities of older adults in California: the role of sexual identity and Latinx ethnicity. Gerontol 2021;61(6):851–7.

58. Goldberg SK, Conron KJ, Halpern CT. Metabolic syndrome and economic strain among sexual minority young adults. LGBT Health 2019;6(1):1–8. Available at: https://home.liebertpub.com/lgbt.

59. Caceres BA, Ancheta AJ, Dorsen C, et al. A population-based study of the intersection of sexual identity and race/ethnicity on physiological risk factors for CVD among U.S. adults (ages 18–59). Ethn Health 2020;27(3):617–38.

60. Kinsky S, Stall R, Hawk M, et al. Risk of the metabolic syndrome in sexual minority women: results from the ESTHER Study. LGBT Health 2016;25(8):784–90. Available at: https://home.liebertpub.com/jwh.

61. López Castillo H, Tfirn IC, Hegarty E, et al. A meta-analysis of blood pressure disparities among sexual minority men. LGBT Health 2021;8(2):91–106. Available at: https://home.liebertpub.com/lgbt.

62. Connelly PJ, Freel EM, Perry C, et al. Gender-affirming hormone therapy, vascular health and cardiovascular disease in transgender adults. Hypertens (Dallas, Tex 1979) 2019;74(6):1266–74.

63. Defreyne J, Van de Bruaene LL, Rietzschel E, et al. Effects of gender-affirming hormones on lipid, metabolic, and cardiac surrogate blood markers in transgender persons. Clin Chem 2019;65(1):119–34.

64. Liu H, Chen IC, Wilkinson L, et al. Sexual orientation and diabetes during the transition to adulthood. LGBT Health 2019;6(5):227–34. Available at: https://home.liebertpub.com/lgbt.

65. Spanos C, Bretherton I, Zajac JD, et al. Effects of gender-affirming hormone therapy on insulin resistance and body composition in transgender individuals: a systematic review. World J Diabetes 2020;11(3):66.

66. Cocchetti C, Castellini G, Iacuaniello D, et al. Does gender-affirming hormonal treatment affect 30-year cardiovascular risk in transgender persons? a two-year prospective European study (ENIGI). J Sex Med 2021;18(4):821–9.

67. Maraka S, Ospina NS, Rodriguez-Gutierrez R, et al. Sex steroids and cardiovascular outcomes in transgender individuals: a systematic review and meta-analysis. J Clin Endocrinol Metab 2017;102(11):3914–23.

68. Salway T, Rich AJ, Ferlatte O, et al. Preventable mortality among sexual minority Canadians. SSM - Popul Heal. 2022;20:2352–8273.

69. Getahun D, Nash R, Flanders WD, et al. Cross-sex hormones and acute cardiovascular events in transgender persons: a cohort study. Ann Intern Med 2018; 169(4):205–13.

70. Dibble SL, Eliason MJ, Christiansen MAD. Chronic illness care for lesbian, gay, & bisexual individuals. Nurs Clin North Am 2007;42(4):655–74.

71. Stewart K, O'Reilly P. Exploring the attitudes, knowledge and beliefs of nurses and midwives of the healthcare needs of the LGBTQ population: an integrative review. Nurse Educ Today 2017;53:67–77.

72. Caceres BA, Turchioe MR, Pho A, et al. Sexual identity and racial/ethnic differences in awareness of heart attack and stroke symptoms: findings from the national health interview survey. Am J Health Promot 2020;35(1):57–67.

73. Caceres BA, Travers J, Primiano JE, et al. Provider and LGBT individuals' perspectives on LGBT issues in long-term care: a systematic review. Gerontol 2020;60(3):e169–83.

74. Mensah GA, Collins PY. Understanding mental health for the prevention and control of cardiovascular diseases. Glob Heart 2015;10(3):221.

75. Rigotti NA, Clair C. Managing tobacco use: the neglected cardiovascular disease risk factor. Eur Heart J 2013;34(42):3259–67.

76. Ronksley PE, Brien SE, Turner BJ, et al. Association of alcohol consumption with selected cardiovascular disease outcomes: a systematic review and meta-analysis. BMJ 2011;342:d671. https://doi.org/10.1136/bmj.d671.
77. The Fenway institute released new tools to help healthcare organizations collect sexual orientation and gender identity data to improve quality of care and reduce LGBT health disparities. Available at: https://fenwayhealth.org/the-fenway-institute-released-new-tools-to-help-healthcare-organizations-collect-sexual-orientation-and-gender-identity-data-to-improve-quality-of-care-and-reduce-lgbt-health-disparities/. Published June 25, 2019. Accessed November 29, 2022.
78. National Academies of Sciences, Engineering, and Medicine; Division of Behavioral and Social Sciences and Education; Committee on National Statistics; Committee on Measuring Sex, Gender Identity, and Sexual Orientation. Becker T., Chin M., Bates N., eds. Measuring Sex, Gender Identity, and Sexual Orientation. Washington (DC): National Academies Press (US); 2022.
79. Lim F, Johnson M, Eliason M. A national survey of faculty knowledge, experience, and readiness for teaching lesbian, gay, bisexual, and transgender health in baccalaureate nursing programs. Nurs Educ Perspect 2015;36(3):144–52.
80. McCann E, Brown M. The inclusion of LGBT+ health issues within undergraduate healthcare education and professional training programmes: a systematic review. Nurse Educ Today 2018;64:204–14.
81. Dorsen C. An integrative review of nurse attitudes towards lesbian, gay, bisexual, and transgender patients. Can J Nurs Res 2012;44(3):18–43. Available at: https://europepmc.org/article/med/23156190. Accessed November 29, 2022.
82. Nursing advocacy for LGBTQ+ populations code of ethics for nurses with interpretive statements. Available at: www.nursingworld.org. Accessed November 29, 2022.
83. National LGBTQIA+ health education center. The Fenway Institute; 2022. Available at: https://www.lgbtqiahealtheducation.org/. Accessed December 1, 2022.
84. Nguyen HB, Chavez AM, Lipner E, et al. Gender-affirming hormone use in transgender individuals: impact on behavioral health and cognition. Curr Psychiatry Rep 2018;20(12):110.
85. Aldridge Z, Patel S, Guo B, et al. Long-term effect of gender-affirming hormone treatment on depression and anxiety symptoms in transgender people: a prospective cohort study. Andrology 2021;9(6):1808–16.
86. Green AE, DeChants JP, Price MN, et al. Association of gender-affirming hormone therapy with depression, thoughts of suicide, and attempted suicide among transgender and nonbinary youth. J Adolesc Heal 2022;70(4):643–9.

Pediatric Murmurs

Rémi M. Hueckel, DNP, CPNP-AC[a],*,
Christy Leyland, MSN, PED-BC, CNL, CPNP-AC[b]

KEYWORDS

- Murmur • Pediatrics • Innocent Murmur • Heart auscultation • Physical exam

KEY POINTS

- Many healthy pediatric patients have murmurs, most are innocent murmurs and not associated with heart disease or defect.
- Innocent murmurs occur independent of other cardiovascular findings, during systole, do not radiate, and often become softer or disappear when the patient moves from supine to sitting position.
- If a murmur is heard during diastole, the patient should be evaluated for cardiac disease or dysfunction.
- Pathologic murmurs, associated with structural cardiac anomalies or cardiac dysfunction, often heard in infants, are frequently associated with other key findings in the patient's prenatal and birth history, history of present illness, physical exam, and growth trajectory.
- All newborns should be screened for critical congenital heart defect(s).

INTRODUCTION

A "normal" cardiac physical exam in pediatric patients includes a regular heart rate and rhythm (S1, S2) without murmurs, gallops, or rubs. However, if a murmur is detected, nurses often ask themselves whether the murmur is "innocent" (benign) or "pathologic" (the result of cardiac disease, dysfunction, or a defect). To determine the answer to this question, the nurse needs to consider the child's clinical history, presentation (reason for the visit), and focused physical exam. In this article, we review resources for nurses caring for pediatric patients and discuss common findings in the history and physical exam of pediatric patients by age-group that will provide context and guidance when a child is found to have a murmur.

---

[a] Duke University School of Nursing, Pediatric Acute Care NP, Duke Children's Hospitals and Clinics, 307 Trent Drive, Durham, NC 27710, USA; [b] Part Time Faculty, Northeastern University Bouvé School of Nursing Charlotte Campus, Pediatric Acute Care NP, Atrium Health Levine Children's, 1000 Blythe Boulevard, Charlotte, NC, 28203, USA
* Corresponding author.
E-mail address: remi.hueckel@duke.edu

Nurs Clin N Am 58 (2023) 475–482
https://doi.org/10.1016/j.cnur.2023.05.013
0029-6465/23/© 2023 Elsevier Inc. All rights reserved.

nursing.theclinics.com

RESOURCES FOR NURSES CARING FOR PEDIATRIC PATIENTS

The American Academy of Pediatrics (AAP) was developed in the 1930s through collaboration among pediatricians who were committed to addressing developmental and health needs unique to children. This organization has grown to over 65,000 physicians and other healthcare providers dedicated to the health and wellbeing of children. Over the decades, the AAP has provided guidance and standards for physical, mental, and preventive care to children from infants to young-adulthood.[1]

Bright Futures[2] and the Periodicity Table[3] are two AAP resources that provide specific guidance for nurses and other healthcare professionals who care for pediatric patients. These are guides for what to expect for preventive care and screening by age-group and are useful resources to review when preparing to see a pediatric patient in the outpatient setting. Bright Futures guidelines outline expected developmental stages, physical exam findings, and provide suggested topics and questions to consider when taking a general history of a pediatric patient.

The AAP has made recommendations, developed screening guidelines, and provided education and advocacy for children who are at the greatest risk for heart disease. There are specific guidelines to screen for congenital heart defects in infants and screen adolescents and young adults to determine their risk of developing sudden cardiac arrest or sudden cardiac death. Congenital heart defects are found in approximately 1% of live births in the United States.[4] Furthermore, one in four infants born with congenital heart defects have a critical congenital heart defect. Despite advances in comprehensive prenatal care and fetal echocardiogram some infants are born with an undiagnosed congenital heart defect. Thus, for over a decade, the AAP has advocated for the use of pulse-oximetry to screen for critical congenital heart defects in newborns before they are discharged from the hospital.[5]

In 2012, the AAP released a policy statement that encouraged providers to evaluate adolescent and young adult athletes for conditions that may lead to sudden cardiac arrest or sudden cardiac death. More recently, the AAP along with multiple other organizations expanded this effort to educate communities, increase awareness of sudden cardiac arrest and sudden cardiac death, and identify and screen for conditions that cause sudden cardiac death in all adolescents and young adults independent of the child's participation in athletics.[6] Recommendations for screening for critical congenital heart defect and sudden cardiac arrest/sudden cardiac death can be found in the Bright Futures guidelines.[2]

REVIEW OF PEDIATRIC CARDIAC PHYSIOLOGY AND TERMINOLOGY

When considering best practices for history taking and performing cardiovascular physical exams on pediatric patients, it is helpful to recall some common terminology, developmental anatomy, and physiology specific to the cardiovascular system.

The Cardiac Cycle

The cardiac cycle consists of systole and diastole. Systole, the contractile part of the cardiac cycle, is created by the closure of the atrioventricular valves (mitral and tricuspid). Systole is synchronous with S1 – the first heart sound and correlates with the pulsation of blood through the arteries. S1 represents the closure of mitral and tricuspid valves and marks the beginning of systole. S1 is best heard along the lower left sternal border. Diastole is the relaxation or filling part of the cardiac cycle. Diastole is created by the closure of the aortic and pulmonic valves, synchronous with S2 – the second heart sound. S2 represents the closure of aortic and pulmonic valves and marks the beginning of diastole. The aortic valve closure is best heard at the second intercostal space (ICS) on the right of the sternum and the pulmonic valve is best heard at the second ICS on the left of the sternum. S1 and S2 are clear, distinct sounds and S1 correlates with the patient's pulse. Extra heart sounds such as a split S2 or S3 are sometimes difficult to discern in infants and young children whose normal resting heart rate is over 100 beats per minute. See **Fig. 1**.

Murmurs

Murmurs are defined as turbulent blood flow and are noted during the auscultation of heart sounds. The turbulent flow of blood causes a distinct swishing sound that occurs within or during the expected sounds of S1 and S2. Murmurs are characterized and described by noting the timing of when they occur in the cardiac cycle (systole or diastole) and the location of loudest sound (**Fig. 2**). Other characteristics of murmurs

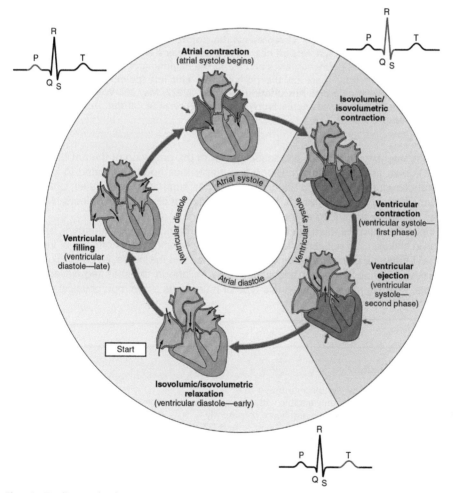

Fig. 1. Cardiac cycle. https://commons.wikimedia.org/wiki/File:Phases_of_the_cardiac_cycle. svg. https://commons.wikimedia.org/wiki/File:2027_Phases_of_the_Cardiac_Cycle.jpg#/media/ File:2027_Phases_of_the_Cardiac_Cycle.jpg. OpenStax College, Anatomy & Physiology, Connexions Web site. http://cnx.org/content/col11496/1.6/, Jun 19, 2013.

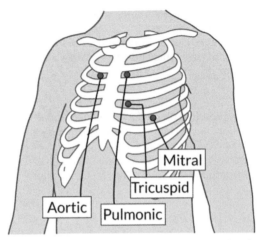

Fig. 2. Areas for auscultation. S1 represents the closure of mitral and tricuspid valves and marks the beginning of systole. Best heard along left lower sternal border. S2 represents the closure of aortic and pulmonic valves and marks the beginning of diastole. S2 is loudest at the second intercostal space on the right (aortic) and left (pulmonic) of the sternum. Theodore Dimitriou, Cardiac Auscultation PNG.png. (2022, May 30). Wikimedia Commons. From https://commons.wikimedia.org/w/index.php?title=File:Cardiac_Auscultation_PNG. png&oldid=660156741.

include intensity and if they are associated with the palpation of the turbulent blood flow known as a thrill (**Box 1**). Blood flow turbulence could be related to increased metabolic states or tachycardia (from conditions such as anemia, fever, pregnancy) or structural changes in the heart (such as congenital or structural defects). Murmurs may be further described as innocent or pathologic.

Innocent murmurs, also referred to as flow-murmurs or benign murmurs, are common in children and not associated with anatomic or functional anomalies of the heart. Small peripheral pulmonary arteries during infancy and the increased cardiac output or increased metabolic states associated with childhood illnesses (eg, fever, tachycardia, anemia) result in having this type of murmur as a common physical finding in

---

Box 1
Murmur intensity

Grading of Intensity: Systolic murmurs 1 to 6
    Grade 1: very quiet, only audible with a quiet patient in a quiet room, intermittent
    Grade 2: easily discernible and heard consistently
    Grade 3: loud, as loud/intense as heart sounds (S1 and S2), no palpable thrill or vibration
    Grade 4: loud, may be heard in more than one location, associated with palpable thrill[a]
    Grade 5: very loud, may be heard over noisy breathing and/or with stethoscope lightly touching chest[a]
    Grade 6: very loud, able to be heard with ear placed on chest[a]

[a] Murmurs grade 4 to 6 are associated with palpable vibration or thrill.

Gonzalez VJ, Kyle WB, Allen HD. Cardiac Examination and Evaluation of Murmurs. *Pediatr Rev.* 2021;42(7):375-382. https://doi.org/10.1542/pir.2020-000604.

patients aged 3 years through teenage years. Characteristics of these innocent murmurs include a low-pitched tone, heard with the patient in a supine position, during *systole* and loudest along the left lower sternal border.[7] Often innocent murmurs become softer or are unable to be heard when a patient sits up or moves from lying down to standing.

Pathologic murmurs are more prevalent during infancy and are associated with changes in blood flow related to congenital heart defects or other anatomic changes in the heart. Some of these are described later in discussion. Often pathologic murmurs are heard in diastole and do not change in character or decrease in intensity with changes in the patient's position.

Foramen Ovale

In utero, fetal blood flows through an intra-atrial connection known as the foramen ovale. In response to a decrease in pulmonary vascular resistance, the foramen ovale often closes in the days to weeks after birth. However, in some neonates the foramen ovale remains open, resulting in a patent foramen ovale (PFO). Blood flow through a PFO may (or may not) result in a soft murmur, heard in systole. Some individuals with a PFO remain asymptomatic. Some older adolescents and young adults, with a PFO may have a soft systolic murmur and symptoms of stroke or migraine.[8]

Ductus Arteriosus

A ductus arteriosus connects the pulmonary artery and aorta in fetal circulation. This connection typically closes within the first week of life in most term newborns. A failure to close results in patent ductus arteriosus (PDA) whereby blood flows from the systemic high-resistance system (aorta) to low resistance system (pulmonary artery). Murmurs associated with a PDA are considered pathologic and are characteristically heard *continuously* throughout the cardiac cycle.[7]

Ventricular Septal Defect

A ventricular septal defect (VSD) is the most prevalent congenital heart defect. A VSD is a disruption in the ventricular septum. In a heart without a VSD, blood is pumped from the left ventricle, through the systemic vascular system and returns to the right atrium, goes through the tricuspid valve then is pumped through the pulmonary vascular system. The systemic vascular system is a high-resistance system and the pulmonary vascular system is a lower resistance system. In the presence of a VSD, blood moves from the left ventricle through the VSD to the right ventricle. This turbulent blood flow through the VSD causes a murmur that is characteristically *harsh, loud,* and heard best along the left lower sternal board during *diastole.*[4,7] Murmurs associated with a VSD are considered pathologic. Patients with this *diastolic,* pathologic murmur will most often also have respiratory symptoms such as tachypnea and rales and crackles on their pulmonary exam.

EVALUATION OF A PEDIATRIC PATIENT WITH A MURMUR
History

Often innocent murmurs occur in young children who have no other concerning vital sign or physical exam findings. Thus, history taking is an important aspect of nursing assessment to help determine if the murmur is innocent or pathologic. Questions in the history help establish the likelihood of cardiac (or pathologic) causes for the murmur. In addition to the history of present illness (why the patient is being seen), the nurse should assess the patient's presenting signs and symptoms, the prenatal history including results of perinatal screening, and the maternal and family history (including any history of sudden death in the family).

Other important aspects of history include maternal exposure to certain medications. For example, one risk factor associated with premature closure of the ductus arteriosus includes the use of non-steroidal anti-inflammatory drugs. Another medication class of concern includes anti-epileptic drugs (eg, valproic acid). In addition, various maternal infections during the first trimester contribute to ventriculo-atrial misalignment and other obstructive pathologies. Finally, stenotic ductus arteriosus and pulmonary artery stenosis have been found with intrautero rubella exposure.[9]

Perinatal screening with ultrasound or fetal echocardiography can identify many cardiac defects. However, for various reasons such as the size or type of cardiac defect or access to fetal echocardiography, some infants may be born with cardiac defects that are not detected prenatally. These patients may present with symptoms (eg, increased metabolic demand with or without feeding – tachycardia, tachypnea, hypoxia, cyanosis, and/or dyspnea) related to the cardiac defect shortly after birth or later in life depending on the severity of the defect.

A history of feeding and activity tolerance in infants and children is also associated with murmurs. For example, a history of difficulty eating, tachycardia, and/or diaphoresis during feeding for an infant may suggest cardiac dysfunction. Another common clinical finding that suggests a cardiac (or pathologic) cause for a murmur may be activity intolerance and inability to keep up with peers. In older children and adolescents, it's important for nurses to ask about palpitations or feeling irregular heartbeats as part of a cardiac-focused history.

Inclusion of questions regarding any recent illnesses and a thorough evaluation of presenting symptoms may also provide insight into the type of murmur the pediatric patient has. As noted, a child's fever and tachycardia may explain an innocent murmur at a particular visit.

Physical Exam

Completing a physical exam on an active or crying infant can be challenging for nurses and other healthcare providers. Determination of positional murmurs, location auscultated best on the chest, and if it radiates are all important aspects of a thorough systematic physical exam – but hearing the murmur at all requires a comfortable, calm, and quiet child. For infants, consider completing the auscultation part of the physical exam while the patient is eating or being held by the caregiver.

Placing patients in particular positions (or doing maneuvers) may help the nurse discern the type of murmur the patient has. For example, some pathologic murmurs increase in intensity (volume) when the patient is sitting upright. Whereas innocent murmurs are loudest when the patient is supine and often quieter with the patient seated, standing, or bearing down (Valsalva).

Once the murmur is located, it is important to listen carefully during the entire cardiac cycle. First, listen to the rhythm of the heartbeat (expectedly faster the younger the patient) and determine if the murmur is during systole (S1) or diastole (S2) or heard continuously throughout the cardiac cycle. A helpful hint to isolate S1 is to palpate the patient's pulse while listening. In infants and young children, the brachial pulse is the easiest to palpate while listening and S1 is synchronous with the brachial artery pulsation.

When describing a murmur, documentation of certain descriptors will aid other examiners when comparing findings from one exam to another. Things like the description of location (where on the chest wall), quality (harsh, blowing), intensity (loudness based on a 1–6 grading system) (see **Box 1**), timing (during systole, diastole or continuously throughout the cardiac cycle), and radiation of the murmur will aid in determining if a murmur might be pathologic or innocent. For example, a benign or innocent murmur may be described as soft, *systolic*, and best heard at the left upper sternal border with no radiation to axillae and not heard posteriorly. *Soft, early systolic* murmurs without radiation or that disappear when the patient stands are most often associated with innocent murmurs.

Beyond the auscultation of heart sounds, other components of the physical exam include growth analysis, vital signs, peripheral pulses, and respiratory and cutaneous findings.[10] Analysis of the patient's growth (height and weight) may give clues if a murmur is associated with cardiac disease, dysfunction, or defect.[3] Many infants and young children with congenital heart defects have challenges with feeding and require more calories to attain steady growth as compared to infants without a congenital heart defect.

Vital signs, such as heart rate, blood pressure, and respiratory rate may also be outside the expected range for age-group in a child with a murmur.[3] Children with innocent murmurs caused by fever or anemia may be mildly tachycardic. An infant or young child with a PDA and a murmur heard throughout the cardiac cycle (also known as a "continuous murmur") may have a widened pulse pressure or diastolic blood pressure lower than expected for age. Infants with harsh, loud diastolic murmurs associated with a VSD are often tachypneic but without signs of increased work of breathing though they may have crackles or rales noted on pulmonary auscultation.

Peripheral pulses should be palpated and compared in all extremities. In addition, consider measuring blood pressures in at least one upper extremity and one lower extremity.[3] Coarctation of the aorta is one type of congenital heart defect that may be diagnosed after infancy. In addition to a loud systolic murmur that radiates to the patient's back, young children with aortic coarctation will very likely be hypertensive, have lower extremity pulses that are difficult to palpate and a 10 mm Hg (or more) difference between upper and lower extremity blood pressures.[7]

Remarkable cutaneous findings associated with a new murmur and fever may include splinter hemorrhages in the nails, erythema (redness) on the palms of the hands and soles of the feet (known as Janeway lesions), and tender nodules on the pads of a child or adolescent's fingers or toes (known as Osler nodes). These findings are characteristic of endocarditis.[10]

SUMMARY

Murmurs in infants and children are relatively common. Up to 8% of infants and approximately 80% of children are found to have a heart murmur early in life. The lifetime incidence of transient and innocent childhood murmurs indicates that most children experience a heart murmur.[9] Whether this murmur is discovered at a routine health maintenance visit or during a focused exam on a child with illness, nurses should keep in mind that a murmur is just one finding. Identification of a murmur must be considered in the overall context of the child's history and other physical exam findings. Identifying characteristics such as timing during the cardiac cycle, location, and radiation of the murmur as well as other history and physical exam findings aide in a thorough evaluation of the child with a murmur. Murmurs associated with a structural or functional defect in the heart occur most often in infancy. Children between ages 3 to 6 years and young adulthoods commonly have innocent (or benign) murmurs which are not indicative of cardiac dysfunction or defect. The key takeaway for nurses is to anticipate what to expect when completing a history and physical exam on pediatric patients. Understanding terminology and utilizing descriptive communication regarding murmurs and the overall cardiovascular exam will facilitate the next steps (if any) toward an additional work up.

CLINICS CARE POINTS

- Many murmurs are 'innocent' and present because of other contributing factors such as fever, anemia, or dehydration.
- A detailed cardiac history and focused physical exam provides context for determining if a murmur may be innocent or pathologic/cardiac related.
- During history, determine if the patient (or caregiver) has been told that the patient has a murmur.
- Consider the child's general appearance in consultation with how caregivers think they look compared to child's baseline.
- To get the best exam, auscultate heart sounds when children are in a position of comfort.
- Positional maneuvers may change in intensity for some murmurs to allow for comparison of heart sounds in varying positions.

DISCLOSURE

The authors have nothing to disclose – no conflict of interest.

REFERENCES

1. Website: American Academy of Pediatrics. https://www.aap.org/en/about-the-aap/. Accessed March 10, 2023.
2. Hagan JF, Shaw JS, Duncan PM. In: *Bright Futures: guidelines for health Supervision of infants, children, and adolescents*. 4th edition. Elk Grove Village, IL: American Academy of Pediatrics; 2017.
3. Website: AAP Preventive Care/Periodicity Schedule https://www.aap.org/en/practice-management/care. Accessed March 10, 2023.
4. Website: Data and Statistics on Congenital Heart Defects. Page last reviewed: January 24, 2022. Accessed March 10, 2023. https://www.cdc.gov/ncbddd/he.
5. Mahle WT, Martin GR, Beekman RH, et al. Endorsement of health and human services recommendation for pulse oximetry screening for critical congenital heart disease. Pediatrics 2012;129(1):190–2.
6. Erickson CC, Salerno JC, Berger S, et al. Sudden Death in the Young: Information for the Primary Care Provider. Pediatrics 2021;148(1). e2021052044.
7. Gonzalez VJ, Kyle WB, Allen HD. Cardiac Examination and Evaluation of Murmurs. Pediatr Rev 2021;42(7):375–82.
8. Teshome MK, Najib K, Nwagbara CC, et al. Patent Foramen Ovale: A Comprehensive Review. Curr Probl Cardiol 2020;45(2):100392.
9. Ford B, Lara S, Park J. Heart Murmurs in Children: Evaluation and Management. Am Fam Physician 2022;105(3):250–61.
10. Zitelli BJ, McIntire SC, Nowalk AJ, et al. Zitelli and Davis' atlas of pediatric physical diagnosis. 8th edition. Philadelphia: Elsevier, Inc; 2023.

Moving?

Make sure your subscription moves with you!

To notify us of your new address, find your **Clinics Account Number** (located on your mailing label above your name), and contact customer service at:

Email: journalscustomerservice-usa@elsevier.com

800-654-2452 (subscribers in the U.S. & Canada)
314-447-8871 (subscribers outside of the U.S. & Canada)

Fax number: 314-447-8029

Elsevier Health Sciences Division
Subscription Customer Service
3251 Riverport Lane
Maryland Heights, MO 63043

*To ensure uninterrupted delivery of your subscription, please notify us at least 4 weeks in advance of move.

Printed and bound by CPI Group (UK) Ltd, Croydon, CR0 4YY

03/10/2024

01040468-0008